BASIC RESUSCITATION

BASIC RESUSCITATION
AND PRIMARY CARE

F. Wilson and W. G. Park
Consultant Anaesthetists

Royal Lancaster Infirmary
Lancaster, UK

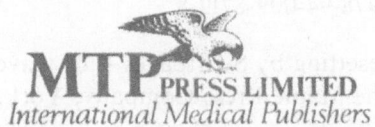

MTP PRESS LIMITED
International Medical Publishers

Published by
MTP Press Limited
Lancaster, England

British Library Cataloguing in Publication Data

Wilson, Frank, *b.1927*
Basic resuscitation and primary care.
I. Title   II. Park, W G
615′ 8043   RC86.7
ISBN-13:978-94-009-8714-2   e-ISBN-13:978-94-009-8712-8
DOI: 10.1007/978-94-009-8712-8

Phototypesetting by Swiftpages Ltd., Liverpool, UK
Printed by The Maple Press Company, York, Pennsylvania

Contents

SECTION II PRACTICAL VENTILATION

SECTION III THE HEART AND CIRCULATION IN HEALTH AND DISEASE

Preface

Provision of efficient resuscitation is mandatory to the successful functioning of all hospital wards and departments. Failure to provide such a service increases morbidity and mortality. Resuscitation falls largely into the domain of the anaesthetist. However, an anaesthetist is not always instantly available and resuscitation has to be initiated by those in other specialities who have had little or no formal training in resuscitation techniques.

The purpose of this book is to guide those involved in resuscitation in the indications and methods of resuscitation. Its creation and contents were stimulated by noting the difficulties encountered in both teaching centres and provincial hospitals.

'Basic' is included in the title to emphasize that, with the exception of 'the acid-base laboratory', the apparatus is simple and available in all hospitals. Furthermore, 'basic' indicates the authors' intention to limit their discussion on resuscitation to that involved in the first hour following the start of treatment. Successful treatment during these 60 minutes, and very often the first few minutes, is often vital in the saving of life. Further management can then be decided by the appropriate specialist.

Basic Resuscitation is written mainly for the newly qualified doctor who has little or no practical experience in resuscitation, and for senior nursing personnel. The authors hope that it will provide some guidance when starting in the wards, casualty department and intensive care unit. They also hope that the potential anaesthetist will find it useful when embarking on his new career.

F. Wilson
W. G. Park

Acknowledgements

We are grateful to Mr John Normanton for producing the diagrams, to Mrs Marjorie Ormsby for her infinite patience and help in preparing the manuscript, to our colleagues for their advice and to Mr David Bloomer and his staff at MTP for their guidance and encouragement at the various stages of publication.

Introduction

General approach to emergency situations

Organs such as the heart and brain are irreversibly damaged by a short period of absent circulation or oxygenation. Therefore, priorities are necessary in the treatment of life-threatening situations such as severe barbiturate poisoning where urgent general measures for circulatory and respiratory support may enable a patient to survive long enough for detoxication and excretion of the poison, and therefore for recovery to take place. There are three stages in the treatment of life-threatening conditions.

STAGE 1

The first stage in resuscitation is to assess the state of both respiration and circulation, ensuring adequate oxygenation and nutrition of all the tissues and the removal from them of waste products. Fortunately the time required for assessment is inversely proportional to the severity of the condition – a patient in cardiac or respiratory arrest needs little time for evaluation! Much more of a problem exists when there is doubt as to whether or not the circulation and respiration are failing, and what degree of support, if any, is required.

STAGE 2

The second stage is to minimize the effects of any depression or arrest of the circulation or respiration on metabolism in general and also on specific organs readily damaged, such as the brain, heart and kidneys, and to monitor any change from the initial assessment. Metabolic acidosis and cerebral oedema, for example, can occur after a relatively short period of anoxia. Therefore, continuing evaluation of the cardiovascular and respiratory systems, cerebral and renal function, and the acid–base status of the body is required for some time after the initially successful resuscitation. The onset or reappearance of circulatory, respiratory, or metabolic failure is often so insidious that the

1

major difficulty is one of recognition before the situation becomes irreversible.

STAGE 3

The third stage is to diagnose the initial cause of the problem, and initiate specific treatment. Correct diagnosis is vital if there is specific treatment for the condition, or it may be useful merely to exclude other differential diagnoses that require more than symptomatic treatment. For example, while the treatment of myocardial infarction is largely symptomatic and supportive, other common causes of sudden collapse and death, such as pulmonary embolus or dissecting aneurysm, require urgent definitive treatment in the form of surgery, thrombolytic or anticoagulant therapy.

The stages can thus be summarized:

(1) Initial assessment and maintenance of the vital functions.
(2) Continuing assessment and treatment of the general condition and support of specific organ function.
(3) Diagnosis and treatment of the underlying cause.

Stages (2) and (3) are normally integrated as a continuing programme of support and therapy; (2) has only been put before (3) to underline the importance of continuing evaluation of all the relevant systems. Cellular metabolism, circulation and lung function are bound together in health and disease; no one system can fail, however marginally, without affecting the others, thereby causing further deterioration in the original failing system. Reassessment should be directed to bodily function and physiology. The rather anatomical approach of the conventional clinical examination can easily miss significant signs such as cold extremities and oliguria.

With each system the questions must be asked:

(1) Is it working efficiently?
(2) If not, why not?
(3) What can be done?
(4) What effects will the treatment have?

This approach does not replace the conventional clinical examination, which should be done as soon as the condition of the patient permits, but establishes the immediate priorities and may occasionally prevent the diagnosis being made *post mortem* rather than *ante mortem*.

Example of this approach to emergency management
Consider two common problems, one of cardiac arrest due to myocardial infarction, and one of mild sedative overdose. In the former, the sequence of treatment might well be:

Step 1   External cardiac massage and artificial ventilation by whatever means is available.

Step 2   (a) Insertion of a venous cannula for
            (i) bicarbonate infusion to offset metabolic acidosis;
            (ii) administration of drugs to establish or maintain more normal electrical and mechanical activity in the myocardium.
            (b) Repeated assessment of circulation and respiration (pulse, blood pressure, peripheral circulation, chest movements, blood gases, etc.), cerebral function (pupil reaction, conscious level, respiratory attempts), acid–base status, and later, renal function.

Step 3   The diagnosis of myocardial infarction.

In a case of mild sedative overdose, the initial assessment may show the circulation and the respiratory exchange to be perfectly adequate and specific treatment of the condition can be instituted forthwith; however, working through the steps systematically as listed above will remind the resuscitator of other possible hazards such as respiratory obstruction from the relaxed tongue or the inhalation of vomit. In the following section, the emergency treatment of specific conditions is described, while in the subsequent sections the various systems, their changes in disease, and their assessment are discussed. Practical techniques are explained where necessary.

SECTION I
SPECIFIC CONDITIONS

1

Cardiac arrest and arrhythmias

Cardiac arrest

The definition of cardiac arrest is sudden cessation of heart function due to any cause.

AETIOLOGICAL FACTORS

1. *Inadequate oxygenation of the myocardium*

This can be due to pre-existing coronary artery disease, producing narrowing of the coronary arteries, or inadequate oxygenation of the blood supplied to the myocardium.

2. *Vagal reflexes*

Vagal reflexes have been implicated in asystole occurring during operations for squint, and surgical manipulations of the heart and biliary tract. Some drowning cases are said to die from vagal inhibition of the heart ('dry drowning').

3. *Electrocution*

Currents as low as 100 microamps can cause ventricular fibrillation if the current source is close to or in contact with the myocardium. Such microshocks can be produced by minor leakage currents from modern invasive monitoring equipment.

4. *Electrolyte disorders and drug therapy*

Hyperkalaemia causes ventricular fibrillation. Infusion of electrolytes and drugs such as calcium chloride ($CaCl_2$), adrenergic stimulants and digitalis, can also induce fibrillation or asystole, particularly if given as a bolus into a central vein.

5. *Mechanical factors*

Obstruction to the right ventricular outflow following a pulmonary

embolus often results in cardiac arrest. Diagnostic procedures such as
cardiac catheterization can also give rise to arrest.

MECHANISMS OF ARREST
The vast majority of patients in cardiac arrest have either ventricular
fibrillation or asystole. About two-thirds of patients in cardiac arrest
following myocardial infarction have ventricular fibrillation. Asystole
is said to be more common in cases of arrest under anaesthesia, particularly at induction of anaesthesia.

Rarely, other rhythms are seen, such as extreme bradycardia or fast
ventricular tachycardia. Sinus rhythm is uncommon, but is occasionally seen in cardiac arrest due to ventricular rupture and as the
result of treatment with antiarrhythmic drugs, but if no cardiac output
is present the outlook is very poor.

DIAGNOSIS
This rests on unconsciousness with absent pulses. No other signs are
necessary; respiration may continue for some minutes after effective
circulation has ceased, and fundal and pupillary examination wastes
time which could be used to initiate resuscitation. However, pupillary
size and reactions are useful later to determine the adequacy of the circulation and oxygenation.

MANAGEMENT
When the diagnosis has been made, no time must be lost. A system
such as the flow diagram Figure 1.1 should be followed. Explanatory
notes to clarify the diagram are given below.

1: *Immediate action*
The individual making the diagnosis should:

    (a) Strike the centre of the chest twice, sharply, with the side of the
        clenched fist. In the first minute following an arrest this some-
        times converts ventricular fibrillation into a more effective
        rhythm.
    (b) Call for assistance.
    (c) With the fingers clear the airway of debris, false teeth and
        vomitus.
    (d) Institute ventilation and external cardiac massage (ECM).

Ventilation by staff unskilled in intubation is best done by gentle inflation with a self-inflating bag and mask (Ambu, or Air-Viva, p. 133).

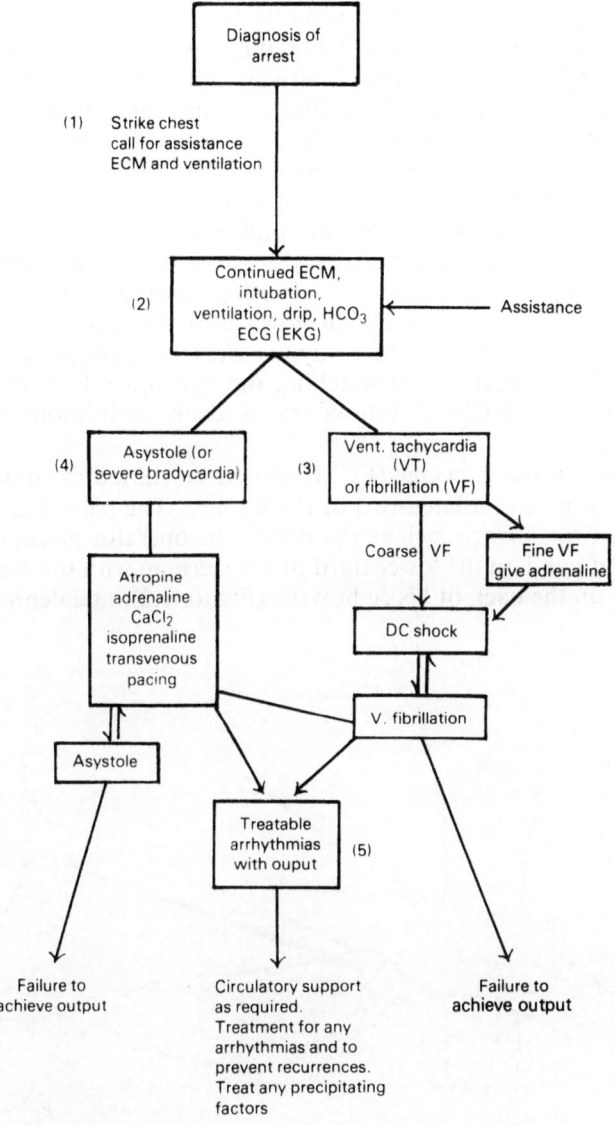

Figure 1.1 Management of cardiac arrest

Added oxygen can be supplied to both these types.

If a bag and mask are unavailable, direct mouth-to-mouth respiration should be started. A Brook airway makes it more aesthetically acceptable. Mouth-to-mouth ventilation, however, will only provide 15 – 16% oxygen which is hardly ideal under the already hypoxic conditions. Whichever technique is used, the patient's head must be in the correct position to maintain a patent airway, that is, with the head extended on the neck and the jaw pulled forwards. The lungs are inflated *gently,* because otherwise gas passes down the oesophagus and the intragastric pressure rises, causing regurgitation of stomach contents; if these are then blown down into the lungs, the outlook for the patient is poor. The best way to assess the adequacy of ventilation breath by breath is by watching the rise and fall of the chest. Intubation and artificial ventilation is dealt with more fully in Section II.

External cardiac massage (ECM) should be started as soon as the patient has been ventilated two or three times. The patient should be on a flat, firm surface such as the floor. The operator places the heel of his right hand on the lower third of the sternum with the heel of his left hand on the back of his right wrist (Figure 1.2), and depresses the

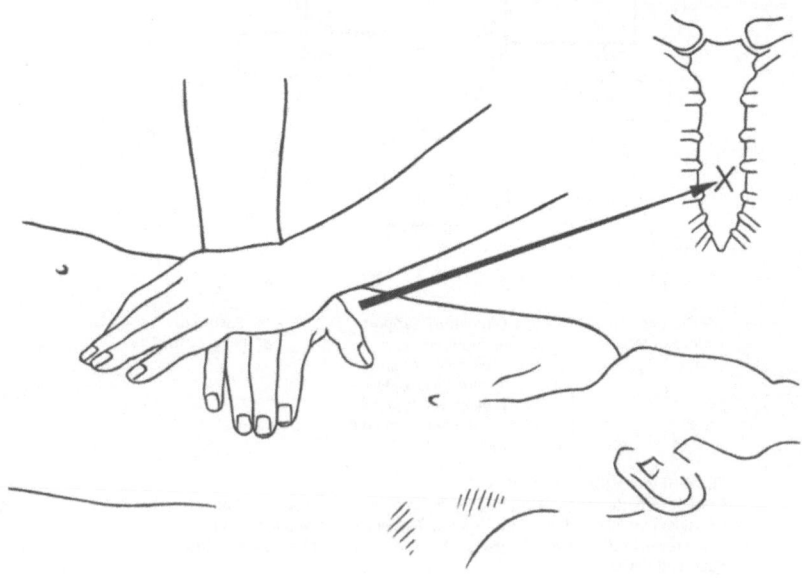

Figure 1.2 Position of hands in external cardiac massage

sternum 4 – 5 cm, taking about 1 sec overall for the compression and relaxation. It is more efficient and less tiring if the arms of the operator are kept straight during ECM, so that the task is performed by his weight. Five or six compressions should alternate with one ventilation. A normal cardiac output cannot be achieved by ECM; a systolic pressure of only about 80 mmHg, with a diastolic as low as 20 mmHg, is produced with well-performed massage. This is unlikely to provide an adequate coronary flow to a compromised myocardium, or to provide adequate cerebral flow for more than a half hour. Thus the time available for resuscitation is very limited. Artificial ventilation and ECM must be continued until either a decision is made to abandon resuscitation, or until the circulation and respiration are adequate.

2: *Adequacy of ECM and artificial ventilation*
If ECM is effective and the lungs are adequately ventilated, previously dilating pupils constrict, the colour of the patient improves, consciousness and respiratory efforts may return, and pulses should be palpable in the carotid and femoral arteries. Later, arterial blood sampling will show:

(1) the metabolic acidosis consequent upon the circulatory arrest,
(2) the adequacy of the minute volume ventilation (from the PCO_2 level),
(3) the adequacy of the arterial oxygenation (from the PO_2 level).

When trained assistance arrives

(1) The patient is intubated and ventilation maintained. This enables the airway to be sealed off from oesophageal and gastric contents, and permits more efficient ventilation with greater concentrations of oxygen.
(2) An intravenous infusion is set up. Although any accessible vein will suffice, the external jugular veins in cardiac arrest are usually distended, easily cannulated, and lead directly to the heart (p. 277). An infusion of 100 mmol sodium bicarbonate solution (that is 200 ml of 4.2% solution, or 100 ml of 8.4% solution) is usually the best initial fluid to combat the metabolic acidosis. This is given over 10 min or so, and followed by a slow infusion of 5% dextrose to keep the vein patent for drug therapy.
(3) An ECG machine is connected to the patient and the nature of

arrhythmia diagnosed. As explained on p. 8, either ventricular
fibrillation or asystole is likely to be present.
(4) Arterial blood is taken for plasma potassium level, blood gas
and acid–base determinations.

3: Treatment of ventricular fibrillation (VF) and ventricular tachycardia (VT)

Adequate oxygenation and bicarbonate therapy increase the chances
of successful defibrillation. If the ECG shows fine fibrillation – that
is, high frequency, low amplitude waves – it should be coarsened with
10 ml of 1 in 10 000 solution of adrenaline (epinephrine) intravenously
before DC conversion is attempted as below.

In ventricular tachycardia or coarse fibrillation, a DC shock of 200
Joules should be given immediately, and repeated if unsuccessful
before increasing it to 400 J (which is probably the largest shock that
can be given without causing damage to the myocardium).

If the dysrhythmia is thought to be digitalis-induced, a shock of 25
or 50 J should be given in the first instance, and the serum potassium
level checked as soon as possible and corrected if necessary.

The defibrillation paddles should be well applied to the chest wall,
with adequate electrode jelly to provide good electrical contact. One
paddle is placed to the right of the sternum below the clavicle, and the
other is placed over the 5th left intercostal space in the anterior axillary line.

Following defibrillation, transient asystole occurs, and then one of
the following is likely to appear on the ECG:

(1) Persistent asystole. This should be treated as under stage 4
below.
(2) Ventricular fibrillation or ventricular tachycardia. This should
again be defibrillated as above.
(3) A rhythm associated with some degree of cardiac output (see
stage 6 below).

4: Treatment of asystole

This is twofold; first of all electrical activity must be induced in the
myocardium, and then the rhythm produced – usually ventricular fibrillation – is converted by DC shock into a rhythm producing effective
ventricular contractions.

Suggested drugs and doses are:

(1) Adrenaline (epinephrine) 1 in 10 000 solution, 5 – 10 ml intravenously.

(2) Calcium chloride ($CaCl_2$) solution 10%, 10 ml intravenously. This should not be mixed with bicarbonate solution, or precipitation occurs.

(3) Isoprenaline (isoproterenol) 50−100 μg intravenously. If severe bradycardia is present atropine 1−2 mg should be given intravenously.

If ventricular fibrillation results from any of the above drugs, DC cardioversion is undertaken as before. If asystole then results from defibrillation the above drugs may be repeated. A transvenous pacing electrode in the right ventricle can be useful to activate the ventricles if asystole persists. If such facilities are unavailable, an infusion of isoprenaline 1−4 μg/min may be useful to maintain spontaneous rhythm, but isoprenaline therapy is not without problems, since other arrhythmias may be induced, and the area of infarcted myocardium may be increased.

5: Therapy following establishment of a cardiac output
If the original arrhythmia was ventricular fibrillation (VF), lignocaine (lidocaine) in an initial dose of 100 mg intravenously, followed by 2 mg/min by intravenous infusion is often used to prevent recurrence of the fibrillation and to suppress extrasystoles. If the extrasystoles are unchanged in frequency or increase, mexiletine 200 mg intravenously given over a period of 3 min followed by an infusion of 3 mg/min for the next hour, reducing to 1 mg/min after 4 hours, is frequently successful.

All drugs used for the treatment of arrhythmias are cardiodepressants, and many clinicians no longer treat patients for arrhythmias before they occur, but monitor the patients carefully and only treat 'warning arrhythmias', that is, frequent, multifocal, or 'R on T' ventricular ectopics (p. 19).

ECM and artificial ventilation must be maintained until the patient is shown to sustain an adequate output (p. 11). Cardiovascular support may be required for some time (pp. 253 and 261). Transvenous pacing may be necessary if heart block or bradycardia persist.

6: Other measures
(1) A steroid such as dexamethasone 8 mg and a diuretic such as frusemide (furosemide) 40 mg are often given in the hope that they protect the brain and kidneys to some extent from the effects of the temporary cessation of the circulation.

(2) Further doses of bicarbonate to offset the metabolic acidosis

may be required if resuscitative efforts are prolonged. Repeated blood gas and acid–base estimations are of value (see p. 318).

(3) Unless the patient is known to the resuscitating team, his notes should be examined, in case he may be an unsuitable candidate for prolonged or repeated resuscitation, or otherwise an obvious treatable precipitating factor may be missed.

(4) The initiating factor in the arrest may require specific treatment, as in pulmonary embolism.

(5) A chest X-ray should be taken after apparently successful resuscitation to show the position of any endotracheal tube, and the tip of any central venous pressure line or pacing electrode. Furthermore, it may show fractured ribs, a pneumothorax, a widening mediastinal or cardiac shadow, or a collapsed lung. An X-ray should always be taken before extubation.

Emergency treatment of arrhythmias

When a patient is found to have an arrhythmia, three questions should be asked:

(1) What is the abnormal rhythm?

(2) Does it require treatment? The arrhythmia may be causing inefficient myocardial activation with cardiovascular deterioration, it may predispose to a more dangerous rhythm, or it may be benign and need no treatment.

(3) How urgently is treatment required? In general, arrhythmias causing rapid deterioration of the patient are best treated by electrical cardioversion rather than drugs.

DC SHOCK

This is generally used to convert to sinus rhythm supraventricular or ventricular tachydysrhythmias which are giving rise to a rapidly deteriorating clinical situation.

Technique

DC shock can either be carried out under full general anaesthesia, or under sedation with an agent such as diazepam, given in 5 mg increments intravenously until the patient no longer responds to vocal or minor painful stimuli. A dose of 20 – 40 mg is usually required, but the requirement for each patient varies markedly. Oxygen should be given before and during the procedure, and the airway maintained.

If the patient is not in cardiac arrest a shock of 100 J should be given by the technique described on p. 12; if unsuccessful this is in-

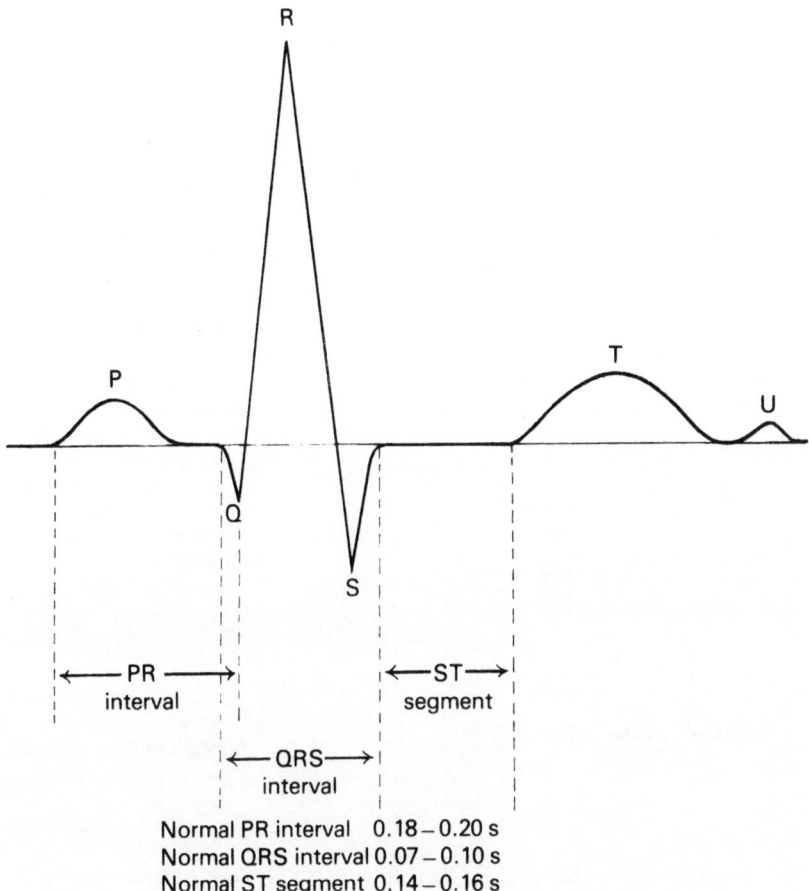

Normal PR interval   0.18 – 0.20 s
Normal QRS interval 0.07 – 0.10 s
Normal ST segment 0.14 – 0.16 s

Figure 1.3 Normal configuration of ECG (EKG)

creased to 200 or 300 J. Synchronized DC shock should be used to prevent the possibility of ventricular fibrillation which may follow a shock given when the patient's ventricles are repolarizing (see R on T, p. 19).

The initial energy level used in patients with digitalis-induced arrhythmia is 25 – 50 J, increasing as before if unsuccessful, but drug treatment is usually preferred in these patients.

SUPRAVENTRICULAR ARRHYTHMIAS
Fast supraventricular arrhythmias usually only demand urgent correction when they are associated with fast or irregular ventricular activa-

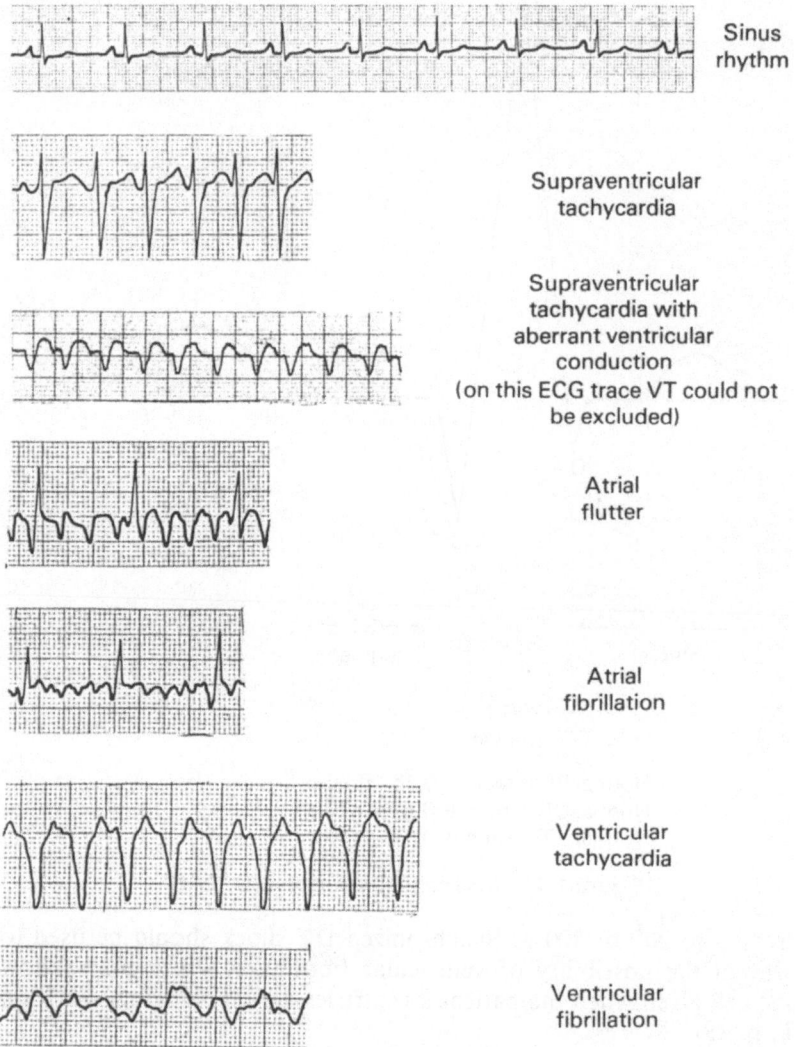

Figure 1.4 Sinus rhythm and common arrhythmias

tion, such as may happen in atrial flutter, paroxysmal supraventricular tachycardia, or atrial fibrillation. A ventricular rate of 160 – 180 or higher leads to inadequate ventricular filling with a consequent fall in output, and may also precipitate myocardial ischaemia with angina or infarction, since coronary flow is maximal during diastole, which is markedly reduced in tachycardia.

Carotid sinus massage should always be tried with fast rhythms unless they are due to digitalis; by increasing vagal tone, sinus rhythm may be re-established, or the ventricular rate may be sharply reduced by increasing the degree of atrioventricular block. If any change in the rate occurs with massage, the arrhythmia is supraventricular. This can be useful diagnostically, as often supraventricular and ventricular tachycardias can be difficult to differentiate even on ECG.

ATRIAL FLUTTER

In atrial flutter atrial activity is fast and regular (200 – 350 beats/min) usually with a 2:1 or 3:1 or varying atrioventricular block and a ventricular rate of 120 – 180 (Figure 1.4).

Treatment

(1) Carotid sinus massage should be tried, although it is usually unsuccessful.

(2) Cardioversion under anaesthesia or sedation is the treatment of choice for most patients. It is most frequently successful in the younger patient in whom the precipitating factor has been or is being treated.

(3) The patient can alternatively be digitalized, which often converts the flutter to atrial fibrillation, and also reduces the ventricular rate by slowing atrioventricular conduction. Verapamil or a beta-blocker may be required with the digoxin for rapid control of the ventricular rate.

ATRIAL FIBRILLATION

In the ECG P waves are absent, and the atria beat at a rate of 300 – 600 beats/min. Second degree atrioventricular block always occurs, and the ventricles beat at an irregular and fast rate. Atrial fibrillation (Figure 1.4) after infarction is usually transient and treatment is rarely necessary.

Treatment

The method of treatment depends on the objective; if the intention is to re-establish sinus rhythm, cardioversion as for flutter is preferred, but often the aim is merely to control the ventricular rate, and then digitalization is the best treatment.

PAROXYSMAL SUPRAVENTRICULAR TACHYCARDIA

This rhythm is often associated with excessive digitalis therapy. The onset and resolution of the arrhythmia can be abrupt. The P waves are different from those of the patient in sinus rhythm, and at fast rates intraventricular conduction block produces widened QRS complexes, which can make the arrhythmia difficult to differentiate from ventricular tachycardia.

Treatment

The aim of therapy is two-fold: firstly to restore sinus rhythm, and secondly to prevent recurrences.

(1) Carotid sinus massage is often effective.

(2) Reassurance, sedation and bed rest often settle the acute attack.

(3) If unsuccessful, verapamil 5 mg over 5 min intravenously may be given, repeated if necessary to a total of 20 mg.

(4) If unsuccessful, or the situation is urgent, cardioversion with DC shock is used.

(5) An alternative drug treatment is digitalization (p. 20), but this takes time, and cardioversion, if it should prove necessary, may be dangerous in fully digitalized patients.

(6) To prevent recurrence, oral verapamil, digoxin, or a beta-blocker can be given.

(7) Another useful drug is disopyramide, 2 mg/kg (but not exceeding 150 mg) given over 5 min intravenously.

TREATMENT OF BRADYCARDIA AND ATRIOVENTRICULAR (AV) BLOCK

On examination of the ECG in bradycardia it should be noted whether the P waves are followed all or most of the time by ventricular activation – that is, QRS complexes – or whether the P waves and the QRS complexes are completely unrelated to one another.

If the former is the case, atropine 0.25 or 0.3 mg should be given, and repeated if necessary.

If the latter is the case, or atropine is ineffective, isoprenaline (isoproterenol) as an infusion of $1-4$ μg/min may improve the rate. Ventricular arrhythmias however may be induced (p. 19). If cardiac output is unsatisfactory, cardiac massage must be maintained until temporary pacing via the subclavian or other suitable vein can be undertaken.

Temporary pacemaker

A temporary pacemaker is often inserted through the subclavian vein and passed under X-ray control to the apex of the right ventricle. A battery-operated demand pacemaker should be used, and the ventricular excitation threshold should not exceed 1 volt.

The main indications for this are:

(1) complete heart block, second degree heart block or severe bradycardia where drugs are contraindicated or the patient is deteriorating.
(2) for the control of some arrhythmias, such as recurrent ventricular tachycardia, by overdrive pacing – that is, initially using an activation rate faster than the intrinsic rate of the ventricle, then gradually slowing.

VENTRICULAR ARRHYTHMIAS

Ventricular ectopics rarely require treatment urgently unless they are frequent (more than 5/min), multiform, in runs of two or more, or occur on the T wave of the previous complex (R on T). In these circumstances ventricular tachycardia or fibrillation often follow, so most clinicians feel that such ectopics should be treated with lignocaine in a loading dose of 75–150 mg slowly intravenously, then 4 mg/min for 30 min, and 2 mg/min thereafter. A beta-blocking drug such as practolol, 5 mg intravenously repeated at 5 min intervals to a maximum of 20 mg, is an alternative which is often successful.

VENTRICULAR TACHYCARDIA (VT)

Ventricular tachycardia (see p. 12 and Figure 1.4) is caused by abnormal impulses arising in the ventricles, and shows wide slurred QRS complexes on the ECG, often similar to fast supraventricular tachycardia.

Cardioversion is the treatment of choice, using an initial shock of 20–25 J, increasing if unsuccessful. Lignocaine (as above) is used to prevent recurrences, and mexiletine may also be used (p. 13). Hypokalaemia may be associated with VT, and require correction.

VENTRICULAR FIBRILLATION

See p. 12.

DIGITALIS-INDUCED ARRHYTHMIAS

Any hypokalaemia must be urgently corrected, and digoxin withdrawn. Beta-blockers are frequently effective in suppressing the ectopic focus (see also ventricular ectopic beats, p. 13). If severe atrioventricular block has occurred with digoxin overdose, ventricular pacing may occasionally be required. To avoid digitalis toxicity, digitalization should be carried out as described below.

Digitalization
Digoxin 0.5−0.75 mg intravenously is given as an initial dose, with one or two further doses of 0.25 mg in the next 24 h, then a maintenance dose of 0.125−0.25 mg per day orally. The biological half-life is long (36 h) and hypokalaemia can induce digitalis toxicity.

Arrhythmias arising during anaesthesia are often due to excessive sympathetic discharge particularly in the atropinized patient, and can often be inhibited by a beta-blocking drug such as practolol 2−10 mg given slowly intravenously. If the arrhythmia is dangerous, such as in ventricular tachycardia, DC shock can be undertaken without delay in the anaesthetized patient.

2

Pulmonary embolism

Massive pulmonary embolism

PATHOPHYSIOLOGY

Before pulmonary embolism can cause serious cardiovascular signs and symptoms, more than half the pulmonary vascular bed has to be obstructed. When the right ventricular outflow is so obstructed, acute right-sided heart failure with right atrial and ventricular dilatation develops, and in the 25% of normal individuals with a patent foramen ovale right-to-left shunting occurs. There are gross abnormalities in lung function, with increased dead space due to absent perfusion in some areas of the lungs, and excessive blood flow in others.

In the systemic circulation there is hypotension with low cardiac output since the obstruction prevents adequate venous return from the lungs, and hypoxaemia from the disordered pulmonary function. ECG signs of left ventricular ischaemia may develop. A reflex increase in sympathetic outflow occurs with peripheral vasoconstriction, sweating and tachycardia, and reflex hyperpnoea with activation of the accessory muscles of respiration.

In emergency situations, pulmonary embolus can easily be confused with such conditions as myocardial infarction, tension pneumothorax, cardiac tamponade, dissecting aneurysm, or lung collapse, so an outline of the diagnostic features is given below.

DIAGNOSTIC FEATURES

(1) Signs and symptoms are distended neck veins, gallop rhythm, cyanosis, respiratory distress, collapse, hypotension and tachycardia.

(2) Predisposing factors may be present, such as a recent operation, pelvic or leg injuries, prolonged bed rest, cardiac failure or malignant disease.

(3) Electrocardiographic changes. The ECG may be normal, or signs of right-sided strain and dilatation may be present (T-wave inversion in the right ventricular leads, atrial flutter or fibrillation, right

21

bundle branch block, axis shift to the right in the frontal plane). Signs of left ventricular ischaemia may also be present in low output states.

(4) A plain chest X-ray is useful mainly to exclude some of the differential diagnoses, and may appear quite normal in massive embolism. However, oligaemic lung fields or distended branches of the pulmonary artery may occasionally be seen. Wedge-shaped opacities are not usually visualized in acute embolism, but may be present from previous embolism.

(5) Blood gas measurements: low PO_2 and PCO_2 values are usually found.

(6) Isotope lung scans and pulmonary angiography are useful to confirm the diagnosis; the latter is also useful in planning definitive treatment.

MANAGEMENT

The pulmonary vascular tree has its smallest cross-sectional area at its origin in the pulmonary trunk and arteries, but the total cross-sectional area becomes much greater as it subdivides into smaller and smaller branches. Therefore, the more distal the embolus can be forced and fragmented, the less obstruction to the pulmonary vasculature.

In massive embolism with collapse, the initial management is directed to (1) forcing the clot distally by external cardiac massage, and (2) ensuring optimum oxygenation and ventilation (p. 236).

A peripheral infusion is set up, and 15 000 units of heparin are given intravenously. This is said to antagonize serotonin-mediated vasoconstriction. ECG monitoring should be instituted as soon as possible.

The left ventricular output is maintained as far as possible:

(1) By maintaining venous return with plasma or plasma substitutes and preventing venodilatation as much as possible (alpha-adrenergic stimulants such as metaraminol may have to be used for a limited period);
(2) By improving myocardial contractility by correcting acidosis and electrolyte disorders, improving oxygenation, and giving agents such as dopamine if required (p. 253).

If the patient is acutely deteriorating despite resuscitative procedures, a modified Trendelenburg operation (which does not need cardiopulmonary bypass) should be considered, or embolectomy with full cardiopulmonary bypass if available.

DEFINITIVE MANAGEMENT

(1) *Embolectomy* for patients with massive embolus and low cardiac output who are deteriorating.
(2) *Thrombolytic therapy* in patients with massive embolus and low but stable cardiac output if no contraindication exists.
(3) *Heparin and oral anticoagulants* in patients with massive embolus, and improving cardiac output.

Thrombolytic therapy
This has been shown to dramatically increase the rate of resolution of embolized thrombus. Very considerable lysis has usually taken place within 72 h with streptokinase therapy, but there is by then very little resolution of the clot in heparin-treated patients.

Contraindications to streptokinase therapy are:

(1) operation in previous 48 h;
(2) bleeding tendency or gastrointestinal ulceration;
(3) hypertension;
(4) previous recent streptokinase therapy.

Sensitivity reactions do occasionally appear, and steroid cover such as hydrocortisone 100 mg should be given; an antihistamine may also be required.

Dose of streptokinase – 250 000 units intravenously in the first half-hour of therapy; then 100 000 units intravenously hourly for 72 h. The thrombin clotting time is used to determine the adequacy of the dose. If the clotting time increases to more than four times the initial value, there is an increased risk of bleeding, and the maintenance dose should be *doubled.* If the thrombin clotting time falls to less than twice the initial value, the dose should be *halved* until the clotting time is again satisfactory.

Heparin therapy
The rationale of heparin therapy is that it:

(1) Limits further clot propagation from the initiating venous thrombosis.
(2) Prevents extension of the clot around the embolus.
(3) Acts as an antiserotonin factor.

Where the latter is the reason for the heparin therapy, doses of 100 000 units/24 h are advocated. Most clinicians, however, use much smaller doses, such as 5000 units every 4 or 6 h intravenously.

Amniotic fluid embolism

Amniotic fluid embolism is caused by the entry of amniotic fluid into the circulation during pregnancy or labour. Although more frequently seen during labour, it has been described following surgical rupture of the membranes. before the onset of labour, during termination of pregnancy when hypertonic saline is injected into the amniotic sac, and even as a spontaneous event in an apparently normal pregnancy.

INCIDENCE AND MORTALITY

The incidence is about 1:30 000 pregnancies, which is fortunate, since a recent review described the mortality at 86%, 25% of whom are dead within an hour of the symptoms presenting.

PATHOPHYSIOLOGY

Acute obstruction to the pulmonary vascular tree occurs as in massive clot embolism (p. 21) with similar effects. Acute right ventricular failure develops with decreased venous return to the systemic circulation. This leads to systemic hypotension, while the obstructed lung vessels cause ventilation/perfusion inequalities and acute hypoxia. Disseminated intravascular coagulation is usually present. Amniotic fluid activates factor X in the clotting cascade, and this may be the initiating factor. Fibrinolysis is also stimulated.

TREATMENT

(1) Cardiopulmonary resuscitation should be commenced (p. 7), care being taken to maintain the blood volume and provide adequate oxygenation.

(2) The bleeding disorder will require blood replacement, and often fresh frozen plasma, fibrinogen, and heparin (p. 271).

3

Management of left ventricular failure

Pulmonary oedema

Acute pulmonary oedema (p. 236) is most often due to increased pulmonary capillary hydrostatic pressure secondary to acute left ventricular failure (LVF), and relatively rarely to other causes such as increased capillary permeability as in bacteraemic shock or inhalation of toxic fumes. If the cause is not LVF, then the most suitable treatment when the condition is severe and the patient hypoxic, is usually intubation and artificial ventilation. While investigations and specific treatment proceed, ventilation will:

(1) Improve the patient's oxygenation.
(2) Relieve him of the considerable increase in respiratory work.
(3) Enable him to be sedated if anxiety is severe.

Treatment of acute LVF (See also p. 57).
(1) Correct any precipitating factor such as a fast arrhythmia.
(2) Give 40–50% oxygen by mask if tolerated.
(3) Give frusemide (furosemide) 80 mg intravenously.
(4) Give morphine 5 mg slowly intravenously over 5 minutes; repeat if necessary. Morphine relieves dyspnoea and anxiety, and reduces pulmonary venous congestion by producing peripheral venous dilatation. Morphine is dangerous to give in bronchospasm due to primary lung disease.
(5) Give aminophylline 250 mg slowly intravenously; repeating after 30 min if necessary. Aminophylline relieves bronchospasm and increases myocardial contractility.
(6) Digitalization may be required to control a rapid ventricular rate in atrial fibrillation or to improve myocardial contractility. Recent treatment with digitalis must be enquired about, before a dose is given intravenously, or death may result.
(7) Intubation and ventilation may, rarely, be required.

Cardiac tamponade

Acute cardiac tamponade develops most commonly following rupture of the ventricular wall in myocardial infarction, or following trauma to the chest. In cases of ventricular rupture, the presentation is usually of circulatory arrest often associated with persisting sinus rhythm. The outlook in these cases is hopeless.

In less desperate circumstances the signs are an elevated jugular venous pressure (or central venous pressure measurement, if available), low blood pressure, and pulsus paradoxus (p. 60) but they may be difficult to elicit in a patient hypovolaemic from haemorrhage.

PERICARDIAL ASPIRATION

If in doubt, and the patient is deteriorating, pericardial aspiration will confirm the diagnosis. A long needle is inserted between the xiphisternum and the left costal margin, pushed deep to the sternum, and then cephalad and just lateral to the midline until the pericardium is penetrated (Figure 12.3). If the aspirating needle is connected to an anterior chest ECG lead, a record similar to a V_4 or V_5 lead will be obtained until the needle touches the surface of the ventricle. The ECG then shows strongly negative QRS deflections with an elevated ST segment, when the needle should be withdrawn slightly, and then aspirated.

Aspiration of blood from the pericardial sac after trauma usually calls for urgent surgical exploration. In other conditions causing pericardial effusion, aspiration may be adequate to reduce cardiac embarrassment. Continuous ECG monitoring should always be used when aspirating a pericardial effusion.

4

Acute self-poisoning, bites and stings

Acute self-poisoning
INCIDENCE AND DIAGNOSIS

It has been estimated that cases of self-poisoning account for up to 30% of all acute medical admissions in the United Kingdom. The mortality of those cases reaching hospital alive is less than 1%. In the absence of head injury or obvious trauma, self-poisoning is the most common cause of coma in the age group 15–55.

It is important during the history-taking to find out if possible:

(1) type of drug and amount ingested,
(2) when taken,
(3) whether alcohol or other drugs were also taken.
(4) if the patient is on any other medication.

Patients themselves are notoriously unreliable as sources of information. Relatives can often help with such information and also with assessments of the patient's previous mental state and intentions. Venepuncture marks and pinpoint pupils may suggest opiate self-administration, and skin blisters on pressure areas are often found in sedative poisoning. Laboratory analysis of samples of urine, gastric aspirate and blood may be required to determine the drug, or mixture of drugs taken. In many cases the analysis does not alter the management of the patient, but in others, such as in cases of paracetamol (acetaminophen) or aspirin poisoning, the serum levels are critically important to determine the appropriate specific therapy.

INITIAL ASSESSMENT AND THERAPY

The treatment of most cases of self-poisoning is supportive; if the vital functions of the body can be maintained the body will detoxify and excrete many ingested poisons over a period of a few days. The initial management is therefore to assess and support the respiratory and

27

cardiovascular systems and maintain fluid and electrolyte balance, kidney and hepatic function. Priorities are assessment and support, if necessary, of:

(1) the airway,
(2) ventilation,
(3) the heart and circulation,
(4) the central nervous system,
(5) other systems where relevant, acid−base and electrolyte balance.

(1) *The airway*

If the patient is unconscious, the reflexes protecting his airway may be obtunded, so that respiratory obstruction or aspiration of acidic gastric contents into the lungs can occur. To prevent this, the patient can either be nursed on his side in the head-down position, with or without an oral airway, or have a cuffed endotracheal tube passed to seal off the airway from the pharynx and prevent aspiration.

(2) *Ventilation*

Ventilation is often markedly depressed in states of sedative or tranquilliser overdose. If the minute volume (p. 124) is less than 4 litres/min measured with a mask and Wright's respirometer (see Figure 18.1), the arterial blood gases should be checked. If oxygenation alone is poor, this may be improved with an oxygen mask, but if the PCO_2 is high, artificial ventilation with a cuffed tube may be required. A chest X-ray should be taken as soon as initial resuscitation has been completed, as inhalation of vomitus often takes place before admission.

Hyperventilation can occur in poisoning with salicylates and is occasionally seen in the syndrome of 'shock lung' which can follow overdose.

(3) *Heart and circulation*

Depression of the heart and circulation can occur, causing low cardiac output and blood pressure, and lead to poor organ perfusion, falling urinary output and a metabolic acidosis.

The depression may be due to:
(a) direct myocardial cell depression (negative inotropism),
(b) depression of the vasomotor centre, with decreased vasoconstriction and venoconstriction, increasing the capacity of the circulation relative to the actual plasma volume,

(c) loss of circulating volume due to increased capillary permeability secondary to hypoxia or drug action.

The logical treatments for (a), (b) and (c) are beta-adrenergic stimulants, alpha-adrenergic stimulants, and plasma expanders respectively, but raising the foot of the bed is often enough to improve the blood pressure and circulation, by increasing the venous return.

Most cases of overdose are not hypovolaemic but have myocardial and vasomotor dysfunction, that is (a) and (b) above. The best treatment for this combination is a mixed alpha- and beta-stimulant such as metaraminol 5 mg intravenously or intramuscularly, repeated up to twice if required. If such a drug is used, the urinary output should be carefully monitored, and the treatment stopped if oliguria occurs.

If an element of hypovolaemia is thought to be present, a plasma expander should be given. If myocardial depression alone is present, then a dopamine, dobutamine or isoprenaline (isoproterenol) infusion is the logical treatment. ECG monitoring should be undertaken in all severely poisoned patients.

(4) *The central nervous system*

The Glasgow coma scale (p. 77) may be used for assessment of conscious level, but the following system based on response to stimuli is more easily remembered and more frequently used.

Four grades of response, and therefore severity, are recognized:

(a) Patient awake but sleepy, responding to vocal commands.
(b) Patient unconscious, responding to minimal painful stimuli.
(c) Patient unconscious, responding to maximal painful stimuli.
(d) Patient completely unresponsive to pain.

The maximal painful stimulus used is rubbing the sternum with the knuckles of the clenched fist.

Except in opiate poisoning, the pupils are of little use in assessing the severity of poisoning.

(5) *Other systems where relevant*

Organ damage occurring in overdoses of particular drugs are discussed on p. 32 *et seq.* Hypothermia is often present, and is best managed by covering the patient with a 'space-blanket' in a warm $(25 - 30\,^{\circ}\text{C})$ environment.

Acid–base and electrolyte balance, and fluid intake and output must be carefully monitored. Convulsions may require intravenous diazepam, titrated against the response (p. 107).

Methods of decreasing absorption and increasing excretion of drugs
GASTRIC EMPTYING BY VOMITING OR LAVAGE
The value of performing gastric lavage or inducing vomiting depends on:

(1) The type and amount of drug ingested. Caustic or oily substances are a contraindication to emesis or lavage due to the risk of aspiration lipoid pneumonia. If the amount of drug ingested is small, and the drug not especially dangerous, the risks of gastric emptying outweighs the possible benefits.

(2) The time since ingestion. If the time elapsed is more than 4 hours, it is unlikely that a useful amount of the drug will be recovered by gastric emptying, except in self-poisoning with:

- (a) tricyclic antidepressants,
- (b) atropine-like compounds, or
- (c) aspirin and other salicylates,

all of which delay gastric emptying.

Induction of vomiting
Vomiting should only be induced in conscious patients, either by physical methods such as stimulating the pharyngeal gag reflex with a suction catheter or by giving an emetic.

The emetic of choice is syrup of ipecacuanha 10−20 ml, followed by 100−200 ml of water. This is particularly useful in children, although there is often a delay of 20 min or so before vomiting occurs.

GASTRIC LAVAGE
If the patient's cough reflex is depressed and the airway therefore unprotected from the dangers of aspiration, a cuffed endotracheal tube must be passed before lavage is carried out.

In an adult, a wide-bore oesophageal tube such as a 30 English gauge Jacques tube should be passed; small-bore tubes are inadequate to remove tablet debris. The patient should be on his side with a slight head-down tilt, unless an endotracheal tube is in place, and 300 ml increments of warm (38 °C) fluid are run into the stomach under gravity through a funnel and connecting tube, and out again by lowering the funnel to below the level of the patient.

Warm tap water is used, except under the following circumstances:

(1) In babies and young children, warm physiological saline is used.

(2) In opiate poisoning, dilute potassium permanganate solution is used.

(3) In iron poisoning, desferrioxamine (deferoxamine) in solution is used (2 g desferrioxamine in 1 litre water). After lavage, 5 g desferrioxamine in 50 ml water is left in the stomach.

(4) In glutethimide poisoning, water and castor oil is used.

Activated charcoal in a dose of 10 − 50 g in water is often given by mouth or nasogastric tube to reduce further absorption of drugs. It is useful particularly in the treatment of poisoning by salicylates, paracetamol, tricyclic antidepressants and barbiturates.

Methods of increasing elimination of poisons
These include:

(1) forced diuresis (acid or alkaline),
(2) peritoneal dialysis or haemodialysis,
(3) exchange transfusion,
(4) haemoperfusion using charcoal or resins.

Only the first method will be described here in any detail.

FORCED DIURESIS
Many drugs are weak acids or bases. The excretion of weak acids is increased in alkaline urine, and the excretion of weak bases in acid urine. Therefore, by manipulation of the urine pH and by increasing the urine output the elimination of some poisons can be enhanced.

In practice, forced alkaline diuresis is only useful for:

(1) salicylate poisoning,
(2) phenobarbitone (phenobarbital) poisoning (it is ineffective in the treatment of poisoning by short or medium-acting barbiturates) and in poisoning by some weedkillers such as 2, 4-D and mecoprop.

Forced acid diuresis is very rarely employed, but it is occasionally useful for:

(1) amphetamine poisoning,
(2) fenfluramine poisoning, or
(3) quinine poisoning.

Technique of forced diuresis
The adequacy of the patient's cardiac, respiratory and renal function must be assessed before and during the procedure. Overhydration and electrolyte disorders readily occur, and careful monitoring of the fluid balance, urea and electrolyte levels, and drug levels in the plasma is required.

(1) *Forced alkaline diuresis* – In the first hour of treatment 1000 – 1500 ml 5% dextrose is given intravenously with 100 mmol sodium bicarbonate. The urine output is maintained at 400 – 500 ml/h by repeated doses of frusemide 20 mg, and the urine pH checked regularly. For effective drug elimination the pH should lie between 7.5 and 8.5 and this may be adjusted if necessary by infusion of further bicarbonate in the replacement fluids, which should also contain enough potassium (usually 20–30 mmol/1) to replace the potassium losses.

(2) *Forced acid diuresis* – Over the first hour 1000 ml of 5% dextrose and 500 ml normal saline are given, followed by 10 g arginine hydrochloride over 20 min to acidify the urine. The pH should be maintained between 5.5 and 6.5 with oral ammonium chloride 4 g every 2 hours. A high fluid output is again maintained with frusemide, and the volume of fluid and the electrolytes which are excreted are replaced.

Specific drugs – their problems and immediate treatment
PARACETAMOL (ACETAMINOPHEN)
Presentation
Often clinical signs and symptoms are delayed. Nausea, vomiting and upper abdominal pain may start 6–12 h after ingestion. Hepatic dysfunction usually becomes apparent about 18 h after taking a serious overdose. If frank hepatic failure develops 2–3 days later, the outlook is poor.

Management
   (1) Measurement of the paracetamol level.
   (2) Gastric lavage if drug ingestion is less than 4 h previously. Lavage should be undertaken even later if any drugs delaying gastric emptying have also been taken, such as aspirin or codeine.
   (3) N-acetyl cysteine (NAC) should be given intravenously to all patients who have ingested a considerable or an unknown quantity of paracetamol within the previous 24 h. If the time since inges-

tion is more than 24 h, NAC will have no beneficial effect; indeed, it is only likely to prevent liver damage if given within 10 h of taking the overdose. Initially, a dose of 150 mg/kg in 5% dextrose is given over 15 minutes, then 50 mg/kg in 500 ml 5% dextrose over 4 h. A further dose of 100 mg/kg in 5% dextrose is given over the subsequent 16 h.

(4) Hepatic and renal failure may require treatment. A bleeding diathesis may require clotting factors and vitamin K.

DISTALGESIC TABLETS

Each Distalgesic tablet contains 325mg paracetamol and 32.5 mg dextropropoxyphene. The latter is a narcotic analgesic, and can cause convulsions, sudden respiratory arrest and death.

Naloxone (1.2−2.4 mg intravenously) reverses the respiratory depression, but it is short-acting, and an infusion may be necessary after the initial dose. The patient must also be treated for the paracetamol component, as above.

Other narcotics, such as morphine, pethidine and dihydro-codeine, and the non-narcotic analgesic pentazocine, are also reversed by naloxone.

SALICYLATES

Presentation

An initial respiratory alkalosis is followed by a severe metabolic acidosis. Although the patient is usually conscious, he may be restless and confused, with overbreathing, roaring in the ears, sweating and vomiting. If the adult patient is drowsy, and no other drugs have been taken, there is usually a severe acidosis present.

Management

(1) Gastric lavage should always be done.
(2) If the serum salicylate level is greater than 50 mg/100 ml in an adult or 30 mg/100 ml in a child, forced alkaline diuresis should be carried out.
(3) The metabolic acidosis may require large amounts of bicarbonate solution. Regular acid−base and blood gas determinations in arterial blood are required.
(4) Artificial ventilation may be required in severe cases.

Other problems with salicylates include haemolysis, hypoprothrombinaemia with gastrointestinal haemorrhage, acute renal failure, pyrexia and convulsions. Death when it occurs is usually due to respiratory arrest or pulmonary oedema.

Sedatives and tranquillisers
There are no specific antidotes for poisoning by these drugs. However, the general supportive measures for poisoning already described (p. 28) usually result in recovery.

TRICYCLIC ANTIDEPRESSANTS
The effects of these drugs in overdose include:

(1) atropine-like effects such as dilated pupils, tachycardia and a dry mouth;
(2) cardiac effects—sinus tachycardia, widening of the QRS and ST segment, T wave changes, ventricular tachycardia and fibrillation can all occur; ECG monitoring is essential;
(3) cerebral effects such as excitement, hallucinations, convulsions and coma.

Management
(1) Gastric lavage in patients seen within 12 h of ingestion.
(2) Instillation of 20 g activated charcoal in 50 ml saline following lavage.
(3) Symptomatic treatment. Particular note should be taken of any acidosis, whether respiratory or metabolic in origin, and this should be treated appropriately. Practolol or another beta-blocking drug is the first-line drug for the treatment of tachy-dysrhythmias in tricyclic drug overdose. A pacemaker may be required for persistent bradycardia. Diazepam may be necessary for the control of convulsions.

PARAQUAT

Management
(1) Gastric lavage.
(2) 250 ml Fuller's Earth and magnesium sulphate mixture is left in the stomach (this is a sterilized mixture consisting of 30 g Fuller's Earth with 5 g magnesium sulphate in 100 ml water). Further doses of 250 ml are given every 4 h for 24–48 h. This reduces absorption from the gut, but does produce severe diarrhoea with fluid and electrolyte loss, which must be monitored and replaced.

(3) Antiemetics may be required for protracted vomiting, and analgesics for burns to the mouth and pharynx; severe metabolic acidosis may require treatment.

LITHIUM

Management
Plasma levels should be taken to confirm the diagnosis.

(1) In severe overdose or poisoning, forced alkaline diuresis is useful.
(2) Supportive therapy (p. 28) may be needed.
(3) Diazepam may be required as an anticonvulsant.

CYANIDE

Clinical presentation
Patients can survive cyanide poisoning without treatment for several hours, contrary to the belief of most people, including doctors. The poison can be inhaled as hydrogen cyanide or taken orally as cyanide compounds. A serious degree of poisoning is indicated by cardio-respiratory depression and coma. The antidotes available are themselves toxic, so the diagnosis should be established beyond reasonable doubt.

Management
(1) Supportive measures for airway maintenance, oxygenation and circulatory depression may be required. Any cyanide on the skin should be washed off.
(2) Inhalation of amyl nitrite (one crushed ampoule every 3 min to a total of six).
(3) Dicobalt edetate 600 mg intravenously, repeated once if improvement does not occur rapidly.

IRON

Clinical presentation
Symptoms and signs may be delayed for some hours after injection. A haemorrhagic gastroenteritis develops, often followed by shock, confusion and coma. Convulsions may occur and in severe cases acute hepatic necrosis. Iron poisoning is often seen in children.

Management
> (1) The plasma iron level should be taken. A plain abdominal X-ray is often useful where the diagnosis is in doubt, as iron tablets remain radio-opaque for several hours after ingestion.
> (2) Gastric lavage with desferrioxamine (deferoxamine) (p.31).
> (3) If the patient is an adult, 2 g desferrioxamine in 10 ml water is given intramuscularly.
> (4) If the plasma iron level is greater than 500 µg/100 ml in children or 800 µg/100 ml in adults, an infusion of desferrioxamine is given (15 mg/kg per h) until the plasma iron level and the general condition of the patient improve.
> (5) Blood loss and shock may require treatment.

Bites and stings in Great Britain

SNAKEBITE

The only venomous snake indigenous to Great Britain is the European adder or viper (*Vipera berus*). Adder venom has principally cardio-toxic and vasculotoxic effects. In Great Britain over the last hundred years only fourteen people have died following adder bites. The mortality from bee and wasp stings is in fact much higher because of the high risk of allergic reactions.

Signs and symptoms
In about one-third of bites venom is not injected by the adder, so fear, anxiety and local discomfort may be the only symptoms. Fingers and toes are most frequently bitten. If venom has been injected, there is local pain and swelling around the wound, and this can spread proximally to involve the whole limb, with bruising and tenderness of the regional lymph nodes. Necrosis does not occur with adder venom.

Systemic signs and symptoms may include:

> (1) colicky abdominal pain, nausea, vomiting and diarrhoea;
> (2) hypotension, ECG changes, and a rise in creatinine phosphokinase;
> (3) a bleeding tendency.

Acute renal failure is occasionally a late manifestation.

Treatment

> (1) *Reassurance* – People with adder bites usually show anxiety and fear – often including fear of death – out of all proportion to their

signs and symptoms, which may be mild, so reassurance is essential.

(2) *Analgesics* – A mild analgesic such as soluble aspirin or paracetamol may be given. Paracetamol elixir is useful for children.

(3) *Local treatment* – The wound is covered without excision or attempts to suck out the poison, and the affected limb rested to reduce lymphatic spread.

(4) *Systemic care and treatment* – Tetanus toxoid is given, the patient admitted to hospital for observation for at least 24 h, and symptomatic treatment given for problems such as vomiting or angioneurotic oedema.

Antivenom should be given to patients with severe systemic signs of envenoming, such as spontaneous bleeding, hypotension or coma. Zagreb antivenom, a highly purified and effective antivenom is used – it must be clear; opacities may mean loss of potency. Two 5.4 ml ampoules are given over 1 h intravenously diluted in 100–200 ml normal saline. This dose can be repeated if no improvement occurs within an hour. Reactions to Zagreb antivenom are rare, but the infusion of the initial dose should be slow for the first 15 min to reduce the likelihood of a severe allergic reaction.

The treatment for bites of snakes not indigenous to Britain is essentially the same as the above, but the clinical presentation may be different and often more severe.

The venom may be:

(1) *neurotoxic* causing ptosis, bulbar palsy, respiratory muscle failure, convulsions and coma;

(2) *necrotizing* causing swelling and blistering locally, with necrosis of superficial tissues;

(3) *myotoxic* causing muscle weakness, and respiratory failure;

(4) *vasculotoxic* causing internal haemorrhage and generalized bleeding.

Systemic envenomation, or the likelihood of local necrosis, are the indications for antivenom. Advice about bites and antivenoms for foreign snake bites can be obtained from: The Poisons Unit, Guy's Hospital, St. Thomas Street, London, SE1 9RT (telephone 01 407 7600)

MARINE STINGS
Jellyfish and Portuguese man-of-war
Bathers coming into contact with these creatures develop lines of weals associated with severe pain. Systemic symptoms include fever,

muscular weakness and paralysis, prostration, vomiting, colic and diarrhoea.

Treatment
   (1) Any remaining undischarged stings in the tentacles are inactivated with alcohol (any spirit is effective) or vinegar, and any tentacles left on the skin are removed after coating them with dry sand.
   (2) Symptomatic treatment with analgesics or antiemetics may be required. Respiratory or cardiovascular support is rarely necessary.

Other marine creatures in British waters have poisonous spines in their tails or dorsal fins, such as the Weever fish, *Trachinus vipera,* which is afforded great respect by the shrimpers of Morecambe Bay. If they are handled or stepped on, intense pain with blistering, swelling and even necrosis of the skin can occur. Systemic symptoms such as collapse, vomiting or diarrhoea are uncommon.

Treatment
   (1) The affected limb should be placed in hot water, or the area infiltrated with lignocaine or other local analgesic.
   (2) Any spines left in the wound must be removed as they may lead to chronic sepsis.

BEE AND WASP STINGS
Local pain is usually the only result of even multiple bee or wasp stings, and a human being can normally survive hundreds of such stings. The main danger of both bee and wasp stings is the possibility of allergic reactions; 0.5% of the British population is hypersensitive to bee or wasp venom, and in this group a single sting can result in death by acute anaphylaxis.

Clinical features of the allergic reaction
The severity of the allergic reaction is indicated by the speed of onset of the symptoms. In the most severe reactions an individual may die within a few seconds of the sting.
   The reaction often begins with tingling of the scalp a few minutes after the sting, followed by generalized urticaria. In the next hour bronchospasm, hypotension, coma, angioneurotic and laryngeal oedema can all develop (p. 262).

Treatment
(1) *For patients not exhibiting allergic reactions*
   (a) Following a bee sting, the barb of the sting remains in the skin, and should be removed by scraping it out with the blade of a knife. The small white sac on the end of the barb – the poison sac – should not be squeezed during removal.
   (b) Domestic meat tenderizer (papain), diluted 1:4 in tap water and rubbed into the area of skin involved is said to remove the pain of both bee and wasp stings. Acid and alkaline solutions are no longer used.
   (c) Mild analgesics can be given, and antiseptics applied locally.

(2) *For patients with allergic reactions*
   (a) An adrenaline (epinephrine) aerosol (Medihaler EPl) provides the most rapid effect.
   (b) Further management is as for other anaphylactic reactions (p. 263). Treatment of bronchospasm or hypertension may be urgently required.
   (c) Local treatment as under (1) above.

5

Disorders of temperature regulation

Hypothermia

Hypothermia is usually defined as being present when the core temperature falls below 35 °C.

To understand the treatment of hypothermia it is important to appreciate the difference between core and shell temperatures.

CORE AND SHELL TEMPERATURES

The abdominal and thoracic viscera, the brain and the spinal cord are at approximately the same temperature. This temperature is known as the core temperature, and is best measured by means of a probe in the upper oesophagus. The core temperature influences the hypothalamus and activates compensatory reflexes if the temperature varies from the normal 37 °C.

The shell temperatures refer to the temperatures in the skin, muscles and limbs. These may vary widely without causing any harm.

MEASUREMENT OF TEMPERATURE

Mistakes are easily made if the method of taking the temperature is not recorded. A thermometer placed in the axilla may give a grossly misleading reading, and one inserted into a mass of faeces in the rectum is little better if sensitive changes during rewarming are to be detected. An intraoesophageal temperature-sensing device is preferred for monitoring the core temperature, but a device inserted in an empty rectum is the next best choice. The diagnosis is often missed by medical and nursing staff not using a low reading thermometer.

Afterdrop

Following exposure to a cold environment a temperature gradient is produced in the body from the cold skin to the warm central core. Even if the patient is warmed externally the cold in the body shell still continues to move inwards and the core temperature continues to drop for the next ½ to 1½ h. This continued fall in core temperature is known as the afterdrop, and is usually 1 °C in the thin patient and 2 °C in the fatter individual. This can be of importance as ventricular fibrillation can occur spontaneously below 28 °C, and a patient with a core temperature of 30 °C when rewarming is commenced may drop his core temperature to 28 °C before it begins to rise.

Groups which develop hypothermia are:

(1) fit young people following immersion or exposure (alcohol or drug overdose may be present);
(2) the very young and the old, due to their poor temperature regulation;
(3) those with a severe debilitating illness such as myocardial infarction or pulmonary embolus;
(4) those with endocrine disorders such as hypopituitarism or hypothyroidism.

REWARMING

There are three different methods of rewarming:

(1) *Internal active rewarming,* by haemodialysis or peritoneal dialysis by giving warm solutions, by warming the inspired air, or even by warm fluids by mouth. Cardiopulmonary bypass has also been used.
(2) *External active rewarming,* by applying warmth to the surface of the body by immersion in warm water, or with a heated mattress or an electric blanket.
(3) *Assisted passive rewarming,* by preventing further heat loss by insulated blankets, (space blankets) in a warm environment. The patient's own metabolism does most of the rewarming, with a contribution from the surroundings.

Problems

(1) Facilities for internal active rewarming are often not available or too complicated to operate, particularly by an emergency rescue team at the site of immersion or exposure. An exception to this is a simple Water's canister device consisting of a mask attached to a sodalime carbon dioxide absorber (p. 159). The patient breathes through this, and the CO_2 and moisture in his expirations (water and CO_2 can also be added directly to the canister) react with the sodalime producing heat to warm his inspirations.

(2) It has been shown that rapid external active rewarming can cause an afterdrop (described above) which may be lethal to the aged. However, good results have been obtained in old people by immersing one forearm in warm water at 40−44 °C while preventing further heat loss by blankets and a warm environment.

(3) The patient's ECG should be monitored since atrial, and more important ventricular, fibrillation can appear without warning. Adequate oxygenation should be maintained, and any acidosis which develops should be immediately treated with bicarbonate. The arterial blood gas results are somewhat misleading when measured at 37 °C, and corrections should be applied; 0.015 pH units should be added for each degree centigrade below 37 °C to correct the pH value. Ventilation is rarely required, and indeed any stimulus such as intubation can result in ventricular fibrillation.

TREATMENT

Young adults
If the patient is young and presumably fit before the episode of exposure or of overdose, rapid rewarming in a bath at 40−44 °C can be undertaken. The afterdrop is said to be reduced when the limbs are not immersed, so only the trunk is submerged. When the core temperature reaches 35 °C, passive rewarming should be instituted.

If exposure occurs in a remote area, a Water's canister as described above (p. 160) can be useful to initiate warming. Hypothermic patients should not be carried in a head-up position, since this may cause postural hypotension.

Hypothermic infants
Hypothermic infants should be rewarmed in a bath only slightly warmer than themselves, and the bath temperature gradually increased every few hours until the temperature is about 35 °C. Again, passive warming is then instituted.

Old people
Old people should be rewarmed slowly, by assisted passive rewarming. A rate of 0.5 − 1 °C/h has been recommended. The rewarming of single limbs by immersion as mentioned previously may be helpful. Often the old have a predisposing condition such as an infection or myxoedema which will require treatment, but acute treatment is rarely required until the general condition of the patient has improved, and the temperature is at least 35 °C. Particular care of the skin especially over

the pressure areas is required, as it is easily damaged in hypothermic comatose patients by pressure or by direct heat.

Care of the unconscious patient
This is dealt with on p. 85.

Malignant hyperpyrexia
Malignant hyperpyrexia is an uncommon condition but in the past 2 years at least two cases have presented in the Lancaster group of hospitals. The following signs and management of malignant hyperpyrexia are those described by Ellis*.

REGIME FOR PATIENTS SUSPECTED OF DEVELOPING
MALIGNANT HYPERPYREXIA

Recognition
The syndrome should be considered with any of the following:

(1) A rise in body core temperature (perhaps with a fall in skin temperature).
(2) Hypertonus (spasm, rigidity) of skeletal muscle
   (a) immediately following suxamethonium;
   (b) with any of the inhalational anaesthetic vapours.
(3) Unexplained tachypnoea, tachycardia, cyanosis, oozing from wound, myoglobinuria, cardiac arrest.
(4) Acute acidosis or acute hyperkalaemia.

Management
(1) Terminate surgery if possible, but in any event discontinue all potent inhalational agents and depolarizing relaxants.
(2) Give 100% oxygen, preferably from an anaesthetic machine without a vaporizer.
(3) Monitor body core temperature (and skin temperature of a limb if possible).
(4) Insert intravenous cannula and take venous blood sample for potassium but retain serum in laboratory for further investigations; start infusion of glucose in water.
(5) Take arterial blood sample for pH, PCO_2, base excess, and PO_2.
(6) Establish ECG.

*Reproduced by kind permission of Dr F.R. Ellis, Reader in Anaesthetics, Malignant Hyperpyrexia Investigation Unit, St James's University Hospital, Beckett Street, Leeds LS9 TTF, England.

(7) Correct electrolyte and pH imbalance on the basis of the results; repeat estimations may be needed. (Hyperkalaemia may be controlled with dextrose 50 g with insulin 20 units.)

(8) Steroid therapy: dexamethasone 1.5−2 mg/kg, or methylprednisolone 7.5−10 mg/kg, or hydrocortisone 30−40 mg/kg; repeat in 15 min if no effect on rate of increase of body core temperature.

(9) Dantrolene intravenously 1 mg/kg up to 100 mg initially.

(10) Give cool 5% dextrose 10−20 ml/kg/1 h intravenously (preferably from a refrigerator or using a blood 'warmer' filled with iced water). Remove all covering from the patient, apply ice to groins and axillae, or use fans in conjunction with cold water, sponging with a wetting agent such as cetrimide.

(11) Consider the following procedures:

    (a) catheterization (save first sample of urine for detection of myoglobin);

    (b) control of cerebral oedema and renal failure with mannitol 1 g/kg;

    (c) diazepam 1 mg/kg;

    (d) droperidol 0.1 mg/kg as alpha-adrenergic blocker;

    (e) practolol 0.1 mg/kg to control arrhythmias;

    (f) isoprenaline 2 mg/500 ml to increase cardiac output.

Heatstroke

AETIOLOGY

Heatstroke occurs when the temperature-regulating mechanisms of the body are overwhelmed, and the diagnosis should be considered whenever collapse occurs during exertion in hot weather.

Competitive walking, jogging or running, when failure will cause loss of face, is particularly associated with heatstroke. The problems are due to:

(1) loss of body fluid and salt.

(2) a rising core temperature.

CLINICAL APPEARANCES

The patient presents in a state of collapse with a history of exertion in a hot environment, often with an inadequate fluid intake. He may be unconscious, or conscious but confused or abusive, and may be vomiting and incontinent.

FINDINGS

The patient appears dehydrated, and may be shocked, with low blood pressure and a fast thready pulse. The core temperature is raised (40–42 °C). The haematocrit may be raised, but the blood urea level is usually normal at the outset, while there is often hypokalaemia and mild hypernatraemia. Urine output is reduced, and may contain protein, blood and ketones. Mild metabolic acidosis is usually present, and the patient may compensate by overbreathing. Damage occurs to various organs and systems.

(1) *The brain*
Damage is usually non-specific and can lead to ataxia and dementia, but localizing signs such as hemiplegia can develop. Death can occur.

(2) *The kidneys and liver*
If treatment, particularly fluid replacement, is undertaken quickly, kidney damage is completely reversible, but renal failure can develop. The potassium and urea levels require close monitoring. Hepatic damage is usually mild and of little consequence.

(3) *The coagulation system*
A consumptive coagulopathy associated with falling platelet levels and fibrinogen, and rising fibrinogen degradation products (FDPs) may appear. Low dose heparin has been used effectively in these circumstances (see also p. 270).

TREATMENT

Cooling
The central temperature must be reduced as soon as possible to less than 40 °C. Immersion in a tepid bath or tepid sponging is helpful.

Giving intravenous fluids
There may be a fluid deficit of 5–10 litres, and the recommended regimen consists of litres of 4% dextrose in 0.18% saline alternating with normal saline or Ringer lactate; 2 litres of fluid should be given in the first hour, and subsequent fluids at a rate of about 1 litre/4 h, depending on the clinical state of the patient. Improvement is assessed by the urinary output, haematocrit and clinical examination of the circulation. Once urinary output is improving, potassium supplements must be added to the regimen. Frusemide can be useful to maintain

urinary output, but correction of the hypovolaemia is the primary consideration.

Using chlorpromazine

This can be given as sedation to reduce excitement and thus physical exertion, and also as a means of increasing peripheral vasodilation and therefore cooling; it should not be used if severe hypovolaemia is present. Intravenous diazepam may be required for convulsions. Heparin and clotting factors may also be necessary (see also p. 270).

6

Endocrine emergencies

Thyroid crisis

This is a life-threatening increase in the signs and symptoms of thyrotoxicosis.

PRESENTATION

Patients with a thyroid crisis often have a history of recent operation, infection or trauma, with pre-existing but untreated or inadequately treated hyperthyroidism. The patient is often prostrated, with profound muscular weakness, extreme tachycardia, hyperpyrexia and cerebral signs such as confusion, delusions or coma.

TREATMENT

This consists of treatment of the thyrotoxicosis and of the precipitating factor, if this is treatable, for example, infection.

IMMEDIATE THERAPY

(1) An intravenous infusion of 5% or 10% glucose is set up; this provides access to a vein for drugs and also provides some energy for the increased metabolic rate.

(2) Propranolol 2 mg (or other appropriate beta-blocking drug) is given intravenously and repeated every 2 h until adequate reduction in the pulse and other signs of sympathetic overactivity occur.

(3) Hydrocortisone 500 mg is given intravenously as a bolus, and 100 mg every 6 h until the crisis is over. There is said to be a relative glucocorticoid lack in thyroid crisis.

(4) Oxygen is given to maintain adequate oxygenation in the face of the increased metabolic rate.

(5) Propylthiouracil 150 mg is given by mouth if possible, and potassium iodide 200 mg by slow intravenous infusion to inhibit

47

further hormone synthesis. Further doses of propylthiouracil
are given every 6 h.
(6) Hyperpyrexia may require tepid sponging and fanning. Chlorpromazine may be helpful to encourage peripheral vasodilatation and reduce shivering.
(7) Sedation with diazepam, chlorpromazine or chlormethiazole
(p. 107) may be necessary to control restlessness and confusion.
Cardiovascular support (p. 253) may also be required.

Addisonian crisis

This is due to acute lack of adrenal cortical hormones, usually both
glucocorticoids and mineralocorticoids.

An Addisonian crisis, or acute adrenal cortical failure, can present
in several ways:

(1) following abrupt cessation of therapy in a patient on long term
steroid treatment;
(2) following stress such as surgery, trauma or infection in a patient
with undiagnosed Addison's disease;
(3) following acute destruction of the adrenal cortices by infection
(classically meningococcal septicaemia) or bleeding, as may happen in anticoagulant therapy.

When faced with an acutely collapsed hypotensive patient in
presumed Addisonian crisis, the practitioner usually has to begin
therapy on clinical suspicion alone.

SIGNS AND SYMPTOMS

These depend on the initiating factor. A patient with undiagnosed Addison's disease may well have a history of insidious ill-health, postural
hypotension, dehydration and vomiting, and may show the
characteristic skin pigmentation on pressure and exposed areas. A patient on previous steroid therapy may have a Cushingoid appearance
and will also have a condition for which steroids are prescribed, such
as asthma or rheumatoid arthritis. Acute destruction of the adrenal
cortices should be considered in patients on anticoagulants who
develop hypotension and abdominal pain, or in patients with septicaemia.

BLOOD INVESTIGATIONS

In the acute situation therapy will be commenced before any results
are available, but before therapy is instituted blood should be taken
for:

(1) urea and electrolytes, including calcium; potassium, calcium and urea levels may be raised in cortical failure;
(2) blood culture;
(3) plasma cortisol level;
(4) blood sugar.

TREATMENT
(1) An intravenous infusion is commenced, and physiological (0.9%) saline run in at a rate depending on the state of hydration and on the patient's age and cardiovascular status; 4 litres may be required in the first 12 h;
(2) Hydrocortisone hemisuccinate 200 mg and aldosterone 1 mg are given intravenously. An alternative for the latter is deoxycorticosterone acetate 5 mg in oil intramuscularly. The mineralocorticoid is not required where the crisis is due to abrupt cessation of glucocorticoid therapy.
(3) hypoglycaemia may require correction;
(4) regular replacement of glucocorticoids and mineralocorticoids must be undertaken.

Acute problems in myasthenia gravis (MG)

Myasthenia gravis is a condition associated with weakness and fatiguability of various muscle groups. Weakness usually involves proximal rather than distal muscle groups, and gradually increases during the day. Muscle wasting may also be present.

The cause of the weakness appears to be abnormal muscle endplates at the neuromuscular junction. The endplates have a reduced response to the release of acetylcholine by the nerve fibres. The medical treatment is normally with anticholinesterase drugs such as neostigmine or pyridostigmine, which increase the amount of acetylcholine available at the endplates, and so improve the chances of nerve impulses causing activation of the muscle fibres.

CHOLINERGIC CRISIS
If an overdose of an anticholinesterase drug is given, the excess acetylcholine at the endplate can lead to a depolarizing or cholinergic block (p. 193) with paralysis of that muscle fibre. One of the major problems in MG is the fact that some muscles appear quite normal, while others are severely affected. Thus if neostigmine, for example, is given to an MG patient in a dose appropriate for his affected muscle groups, a cholinergic block may develop in the normal muscles as the excessive

accumulation of acetylcholine at the endplates causes a relative overdose. An absolute or relative overdose of an anticholinesterase drug leading to widespread depolarizing block is termed a cholinergic crisis, and may require assisted ventilation if the respiratory muscles are involved. Atropine may be necessary to reduce the muscarinic effects of the neostigmine or pyridostigmine, such as salivation, bradycardia and pupillary contraction.

MYASTHENIC CRISIS

This arises when a dramatic increase in the weakness and fatiguability of muscle groups occurs, frequently in the bulbar or respiratory muscles, and it is often precipitated by an infection or other illness. The treatment is to increase the anticholinesterase medication, but as myasthenic crisis can readily be confused with cholinergic crisis, a diagnostic test using a short-acting anticholinesterase drug, edrophonium, is often carried out first; 2 mg edrophonium is given intravenously, followed by a further 8 mg if the condition of the patient improves or is unchanged. If the patient becomes weaker, he is suffering from a cholinergic crisis; if stronger, a myasthenic crisis is the diagnosis, and longer-acting agents can be given. Prolonged and severe weakness of the respiratory and bulbar muscles may require intermittent positive pressure ventilation (IPPV) often with a tracheostomy or endotracheal tube to prevent inhalation of saliva and food material.

Sometimes the patient alternates between cholinergic and myasthenic crisis in a so-called 'brittle crisis', and here anticholinesterase drugs are relatively ineffective. IPPV is often required to maintain adequate pulmonary function until the situation is clarified.

Diabetic ketoacidosis

Patients in diabetic ketoacidosis usually have overall deficits of the following:

(1) body fluid (mainly extracellular fluid);
(2) electrolytes, especially potassium;
(3) insulin activity.

Water, sodium and potassium are lost in the urine in diabetic ketoacidosis due to the osmotic diuresis caused by excessive plasma glucose levels. Since both water and electrolytes are lost in similar relative amounts the plasma electrolyte levels are often within normal limits on admission. The lack of insulin activity encourages the production of glucose, with increased formation of ketone bodies and a metabolic acidosis.

PRESENTATION AND DIAGNOSIS
Although patients with diabetic ketoacidosis may present in coma, more frequently they are conscious. Typical 'air hunger' due to the ketoacidosis may be present, and the smell of acetone may be detectable in the patient's breath. Dehydration, with inelasticity of the subcutaneous tissue, dry buccal mucosa and sunken eyes, may be severe, and there may be a fluid deficit of 5−6 litres. Diagnosis is confirmed by urinalysis, which shows sugar and ketones, and by a plasma glucose estimation.

MANAGEMENT
(1) If the patient is unconscious, the airway must be maintained and protected from aspiration of stomach contents (p. 85).
(2) Blood samples are taken for the following tests:
(a) haemoglobin and haematocrit; results may be high initially due to haemoconcentration;
(b) urea and electrolytes; these are often normal on admission;
(c) plasma glucose;
(d) blood culture; the precipitating event in diabetic ketoacidosis is often an infection;
(e) arterial blood is taken for blood gas and acid−base determinations.
(3) A peripheral infusion is set up. If the patient is severely hypovolaemic with impending circulatory collapse, a central venous catheter may be easier to insert, and will be useful in determining how much fluid should be given.
(4) In the first hour of treatment of an adult patient 2 litres of normal saline should be given, each with the addition of 20 units soluble insulin. If the initial serum potassium level is less than 4 mmol/l, 20 mmol/l potassium as chloride are added to the second litre. At the end of the first hour, the plasma glucose and potassium levels should be checked again. Since potassium moves into the cells with glucose under the action of insulin, the serum potassium level falls, and potassium supplements of 20−40 mmol are required in subsequent litres of fluid to maintain the plasma level.
After the initial 2 litres, the fluids are given more slowly. Further litres of normal saline with insulin and potassium supplements are

given approximately every 2 h until the blood glucose level falls below 15 mmol/l (270 mg/100 ml). The plasma glucose, potassium and sodium levels are regularly checked, and the supplements adjusted appropriately. Once the blood glucose is less than 15 mmol/l, the infusion is changed to 5% dextrose with potassium additions depending on serum levels, and insulin additions to provide 4−8 units/h of the infusion.

(5) Acidosis will require treatment if severe. If the initial base deficit is greater than 10 mmol/l, 100 mmol bicarbonate solution is given (p. 251). As rehydration and insulin infusion continue, repeated arterial samples will show maintained improvement in the acid−base status.

(6) Lactic acidosis can occur in association with the oral hypoglycaemic agent, phenformin. A severe acidosis is found in the absence of marked ketosis. High plasma lactate levels are diagnostic. Treatment with insulin and large amounts of bicarbonate is often unsuccessful.

(7) If the initial serum sodium is above 155 mmol/l, the fluid regimen is modified by giving litres of dextrose 4% in 0.18% saline, with the additives as before, until the serum sodium returns to normal.

Hypoglycaemic coma
There is rarely any difficulty in differentiating hypoglycaemia from hyperglycaemia.

The symptoms and signs in hypoglycaemia are due to:

(1) excessive sympathetic activity such as sweating, tremor, palpitations and apprehension;
(2) lack of glucose in the brain, producing abnormal behavioural patterns, headaches, aphasia, fits and coma.

In contrast to the patient in diabetic ketoacidosis, the patient is usually well-hydrated, his breath does not smell of acetone, and he is not hyperventilating. The clinician, however, may be misled by the presence of sugar in the urine, although this urine may well have been passed into the bladder some hours before the onset of hypoglycaemia. The diagnosis is best confirmed by a plasma glucose estimation, but a glucose oxidase reagent strip such as Dextrostix is helpful in the acute situation to give an estimate of the blood sugar. The strip should be from a recently opened box and its expiry date must not have passed otherwise it may be inaccurate.

TREATMENT

This poses few problems. If the patient is conscious, 20–30 g glucose or sucrose is taken by mouth; if unconscious, 20–50 ml 50% glucose is given intravenously. To reduce the very high incidence of thrombophlebitis, the largest vein available should be used, and the glucose flushed in with 10–20 ml 0.9% saline. If no vein can be found, or the patient is restless or aggressive, glucagon 1 mg intramuscularly can be given to stimulate a rise in plasma glucose levels. Glucose is, however, much more satisfactory. If the hypoglycaemia has been present for some time before therapy begins, the patient may have permanent neurological damage or cerebral oedema. If intravenous glucose does not produce normal conscious levels—and the diagnosis is correct—the patient should be treated for cerebral oedema (p. 84).

7

Status epilepticus and the control of violent patients

Status epilepticus

Status epilepticus is present when epileptic seizures occur continuously without intervening periods of recovery. It constitutes an immediate threat to life, since the patient may suddenly develop airway obstruction, may vomit and inhale gastric contents, and also become hypoxic from exhaustion or suffer cardiorespiratory collapse.

MANAGEMENT

(1) As in other life-threatening emergencies, the immediate concern is the airway (p. 28).

(2) The adequacy of respiratory exchange is then assessed by the patient's colour and his chest movements. If inadequate, oxygen by mask or IPPV may be required.

(3) The patient is restrained as necessary to prevent injury, and all hard, sharp or hot objects removed from the area. The tongue is frequently bitten, and may be bleeding profusely, causing a degree of respiratory obstruction. Until skilled assistance arrives, the patient is best held on his side in a head-down position.

(4) Drug treatment should be given as soon as possible, as the sooner the seizures are controlled, the less likelihood of neurological sequelae. Drugs should be given intravenously wherever possible, since a more rapid action is then obtained, and the dose may be titrated directly against the response.

Diazepam is probably still the drug of choice, and is particularly useful for initiating treatment outside hospital. It is given in a dose of 0.25 mg/kg intravenously, half over 60 s, and the effect after 5 min noted, the rest of the dose is then given, if required, over a 5 min period to minimize respiratory depression. Individual response is rather variable, and more or less may have to be given. The effects of the dose will only last 30–60 min, so if transfer to hospital is delayed a second dose may have to be given, or 100 mg phenobarbitone can be given intramuscularly to give a prolonged anticonvulsant action.

Continuing control of the seizures can be achieved by a diazepam drip, 200 mg diazepam in a litre of normal saline; this is given at an initial rate of 60 drops per minute (4 ml/min), reducing or increasing the rate depending on the response.

USE OF OTHER DRUGS
Chlormethiazole is an effective anticonvulsant and is given as an infusion of 0.8% solution (p. 107).

Clonazepam, 1 mg for adults and correspondingly less for children, is given slowly intravenously over 60 s, and is very effective.

Phenytoin, 2 – 4 mg/kg over 5 min is given intravenously. Cardiovascular and respiratory depression may be produced. The solution must not be given extravenously as sloughing of the tissues may occur. High blood levels may exacerbate seizures.

Thiopentone, (p. 187) 2–4 mg/kg by slow intravenous injection is an excellent anticonvulsant, but again cardiovascular and respiratory depression may be produced, and it is best administered by an anaesthetist. The length of action is short unless a continuous infusion is maintained.

Phenobarbitone is a useful anticonvulsant which may be given 50–100 mg intravenously concomitantly with other drugs.

Paraldehyde is now rarely used, as it can produce sterile abscesses, cause sloughing of tissues, may deteriorate in storage, is painful on injection, and must be given with a glass syringe.

If all else fails, the patient may require intubation and artificial ventilation while investigation and treatment of the epilepsy continues.

Adequate hydration and nutrition must be maintained for prolonged status epilepticus.

Febrile convulsions in children
The treatment of febrile convulsions has three aims:

(1) to reduce the temperature, by tepid sponging or bathing, and by antipyretics.
(2) to maintain the airway and control the convulsions with
    (a) intravenous diazepam as described on p. 54, or
    (b) intramuscular phenobarbitone 5 mg/kg, or
    (c) intravenous thiopentone 2–4 mg/kg, given by an anaesthetist,
(3) to treat the cause of the febrile illness.

Control of the violent patient
The aetiology of violent or aggressive patients is:

(1) Personality disorders, often associated with alcohol or drugs.
(2) Psychoses, such as acute schizophrenia or mania, often with hallucinations or delusions.
(3) Organic brain diseases, toxic confusional states or epilepsy, particularly temporal lobe epilepsy.
(4) General medical conditions such as hypoglycaemia or, rarely, myxoedema.
(5) Ingestion of drugs such as amphetamines or lysergic acid diethylamide (LSD); alcohol may also contribute to the aggression.

MANAGEMENT

Psychological approach
An immense amount of diplomacy, patience and self-control may be required for the management of these patients. No hostility should be shown towards them. Reassurance about their problems or delusions may have a calming effect. However, this approach frequently does *not* have the desired result.

Drug therapy
Drugs to produce initial control usually have to be given by deep intramuscular injection rather by intravenous injection, which can be impossible in a struggling, violent patient.

(1) Haloperidol or droperidol, 10 mg, is usually effective in producing tranquillity and sedation after about 30 min. These drugs are said to be particularly useful in both manic and old, confused patients.

(2) An alternative is the well-tried and deservedly popular chlorpromazine, 25–100 mg intramuscularly, depending on the age and general condition of the patient. All these drugs should be given with caution to patients with suspected drug or alcohol ingestion, as they may potentiate the effects of both alcohol and drugs. Once control of the aggression has been established, further doses of the above drugs may be given, or a 0.8% solution of chlormethiazole may be used to maintain drowsiness (p. 107).

(3) Investigations for suspected medical conditions may be required.

8

The rapid reduction of hypertension (high blood pressure)

Treatment of hypertension

Hypertension is treated for two reasons, firstly to reduce the symptoms of present disease, and secondly to prevent the consequences of hypertension such as cerebrovascular, myocardial, or renal insufficiency. The rate at which an elevated blood pressure should be reduced, and the level to which it should be lowered, depends both on clinical indications and on the adequacy of organ function. An elderly asymptomatic hypertensive may be precipitated into renal failure or a stroke by an excess of zeal and medication.

However, such conditions as hypertension causing acute left ventricular failure, hypertensive encephalopathy, or hypertension due to monoamine oxidase inhibitors (MAOIs), clonidine withdrawal or a phaeochromocytoma may demand urgent reduction in blood pressure by intravenous agents, changing to oral therapy when the diastolic pressure is falling towards safer levels and the general condition of the patient is improving.

When deciding which drug or drugs to use for a particular condition it is important to think of the pathophysiology of the circulatory disorder, how best the disorder can be reversed, and what are the drug's pharmacological actions.

Hypertensive conditions

ACUTE LEFT VENTRICULAR FAILURE DUE TO HYPERTENSION

In treating hypertension causing acute left ventricular failure (LVF) with pulmonary oedema, the aim is to reduce both the afterload on the heart (the peripheral resistance) and also the effective circulating blood volume by promoting venous pooling and diuresis. No agent which depresses myocardial contractility should be used.

Sodium nitroprusside, which produces both arteriolar and venous dilatation and is given as an intravenous infusion of 500 mg in 500 ml dextrose, is a useful drug. An initial dose of $0.5 - 1$ (μg/kg)/min is given, and slowly increased, and the blood pressure carefully monitored, preferably by an intra-arterial cannula. The instructions as to the total dose which may be given and the preparation and care of the solution must be carefully followed. The effects of the drug pass off very quickly on discontinuing the infusion, so other drugs must be given orally to maintain the effect.

Frusemide (furosemide) is usually also given intravenously at the initiation of treatment. If diazoxide or hydrallazine are given to the patient with a decompensating left ventricle, reflex tachycardia and angina may be precipitated. Other agents such as phentolamine (p. 251) may also be used to reduce the left ventricular afterload.

HYPERTENSIVE ENCEPHALOPATHY
The cerebral blood flow (CBF) is normally maintained at a steady level, irrespective of the blood pressure, until the mean blood pressure falls to about 60 mmHg; the CBF then declines. In hypertensive patients, this autoregulation fails at a higher pressure when their blood pressure is reduced, so a sudden drop in blood pressure can precipitate cerebral ischaemia. Despite this, some reduction in the blood pressure of these patients must be urgently made. The drugs of choice here are labetalol, diazoxide, hydrallazine or nitroprusside. Frusemide (furosemide) should also be given at the outset.

Labetalol
This drug has both alpha and beta-adrenergic blocking effects, and is given in increments of 50 mg/5 min until a suitable effect is obtained. It is much easier to control and much longer lasting than a nitroprusside drip.

Diazoxide
This drug has a direct effect on arteriolar muscle; it also has hyperglycaemic and antidiuretic effects, so a diuretic should be given with it.

A dose of 300 mg is usually given by rapid injection over 10 s. Many clinicians are unhappy about giving a potent drug at this rate rather than titrating the dose against the response, but the best and most predictable results are obtained only by rapid injection. If the clinician is worried about producing hypotension, half the dose should be given, but at the same speed. If no left ventricular failure is present, the patient can be pretreated with intravenous propranolol 0.1 mg/kg to prevent undue tachycardia.

Hydrallazine

This drug is a potent vasodilator, and causes reflex tachycardia which may precipitate angina; these side-effects can be attenuated with propranolol. Headache may be a problem, due to cerebral vasodilatation, when hydrallazine is used for other conditions besides encephalopathy, but the lupus syndrome is not seen when the drug is given for a short time.

It is best given in increments of 5 mg/5 min until control is achieved (20−40 mg may be required).

PHAEOCHROMOCYTOMA

This sympathetic amine-secreting tumour requires both alpha and beta sympathetic blockers for control of the often episodic hypertension. Labetalol has recently been shown to be effective.

MAOI INTERACTIONS WITH AMINES, AND HYPERTENSION DUE TO CLONIDINE WITHDRAWAL

These drug actions are best treated with an alpha-blocker such as phentolamine (p. 251).

9

Pulmonary emergencies

Acute asthma

The treatment depends on the urgency of the situation, the recent medication and the past history of the illness in each individual patient. As in so many conditions, circulatory and respiratory support may be required in the very ill patient to permit him to survive long enough for the therapy to be effective. This is less likely to be necessary if treatment is maximal at the outset, and the intensity reduced as the patient improves, rather than half-hearted at the start followed by a dramatic build-up as the patient worsens.

ASSESSMENT OF SEVERITY

The adequacy of the respiration and the circulation have to be considered. The most useful assessments to be made in status asthmaticus are the amount of work being done by the patient to achieve gas exchange, how he is coping with the added work and the results as measured by arterial blood gas analysis. In the normal individual (at rest) the work of breathing requires about 3% of the total oxygen uptake; this can rise to more than 50% in severe asthma.

Signs of increased respiratory work are:

(1) flaring of the alae nasae;
(2) increasing use of the sternomastoid muscles and other accessory respiratory muscles in inspiration and abdominal muscles in expiration;
(3) mouth opening with each breath, breathing with pursed lips, inability to talk easily or eat.

CIRCULATORY SIGNS

In asthma uncomplicated by right ventricular failure, the circulation usually copes well despite the enormously increased respiratory work and cardiac output. Pulsus paradoxus (where the pulse volume increases in expiration, and decreases in inspiration) occurs in severe asthma due to the considerable intrathoracic pressure changes; reducing pulsus paradoxus is usually a sign of improvement but can also be a sign of impending respiratory failure. Tachycardia and tachydysrhythmias may be present due to both endogenous and exogenous sympathomimetic stimulation, hypoxia and hypercarbia. Cooling extremities and oliguria in the absence of dehydration are ominous signs.

CONSCIOUS LEVEL

If the respiratory distress increases, the alert anxious patient becomes apathetic, drowsy and finally comatose. These changes are usually initially unrelated to the blood gas values, which often remain within acceptable limits until cardiorespiratory collapse is about to occur.

IMMEDIATE ACTION

This, of course, is modified by the mildness or severity of the condition. Immediate intubation and ventilation are rarely required.

(1) Give 40–50% oxygen by MC or similar mask at a flow rate of 4–5 litres/min oxygen.
(2) Set up an intravenous infusion of 5% dextrose.
(3) Give hydrocortisone 500 mg intravenously immediately and aminophylline 250 – 500 mg slowly intravenously over 10 – 15 min.

INVESTIGATIONS

(1) *Blood gases.* Absolute values for PO_2 and PCO_2 are less useful than trends. The PO_2 is likely to be low when the patient is breathing air due to the ventilation/perfusion abnormalities in asthma, and oxygen as suggested above should be given if the PO_2 falls to below 60 mmHg (8 kPa).

The PCO_2 is often 30–35 mmHg (4–4.5 kPa) in acute attacks particularly in young asthmatics, but may be normal or elevated. Again, the trend of the PCO_2 is more important than the individual value. A rising PCO_2 associated with a deteriorating, exhausted patient is a bad omen, and usually means that ventilation will be necessary.

(2) *Erect chest X-ray* is useful largely to exclude acute pneumothorax, which is the major differential diagnosis. In uncomplicated asthma the chest X-ray is normal, or shows hyperinflation of the lung fields.

(3) *Peak expiratory flow rate* is a useful indication of progress when measured every 4 h or so for the first 24 h.

(4) *ECG.* If the pulse is fast or irregular, continuous ECG monitoring should be undertaken while infusing agents such as beta-2 agonists and aminophylline.

(5) *Plasma electrolytes, urea,* and *haemoglobin* should also be measured.

GENERAL MANAGEMENT

Reassurance

The patient often has a feeling of impending doom, which unfortunately is sometimes justified. After the initial assessment and following institution of treatment, the patient should be reassured that the symptoms should ease in the following few hours, and then be left in the able care of the nursing staff. A physician hovering about – waiting for something to go wrong – does not increase patient confidence. There is no place for sedatives, tranquillisers or narcotics.

Rehydration

Patients with acute exacerbations of asthma often become dehydrated. This is due to increased insensible loss from the lungs, to perspiration from the increased work done, and also to decreased fluid intake; a litre of 5% dextrose every 8 h will improve this, and can also be used as a vehicle for drug infusions. Humidification of the inspired gases can be very helpful in loosening inspissated secretions.

Steroids

It is best to err on the side of excessive dosage in the acute situation, and start with 500 mg hydrocortisone hemisuccinate or equivalent, repeated every 4 h until improvement occurs. Several hours will elapse before the effect of the dose becomes apparent.

Aminophylline

Initially this is best given by slow intravenous injection of 7 mg/kg (250–500 mg for most individuals) over 10–15 min to obtain a reasonable plasma level, which can then be maintained either by repeating the initial dose intravenously every 4–6 h or by infusion of 500–1000 mg/8 hourly in the dextrose solution.

Beta-2-adrenergic agents
On arrival the patient may already have had considerable and often excessive self-medication with these drugs from pressurized inhalers, and be exhibiting tachycardia and often arrhythmias. Hypoxia, hypercarbia, and metabolic acidosis tend to increase the incidence of such arrhythmias, which limit the use of such drugs as salbutamol (albuterol), terbutaline. However, when cardiac rate and rhythm permit, these may be given intravenously or preferably nebulized and inhaled (a Bird respirator is very useful here).

Appropriate doses are: salbutamol $5-20$ $\mu g/min$ as an intravenous infusion or $1-2$ mg/h in a concentration of $50-100$ $\mu g/ml$ for nebulization; terbutaline $2-10$ $\mu g/min$ as an intravenous infusion or $1-2$ mg/h in a concentration of 100 $\mu g/ml$ for nebulization.

Oxygen
This should be given if the PO_2 is below 60 mmHg (8 kPa), and is best given by an MC-type mask. If the patient's history or a rising PCO_2 suggests liability to CO_2 retention the MC mask should be replaced by a Ventimask (p. 69), and the inspired oxygen tension slowly increased until the highest possible PO_2 is obtained without CO_2 retention.

Treatment of acidosis with bicarbonate
This is rarely necessary. A mild acidosis improves tissue oxygenation, while a severe and increasing acidosis implies deteriorating circulatory and lung function and probably impending collapse. Ventilation may then be necessary (see also p. 251).

Physiotherapy
This is of no value in the emergency situation.

Ventilation
The main indications for ventilation in patients with acute obstructive airways disease are:

(1) Clinical deterioration and exhaustion, often associated with deterioration of the conscious level, loss of cooperation, and inability to clear secretions from the airways.
(2) High and rising PCO_2 levels despite treatment. Adequate PO_2 levels are irrelevant. Ventilation is best instituted earlier rather than later. Clinical signs of imminent collapse are usually present before blood gas changes become significant.

Near drowning

Near drowning is a term used to describe the condition of a person who has lost consciousness following immersion in water but is rescued before death.

Loss of consciousness due to hypoxia may occur without the aspiration of water and causes a low PO_2, high PCO_2 and acidosis. Additional effects (Tables 9.1 and 9.2) manifest themselves after the aspiration of water, depending on whether it is fresh or salt.

Table 9.1 Blood changes after aspiration

Fresh water	Salt water
Hypervolaemia	Hypovolaemia
Haemodilution	Haemoconcentration
Haemolysis	
Haemoglobinaemia	

Table 9.2 Electrolyte changes after aspiration

Fresh water	Salt water
Hyponatraemia	Hypernatraemia
Hypochloraemia	Hyperchloraemia
Hyperkalaemia	Hypokalaemia

Table 9.3 Blood gas values after near drowning

	Interpretation
*pH 7.219 PCO_2 35.5 mmHg (4.7 kPa) PO_2 43.8 mmHg (5.8 kPa) HCO_3^- 14.0 TCO_2 15.0 BE 13 Sat 69 SBC 13.9	PO_2 is low. The hypoxaemia is associated with hyperventilation which lowers PCO_2; however, pH is low indicating an acidosis. The low HCO_3^- and the negative base excess denotes that the acidosis is metabolic in origin.

*For meaning of abbreviations see p. 290.

Clinical manifestations following aspiration include pulmonary oedema, tachycardia and hypotension. Hypothermia may be profound. Respiratory movements may be deep and rapid, or shallow or absent; cardiac arrest may occur due to ventricular fibrillation.

Different clinical pictures present, but one pitfall is to believe that the presence of deep and rapid respiration guarantees adequate oxygenation. Table 9.3 shows the blood gas analysis of an unconscious fresh water near-drowning victim who was hyperventilating on admission to the Royal Lancaster Infirmary.

The patient's hypoxia was treated by IPPV with 50% oxygen which raised his PO_2 to 69 mmHg (9.2 kPa); 200 mmol of 8.4% sodium bicarbonate solution were given intravenously to help combat his acidosis. Vast quantities of pink froth poured out of his bronchi; this can occur within minutes after aspiration but may be delayed for up to 3 days. Grossly abnormal radiological changes in the lung rapidly disappear within a few days.

Remarkable and complete recoveries from near drowning are recorded in the literature. One of the authors (FW) and his colleagues successfully revived an adult who had been submerged for at least 8 minutes in fresh water at a temperature of 6 °C. Many other listed successes such as 20 min immersion in liquid manure at 4 °C with no apparent after-effects in a child aged 6 years illustrate the importance of instituting and persevering with resuscitation measures in those apparently dead, especially if the victim has a low body temperature.

TREATMENT

This depends on the state of consciousness, type of near drowning, body temperature, and presence of carotid pulse.

Absence of respiration and carotid pulse demand treatment as for cardiac arrest with ventilation and external cardiac massage.

In the following routine it is understood that the patient has a carotid pulse and his upper respiratory passage is free of debris.

(1) Give a high concentration of oxygen by face mask.
(2) If condition deteriorates, intubate, suck out bronchi and start IPPV with 100% oxygen.
(3) Take blood gas readings; try to maintain PO_2 at a minimum of 60 mmHg (8 kPa).
(4) If pH is less than 7.2 give $NaHCO_3$ 1 mmol/kg body weight as 8.4% solution. Repeat every 10 min until the acid-base status is satisfactory. Some authorities give an initial dose of $NaHCO_3$ 150–200 mmol to the adult patient.

(5) Check electrolytes; set up CVP line; record temperature (p. 40).
(6) Support circulation with
  (a) normal saline for fresh water drowning,
  (b) 5% dextrose for salt water drowning,
  (c) plasma or a plasma expander if above fail to maintain blood pressure; all intravenous fluids should be warmed in a blood warmer.
(7) Give broad-spectrum antibiotics.
(8) Give dexamethasone 4 mg twice daily.
(9) Warm with blankets (p. 41).

If a PO_2 of 60 mmHg (8 kPa) cannot be maintained, PEEP (positive end expiratory pressure), starting at 2.5 cm water (0.25 kPa) and if necessary rising to 10 cm water (1 kPa), may maintain oxygenation at a lower FIO_2 (p. 209). The use of PEEP usually requires the services of an anaesthetist.

The consensus of opinion that positioning the patient head down to drain fluid from the lungs is only of use in salt water drowning should not distract the resuscitator from his prime aim which is to maintain adequate oxygenation and circulation.

Treatment of inhalation of gastric contents

(1) Place the patient in the head-down lateral position.
(2) Aspirate the mouth and pharynx.
(3) If the patient is
  (a) breathing, coughing and pink in colour – give oxygen and observe;
  (b) breathing and cyanosed – give oxygen by face mask and prepare to intubate. For intubation give suxamethonium 50 mg intravenously, insert airway, give IPPV with oxygen and face mask, then intubate and continue to give oxygen; this method demands skill in ventilating the paralysed patient (p. 194).
  (c) not breathing or remains cyanosed – intubate and aspirate; if solid material is suspected of being aspirated, bronchoscopy is advisable;
(4) Bronchial lavage consists of the installation of 10 ml normal saline into the trachea followed by aspiration, repeated several times. This method has its advocates, but others think it may spread the foreign material further into the lungs.
(5) Drugs used are:

(a) hydrocortisone 500 mg intravenously followed by 250 mg intramuscularly every 4 h for 24 h.
(b) adrenaline 1:1000, 0.5 ml subcutaneously, and aminophylline 250 mg intravenously over 5 min.

Oxygen therapy

The aim of oxygen therapy in general is to produce adequate oxygenation of the tissues while maintaining a normal or almost normal level of carbon dioxide in the blood. With most people there is little difficulty in maintaining a normal PCO_2. In the normal individual respiration is controlled by the partial pressure of carbon dioxide in the blood and this is held remarkably constant in health at 40 mmHg (5 kPa) under widely varying conditions. If the carbon dioxide level in the blood should tend to increase, for example due to exercise or perhaps due to decreased lung efficiency after an operation, ventilation is stimulated, and the PCO_2 returns to normal.

The PCO_2, indeed, is much less variable than the PO_2, which in health falls slowly over a person's lifetime. An educated guess – no more – of what a person's PO_2 should be in health can be obtained from the formula

$$PaO_2 = 102 - 0.33 \text{ (age in years) mmHg} \quad \text{or}$$
$$PaO_2 = 13.6 - 0.044 \text{ (age in years) kPa}$$

that is, an 80-year-old man cannot expect to have a PO_2 much above 80 mmHg (10 kPa). The PO_2 of the arterial blood has normally little effect on ventilation until it drops to 60 mmHg (8 kPa) or below, when ventilation is considerably stimulated ('hypoxic drive'). This fall can happen when climbing a mountain due to a fall in the inspired oxygen tension, or, more commonly, when the lungs are inefficient due to some lung condition such as emphysema. Some people with lung disease have lungs so inefficient at gas exchange that they cannot cope with the increased ventilation required to maintain a normal PCO_2, so the PCO_2 drifts upwards, no longer acts as an effective stimulus to ventilation, and may eventually rise to a level which actually depresses ventilation. These people inevitably have low PO_2 levels breathing air due to their poor lung function, and depend on this hypoxic drive for their very survival. If they are given high oxygen concentrations, the hypoxic drive is removed, respiration is depressed, and the PCO_2 rises further depressing ventilation (CO_2 narcosis). Finally apnoea supervenes. These patients, however, form a relatively small if important group, and in the past the fear of CO_2 narcosis has led many a patient to have either no added oxygen, or an oxygen concentration inadequate for his needs. The advent of readily available blood gas measurements in most hospitals should have removed both the fear and the mystique of CO_2 narcosis.

TREATMENT OF PATIENTS LIABLE TO CO_2 NARCOSIS
Any patient who presents with an exacerbation of a chronic obstructive airways disease such as chronic bronchitis, particularly if right-sided heart failure is present ('blue bloater') should have blood gases taken before oxygen is given. These will give a baseline for later comparison, and will also show if CO_2 retention is present, and also the level of oxygenation on air.

It is difficult to give the levels of PO_2 below which treatment is required, as the individual variation in patients is immense, and patients with severe obstructive airways disease may have a PO_2 of 60 mmHg (8 kPa) when they feel well. The patient must be considered as a whole, and assessment and reassessment at short intervals of his conscious level, respiratory effort, acid–base balance, and renal output must be undertaken, as well as trends in his PCO_2 and PO_2 levels. Oxygen is best given to these patients by masks using the HAFOE principle (High Air Flow with Oxygen Enrichment) such as Ventimasks; these provide accurate oxygen concentrations, and five different ones are available – 24%, 28%, 35%, 40%, and 60%. It is best to start with a 24% or at most a 28% Ventimask, and repeat the blood gases after 1 h. If the PCO_2 is stable, a 28% or 35% mask may be substituted and the PCO_2 and the PO_2 checked again after another hour. If the PCO_2 is rising even with the 24% mask, it is likely that controlled ventilation will be necessary. In this situation respiratory stimulants such as doxapram merely delay the inevitable and have little place in treatment.

OXYGEN THERAPY FOR PATIENTS NOT LIABLE TO CO_2 NARCOSIS
For patients who maintain normal PCO_2 levels irrespective of the inspired oxygen concentration (the vast majority of individuals requiring oxygen therapy) there is no problem and added oxygen can be given by a variety of devices. With masks and catheters, oxygen concentrations up to about 50% can be produced. There is little danger of oxygen toxicity with such concentrations in adults, even if a concentration of 50% is maintained for several days. Humidification of the inspired gases is useful and may prevent excessive drying of the secretions, particularly if the patient is mouth-breathing and so bypassing the normal humidifying effect of the nose.

MASKS

A mask is the most commonly used method of oxygen administration. They are particularly useful when a moderately predictable oxygen concentration is required, and when a patient is mouth-breathing. Some patients, however, tolerate masks poorly.

There are three groups of masks:

(1) *HAFOE type (High Air Flow with Oxygen Enrichment)*

These have a high air flow, usually produced by a venturi, no rebreathing occurs, and an accurately known inspired oxygen concentration can be produced. The best known example of these is the Ventimask (Figure 9.1). As previously mentioned, they are particularly valuable in patients thought to be retaining carbon dioxide.

(2) *Moderate flow but with very little rebreathing*

These can give concentrations of oxygen up to about 60%, depending on the type of mask and the minute volume of added oxygen, and are used for patients requiring improved oxygenation who are unlikely to develop carbon dioxide retention, such as postoperative patients or those with pulmonary embolus or pulmonary oedema. The MC mask is a commonly used disposable mask of this type. The concentration of oxygen obtained by an MC mask is less predictable than the HAFOE type, as it depends more on the patient's characteristics, but this is unimportant. With 4−8 litres/min oxygen an MC mask will deliver 40−50% oxygen.

(3) *Moderate flow with some rebreathing*

With this type a higher oxygen concentration can be obtained at the cost of some rebreathing, so they are unsuitable for patients liable to CO_2 narcosis. Disposable masks of this type are the Pneumask and the Polymask.

OTHER DEVICES

Neonatal incubator

These may be used to provide neonates with up to 40% oxygen in a controlled environment. Concentrations greater than 40% in neonates can cause retrolental fibroplasia, with permanent blindness.

Croup tent

This is a tent providing moderate humidity with added oxygen for children with upper respiratory tract disorders, especially acute laryngo-tracheo-bronchitis. Minute volumes of up to 10 litres are used, and concentrations of up to 80% oxygen can be obtained.

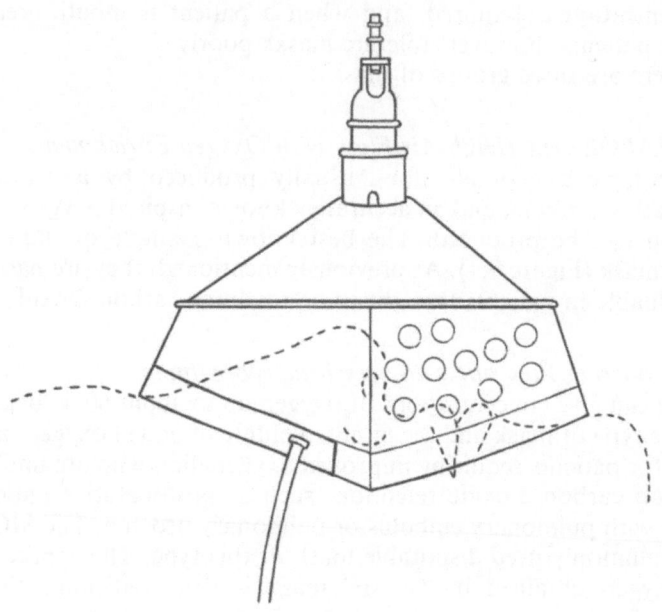

Figure 9.1 Equipment for oxygen therapy – the Ventimask

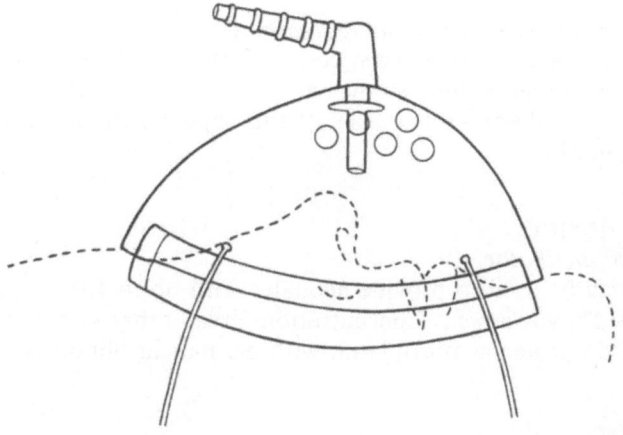

Figure 9.2 Equipment for oxygen therapy – the MC mask

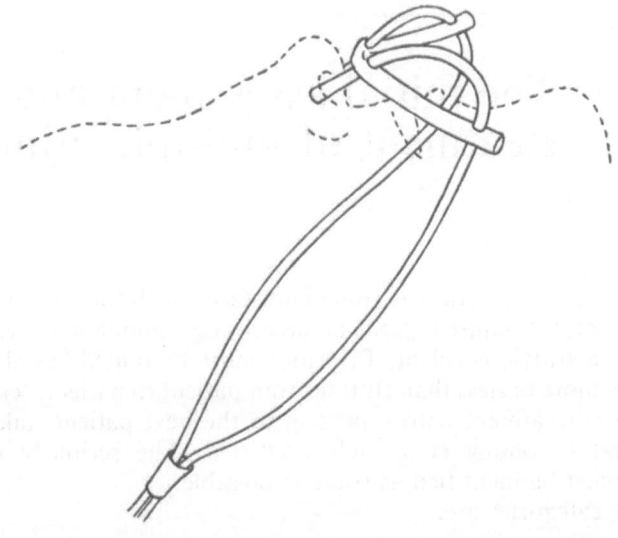

Figure 9.3 Equipment for oxygen therapy – nasal cannulae

Nasal catheters and nasal cannulae

These devices are useful for oxygen enrichment in patients not mouth-breathing and in those who will not tolerate a mask. They are also useful – and more comfortable – once the patient's status is improving and enable him to eat and drink without discontinuing the oxygen therapy. The nasal cannulae (Tudor Edwards) are inserted in the anterior nares, while if a catheter is used it is lubricated with local anaesthetic gel and passed along the floor of the nose to the naso-pharynx. With an oxygen flow of 2–4 litres, 30–50% oxygen is provided.

INDICATIONS FOR VENTILATION

These are discussed on p. 63 in the treatment of asthma.

10

The initial assessment and treatment of multiple injuries

A casualty officer is sometimes faced with the daunting problem of several injured patients presenting simultaneously, often following a traffic accident. Priorities must be quickly established; nothing is more useless than flitting from patient to patient, tentatively initiating treatment before passing to the next patient, taking no notes, and becoming completely confused. The seriously injured patients must be identified as soon as possible.

Patient categories are:

(1) Dead
(2) Critical
    (a) will die
    (b) may survive
(3) Serious
(4) Minor
(5) Sorrowful.

There must be a fast initial assessment of all the injured to decide on the appropriate category for each patient, and to identify immediately life-threatening problems, such as airway obstruction, crushed chest, or exsanguination. (It is said that this is as easy as ABC – airway, breathing, circulation.)

Airway

The airway is always the primary consideration, and is endangered in unconscious patients (especially lying supine), in patients with face or neck injuries, or in patients who are vomiting. Head injuries may be made much worse by hypoxia or straining. Often simply lifting the jaw forward is enough to relieve respiratory obstruction, but intubation, tracheal puncture (p. 97) or even tracheostomy may be required if the airway remains obstructed or unprotected.

Breathing

The adequacy of the patient's ventilation must be assessed. If the patient is conscious he can be questioned about breathing difficulties or chest discomfort, but the chest should be examined in every case.

If the patient has no respiratory distress, the chest moves well and equally on both sides with no obvious flail segment or surgical emphysema, the trachea lies in the midline, and the colour of the patient remains good, there is unlikely to be any major respiratory problem. The two conditions which may be present and need urgent treatment are tension pneumothorax and a flail chest (see p. 88). A ruptured diaphragm can also cause respiratory distress, but is more frequently discovered as a chance finding during exploration of the abdomen for suspected liver or splenic rupture.

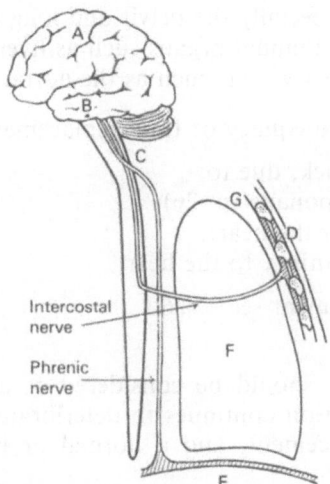

Figure 10.1 Causes of inadequate gas exchange after trauma

(A) Severe cerebral injury or raised intracranial pressure.
(B) Medullary damage involving respiratory centres.
(C) Spinal cord transection – if above C3, the tracts to the phrenic and intercostal nerves are divided.
(D) Fracture or flail segment of bony thoracic cage.
(E) Rupture of diaphragm with abdominal contents in thorax.
(F) Pulmonary contusion, oedema or haemorrhage.
(G) Pneumothorax.

CAUSES OF INADEQUATE GAS EXCHANGE FOLLOWING TRAUMA

Medical causes of inadequate ventilation such as muscle weakness due to myasthenia gravis or muscle relaxants, nerve disorders as in

Guillain–Barré syndrome or poliomyelitis, or cerebral depression following self-poisoning are considered elsewhere.

Circulation

Following trauma, external blood loss is less common than internal bleeding, which is frequently either unrecognized or underestimated. Patients in shock should have intravenous infusions started as soon as possible, preferably via two large cannulae. Plasma or plasma substitutes should be given until cross-matched blood becomes available (p. 272).

Two types of shock found after trauma are:

(1) Hypovolaemic, due to blood loss from:
    (a) fractures, especially the pelvis and long bones,
    (b) ruptured abdominal organs such as liver and spleen,
    (c) ruptured great vessels such as the aorta.

For assessment of adequacy of fluid replacement, see p. 247.

(2) Cardiogenic shock, due to:
    (a) cardiac tamponade (p. 26),
    (b) contusion of the heart,
    (c) penetrating injury to the heart.

For details of treatment see p. 260.

Cardiogenic shock should be considered as a possible diagnosis whenever the circulation continues to deteriorate despite apparently adequate fluid replacement, and a normal or high central venous pressure.

11

Head injuries and the unconscious patient

Pathology and clinical features
CONCUSSION

This is a temporary self-limiting inhibition of cerebral function due to injury to the head. Although the individual is rendered immediately unconscious, steady improvement tends to take place from then on. A useful guide to the severity of concussion is the duration of the post-traumatic amnesia.

CEREBRAL CONTUSION OR LACERATION WITHOUT
COMPRESSION

This is a more severe injury to the brain, but one in which cerebral compression does not occur, either because there is neither intracerebral bleeding nor severe oedema within the skull, or because the injury is decompressed by a skull fracture. Again the level of unconsciousness tends to be maximal at the time of injury, but recovery is likely to be slower, and often incomplete, when there may be signs of localized damage to areas of cerebral cortex causing aphasia or hemiplegia.

INJURIES WITH COMPRESSION

Compression of the brain substance can be due to acute haemorrhage, oedema, or a more slowly developing haematoma, and occurs most often in the anterior or middle cranial fossae, and relatively rarely in the posterior fossa.

Extradural haemorrhage

This is due to torn meningeal arteries usually associated with skull fractures. It commonly causes rapid deterioration of consciousness, often after a period of apparent improvement in the conscious level, usually called the 'lucid interval'. Rapid expansion of a blood clot

75

shifts the cerebral hemispheres to the side opposite the bleeding, distorting them and the brain stem, and producing in the untreated case a deepening level of unconsciousness, a slowing pulse, a rising blood pressure, fixed dilated pupils, and finally death. These patients have often not sustained severe brain injury at the time of the accident, and in general have a good prognosis if there is early surgical intervention.

Acute subdural haemorrhage
This usually implies a severe brain injury, with a poor prognosis.

Chronic subdural haematoma
This can occur in the elderly after apparent trivial injury, particularly in alcoholics or patients with some degree of cortical atrophy. The signs and symptoms are slow in onset, and a diagnosis of dementia is often wrongly made.

Cerebral oedema
It can be difficult to differentiate cerebral oedema from other causes of cerebral compression which require urgent surgical intervention. An absence of focal neurological signs may point to cerebral oedema, but this is by no means necessarily true (see p. 84 for treatment of cerebral oedema).

The emergency care of head injuries involve two main priorities:

(1) To provide the best conditions for recovery.
(2) To recognize deterioration or rising intracranial pressure as early as possible.

The optimal conditions for recovery include:

(1) An adequate airway and adequate oxygenation.
(2) Maintenance of the circulation.

ADEQUATE AIRWAY AND ADEQUATE OXYGENATION
Obstruction or partial obstruction of the airway is the commonest preventable cause of deterioration in head injury. Straining to breathe through an obstructed airway, hypoxia, and hypercarbia all increase intracranial pressure (ICP) which may remain elevated in head injury even after the precipitating cause is no longer present, in contrast to the normal patient whose ICP quickly returns to normal. Often a simple oral airway with the patient on his side with his jaw pulled forward

is enough to ensure adequate oxygenation, but if injuries to the chest or face are present, an endotracheal tube, or even a tracheostomy tube may have to be inserted and intermittent positive pressure ventilation (IPPV) instituted.

MAINTENANCE OF THE CIRCULATION

The circulation must be maintained and hypovolaemia avoided. Shock is very rarely produced by head injury; its presence suggests other causes, such as thoracic, abdominal or pelvic injuries; 30% of head injuries have these.

If transfer to a neurosurgical centre is to be undertaken, the adequacy of the airway and the circulation must be ensured throughout the journey.

Assessment of head injuries

A useful reproducible assessment of patient response in head injuries, or indeed in altered consciousness of any kind, is the Glasgow coma scale. It is particularly useful if transfer to a neurosurgical centre is contemplated. Three aspects of function are considered on the scale: eye opening, motor response, and verbal response to various stimuli. Points are awarded depending on the responses, from a minimum of three points for an unconscious patient without any responses to pain, to a maximum of fifteen points for an awake and orientated patient with normal motor responses (see Table 11.1).

Table 11.1 Glasgow coma scale

Eye opening	spontaneous	4
	to speech	3
	to pain	2
	nil	1
Best motor response	obeys	6
	localizes	5
	withdraws	4
	abnormal flexion	3
	extends	2
	nil	1
Verbal response	orientated	5
	confused conversation	4
	inappropriate words	3
	incomprehensible sounds	2
	nil	1

Good baseline assessment of head injuries is essential if any later deterioration is to be diagnosed early. The following should be noted:

(1) A description of the level of consciousness, based on the above scale, but the responses should be described in the case notes.
(2) Blood pressure, and pulse rate.
(3) Respiratory rate and whether respiration is regular.
(4) Pupillary size and reactions to light.
(5) Localizing signs such as hemiplegia; a full neurological examination should be done as soon as possible.
(6) Other injuries, such as neck or spinal injuries, fractured ribs, pneumothorax, ruptured viscera, fractured pelvis and long bones.

SIGNS OF RISING INTRACRANIAL PRESSURE
(1) Deterioration in the level of consciousness; this is usually the first and the most important sign.
(2) Rising systolic pressure, and widening pulse pressure.
(3) Progressively slowing pulse.
(4) Respiratory changes; breathing may become irregular or the rate may decrease.
(5) The appearance of localizing signs such as hemiplegia.
(6) Pupillary changes; the pupils eventually become non-reactive and dilated, but treatment must be undertaken before this occurs.

Patients with expanding haematomata in the posterior fossa are rare, but sometimes present with respiratory and cardiovascular abnormalities, as described above, rather than with deteriorating conscious levels, which may be relatively late in appearance. An occipital fracture is usually seen on a skull X-ray (which should always be taken after head injury, and examined for foreign bodies as well as fractures). A calcified pineal gland can often be visualized on Towne's X-ray view, and any displacement from the midline will indicate an expanding lesion.

Surgical decompression by burr holes or craniectomy will not be discussed here.

Pupillary changes in head injury
NERVE SUPPLY TO THE EYE
The nerve supply to the eye is complicated and is the source of much confusion. However, knowledge is essential because much reliance is

rightly placed on the size of the pupils and their response to light in determining the extent and deterioration of a head injury. Such deterioration may call for urgent surgery. The pupillary signs are often useful in deciding the site of surgical intervention.

PUPILLARY REACTION

The size of the pupil is determined by the muscles in the iris which are arranged circularly and radially around the pupil. Contraction of the circular muscle (sphincter pupillae) constricts the pupil, whereas contraction of the radial muscle (dilator pupillae) causes its dilatation.

Normally there is a balance between the activities of the two types of muscle due to the balance between their different nerve supplies, namely the parasympathetic system which constricts the pupil and the sympathetic system which causes dilatation.

Parasympathetic fibres

The constrictor parasympathetic fibres have their cell bodies in the Edinger–Westphal nucleus in the midbrain. Their fibres pass along with the oculomotor nerve and its branch to the inferior oblique muscle to enter the ciliary ganglion. Short ciliary nerves leave this ganglion to enter the eye.

These parasympathetic fibres 'hitchhike' along the oculomotor nerve. If, therefore, the oculomotor nerve is damaged so too are the parasympathetic fibres. As a result the pupil cannot maintain its constrictor tone, the sympathetic system is unopposed and the pupil dilates.

In order to understand pupillary reflexes it is essential to remember that parasympathetic fibres run with and are intimately associated with the oculomotor nerves. Although they are entirely separate functionally damage to one results in damage to the other.

Sympathetic fibres

The pupillary dilator sympathetic fibres have their cell bodies in the interstitial nucleus of the midbrain. Their fibres pass downwards to leave the spinal cord at the level of T1 or T2 on their way to the superior cervical ganglion. From here they 'hitchhike' along the internal carotid artery and its branches, some becoming intimately associated with the nasociliary branch of the ophthalmic nerve and eventually entering the long ciliary nerves and the eye. However, sympathetic fibres enter the pupil from a variety of different routes, and damage to one route usually leaves the others unaffected. As a result head injury is not usually associated with pupillary constriction due to intracranial sympathetic paralysis. It is, however, seen in Horner's syndrome (p. 84).

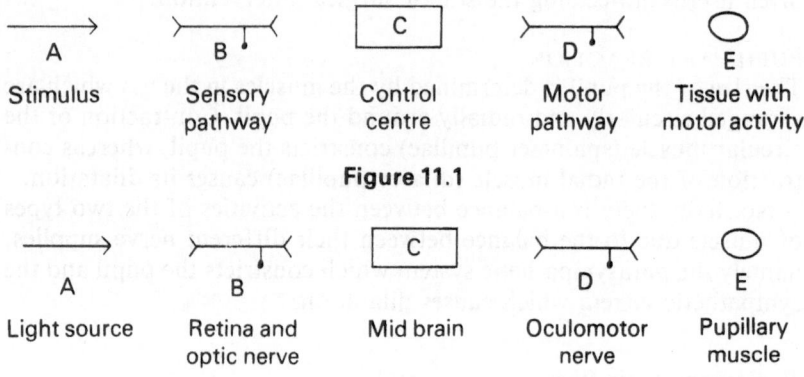

Figure 11.1

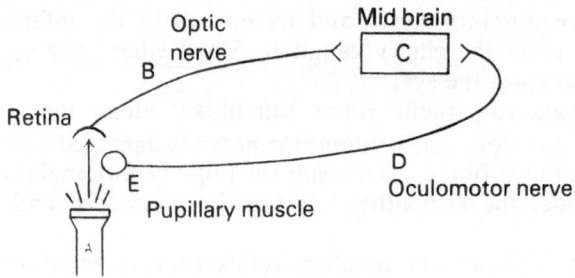

Figure 11.2

Optic
nerve

Mid brain

Retina

Pupillary muscle

Oculomotor nerve

Figure 11.3

THE PUPILLARY REFLEX
Figure 11.1 shows that a single reflex consists of a stimulus (A), a sensory pathway along which the stimulus travels (B), and a control centre (C) where the stimulus is received and interpreted, and where a decision is made regarding any reaction that might be necessary. Finally there is the motor pathway (D) which conveys this reaction to the tissue (E) which carries it out. Figure 11.2 shows the pupillary reflex redrawn.

Figure 11.3 shows how the pupillary reflex can now be coiled on itself. Normally, the light shone into an eye stimulates the retina and the impulse passes along the optic nerve to the midbrain. Then the impulse passes out along the oculomotor nerve to cause constriction of the pupil. However, the midbrain does not restrict its activity to the oculomotor nerve (D) on the same side (ipsilateral side) as that to which the light is directed. It also sends messages out along the other oculomotor nerve D_1 (contralateral side) to the other pupil (E_1) and the reflex is redrawn in Figure 11.4

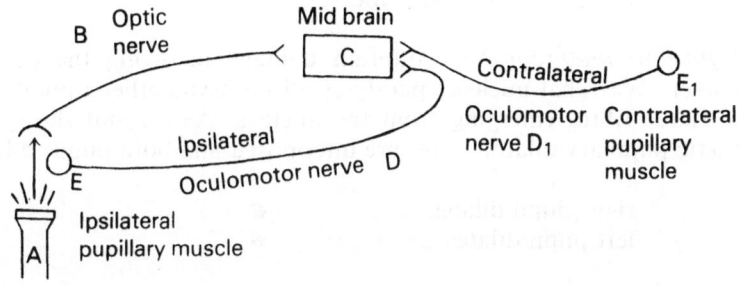

Figure 11.4

Constriction of the same pupil is known as the pupillary light reflex, and of the opposite pupil as the consensual reaction.

Abnormal light reflexes in response to a torch directed towards the right eye (Figure 11.5) produce typical signs, the causation of which is predictable on anatomical grounds.

Normal reaction: Torch at A causes

    right pupil to constrict   •
    left pupil to constrict   •

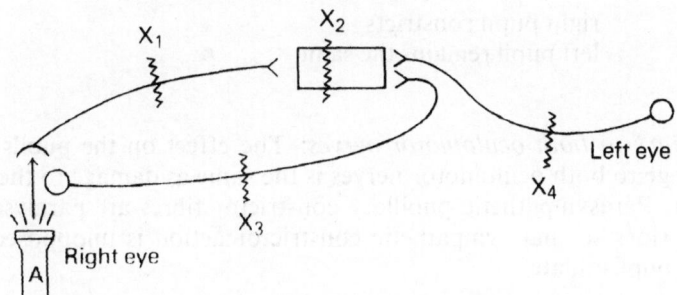

Figure 11.5

Division of right optic nerve at X_1: Optic nerve lesion at X_1 prevents light stimulus reaching midbrain which, therefore, is unable to transmit along the oculomotor nerves. Neither pupil reacts. The patient is blind in the right eye.

        right pupil stays the same   ●
        left pupil stays the same   ●

Injury to midbrain X_2: Midbrain damage involving the centre (Edinger–Westphal nucleus) paralyses all parasympathetic pupillary constrictor fibres emerging from the nucleus. As a result the sympathetic pupillary dilator fibres are unopposed and both pupils dilate

        right pupil dilates   ⬤
        left pupil dilates   ⬤

Injury to right oculomotor nerve at X_3: Ipsilateral oculomotor nerve damage impedes impulses passing from midbrain to pupil so that the pupil fails to constrict on the same side. However, unimpeded impulses pass along the contralateral oculomotor nerve causing pupillary constriction of the contralateral side

        right pupil remains the same ●
        left pupil constricts   •

Injury to left oculomotor nerve at X_4: Contralateral oculomotor nerve injury prevents impulses passing from midbrain to the opposite pupil which remains unchanged. Uninterrupted impulses pass down the ipsilateral oculomotor nerve and cause pupillary constriction on the same side

        right pupil constricts   •
        left pupil remains the same ●

Injury to both oculomotor nerves: The effect on the pupils after damage to both oculomotor nerves is the same as damage to the midbrain. Parasympathetic pupillary constrictor fibres are paralysed on both sides so that sympathetic constrictor action is unopposed and both pupils dilate

        right pupil dilates   ⬤
        left pupil dilates   ⬤

Relating signs of injury

Although anatomical knowledge is essential to account for the origin of abnormal pupillary reflexes, the clinician sometimes finds difficulty in translating the signs into an accurately localized clinical diagnosis unless he deals daily with head injuries. In head injury it is important to act on changes in pupillary size and reaction as soon as possible. If the clinician waits for one or both pupils to be fixed and dilated, unnecessary and usually irreversible brain damage will have been caused. It is useful to record the possible pupillary reactions and by reference to the figures deduce the site of the lesion (Table 11.2)

Table 11.2

	Shine torch into right eye	Diagnosis
(1)	Right pupil constricts •	Normal
	Left pupil constricts •	
(2)	Right pupil stays the same ●	Right optic nerve lesion
	Left pupil stays the same ●	
(3)	Right pupil remains dilated ●	Midbrain lesion, or
	Left pupil remains dilated ●	right and left oculomotor nerve lesion; often severe irreversible brain damage is present
(4)	Right pupil stays the same ●	Right oculomotor nerve lesion
	Left pupil constricts •	
(5)	Right pupil constricts •	Left oculomotor nerve lesion
	Left pupil stays the same ●	

	Shine torch into left eye	Diagnosis
(1)	Left pupil constricts •	Normal
	Right pupil constricts •	
(2)	Left pupil stays the same ●	Left optic nerve lesion
	Right pupil stays the same ●	
(3)	Left pupil remains dilated ●	Midbrain lesion, or
	Right pupil remains dilated ●	left and right oculomotor nerve lesion; often severe irreversible brain damage is present

Table 11.2 (Continued)

Shine torch into left eye		Diagnosis
(4) Left pupil stays the same Right pupil constricts	● ●	Left oculomotor nerve lesion
(5) Left pupil constricts Right pupil stays the same	● ●	Right oculomotor nerve lesion

Pitfalls
The glass eye – This is an obvious source or error.

Horner's syndrome – Interruption of sympathetic impulses due to injury or surgery of the superior sympathetic cervical ganglion causes constriction of the pupil; the contralateral pupil is thus relatively . dilated and may falsely suggest intracranial damage.

Miotics and mydriatic drugs – Parasympathomimetic drugs in the form of physostigmine or ecothiopate eye-drops are used in the treatment of glaucoma. As they are miotics they constrict the pupil.
Parasympatholytic drugs in the form of eye-drops such as atropine or cyclopentolate are used in treating iritis and iridocyclitis and are sometimes used to facilitate examination of the pupil. The dilatation they cause can be wrongly diagnosed as oculomotor nerve damage.

Cerebral oedema
Without fairly specialized equipment in cases of head injury it is difficult or impossible to differentiate cerebral oedema from rising intracranial pressure (ICP) due to intracranial bleeding. If there is any doubt as to which is responsible, surgery must be undertaken, as treatment for cerebral oedema by hyperosmolar solutions when the actual pathology is bleeding can encourage further expansion of an intracranial clot with further deterioration of the patient.
Treatment for cerebral oedema should thus be limited to:

(1) medical causes of cerebral oedema such as hypoxia, cardiac arrest and cerebral tumours;
(2) reduction of intracranial pressure while preparations for surgery are being made;
(3) postoperative head injury patients.

TREATMENT
Steroids
Dexamethasone can be given 4–8 mg intravenously thrice daily for 2 or 3 days; this is probably of limited effectiveness, except in oedema secondary to cerebral tumours.

Hyperosmolar solutions
Mannitol is the most frequently used solution. In the presence of good renal function, 1.5 g/kg can be given intravenously, but it is only effective if the blood – brain barrier is impermeable to the solution. Rebound cerebral oedema can occur.

Controlled hyperventilation
Reduction of the PCO_2 by controlled hyperventilation following endotracheal intubation and muscle relaxation is an effective way of reducing intracerebral pressure. A PCO_2 of between 25 and 30 mmHg (3–4 kPa) is ideal. Treatment in the head-up position also helps reduce intracranial pressure provided that the blood pressure is adequate for cerebral perfusion.

Care of the unconscious patient
The airway is always the priority. Unconscious patients can often be safely nursed on their sides if they are breathing adequately with intact protective reflexes. Such patients should never be laid supine unless the airway is secured by either a cuffed endotracheal tube or a tracheostomy. If the upper airways are bypassed by either an endotracheal tube or a tracheostomy, the gases supplied to the lungs must be adequately humidified. Physiotherapy and suction are required to prevent accumulation of secretions and hypostatic pneumonia.

Other problems in prolonged unconsciousness are: pressure and positional problems, nutritional problems, temperature control, and dangers of nasogastric tubes.

PRESSURE AND POSITIONAL PROBLEMS
These can lead to:

(1) bedsores in the sacral region, heels and other pressure areas;
(2) nerve injuries, such as radial or ulnar nerve damage following prolonged pressure;

(3) an increased risk of deep venous thrombosis;
(4) corneal abrasions.

These problems are usually minimized by good nursing care with regular turning of the patient and passive movements of the limbs.

NUTRITIONAL PROBLEMS
The patients are usually best fed by nasogastric tube in the long term, but in the short term or where aspiration of stomach contents is likely, an intravenous drip to provide essential fluids and electrolytes may be safer. Intravenous nutrition is rarely needed before several days have passed, by which time the gut is usually functioning. A urinary catheter is necessary both to provide accurate measurement of urinary output and to protect the patient's skin from irritation.

TEMPERATURE CONTROL
A raised temperature often occurs in head injury and may require control by fanning or tepid sponging. Chlorpromazine may be used to depress the temperature-regulating centre and prevent shivering while the cooling is being carried out.

DANGERS OF NASOGASTRIC TUBES
Introduction of a nasogastric tube is often difficult in the unconscious patient, especially through the nose. If the patient is comatose it is easy to pass the nasogastric tube accidentally through the vocal cords and into the trachea without causing him to cough. The small baby is especially tolerant to such circumstances and apart from the occasional cough it soon settles down and behaves as if the tube were non-existent. Attempted stomach washout or introduction of a milk feed then has disastrous results. Any coughing episode during the passage of a nasogastric tube in a baby should arouse suspicion, and calls for careful aspiration of the tube to confirm the presence of gastric contents. If these are unobtainable 0.5 ml water should be injected down the tube. Any resultant coughing demands withdrawal of the tube.

If the nasogastric tube is left in the trachea difficulties can arise during IPPV. First the nasogastric tube lies between the cuff of the endotracheal tube and the trachea and allows air to escape through the cords during inspiration. Usually the leak is audible at the mouth or at the proximal end of the nasogastric tube. If the tube is connected to an airtight plastic bag for the collection of gastric contents, then during inspiration air is forced from the trachea up the nasogastric tube, causing the plastic bag to distend.

If a tube is necessary in an unconscious patient, the airway must be adequately protected during its insertion, as vomiting often follows stimulation of the pharyngeal wall. Endotracheal intubation is often required.

12

Chest and other injuries

Flail chest and chest injury

Spontaneous breathing is dependent on the integrity of the bony thorax. Muscles acting on the rib cage increase the intrathoracic volume during inspiration, producing a fall in intrathoracic pressure, and air is drawn into the lungs from the atmosphere. If part of the chest wall loses this rigidity by reason of multiple rib fractures, it is sucked in during inspiration by the fall in intrathoracic pressure when the rest of the chest wall is expanding outwards, and is similarly pushed out in expiration. This is called a flail segment, and implies that double fractures of three or more adjacent ribs are present. The mechanical inefficiency of the chest wall if the segment is large leads

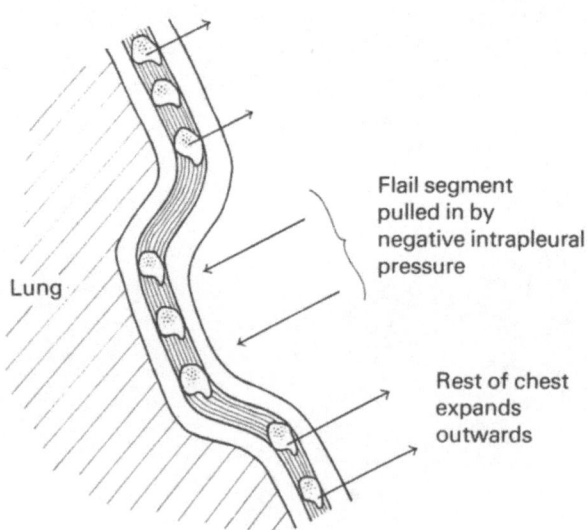

Flail segment
pulled in by
negative intrapleural
pressure

Lung

Rest of chest
expands
outwards

Figure 12.1 Flail chest in inspiration

to respiratory embarrassment and hypoventilation. There are three types:

(1) *Lateral.* This is commonest type; the 5th to the 9th ribs are most often involved.
(2) *Anterior.* In this type the sternum is separated from the ribs and acts as the flail segment.
(3) *Posterior.* This usually causes few problems since the muscle mass of the back tends to prevent undue movement of the flail segment.

Besides the hypoventilation and respiratory distress consequent upon a large flail segment, respiratory function is also impaired by direct trauma to the lung, the pain of the fractures inhibiting adequate chest movement, any pneumothorax or haemothorax which may be present, and the inability to cough adequately to clear secretions. These may lead to a slow but progressive deterioration in lung function.

Cardiovascular problems can also develop; the great vessels may be kinked by the movement of the mediastinum from side to side with respiration when a lateral flail segment is present, while an anterior flail segment can press directly on the heart and great vessels during inspiration, reducing venous return and cardiac output. The situation may be made worse by cardiac tamponade due to the chest injury, or by hypovolaemia due to blood loss.

MANAGEMENT

A tension pneumothorax frequently coexists with the flail chest, and requires urgent treatment as a priority (p. 92). A flail chest does not usually cause sudden unexpected deterioration, whereas a tension pneumothorax frequently does. Patients with a pneumothorax must never undergo intermittent positive pressure ventilation (IPPV) before an intercostal drain is inserted, or a rapidly expanding tension pneumothorax may develop.

The management of a flail chest depends on the degree of respiratory impairment. Mild cases can often be treated conservatively, with adequate pain relief and oxygen, but more serious cases will require IPPV for 10—14 days following an elective tracheostomy. Treatment with IPPV is required if there is evidence of respiratory embarrassment, with

(1) an obvious flail segment with paradoxical movement,
(2) inability to cough adequately,

(3) low PO_2 level,
(4) high PCO_2 level; this is ominous and presages collapse,
(5) rapid, shallow, painful breathing.

Chest radiography

Chest X-rays are essential for proper assessment of any chest injury, and should be undertaken as soon as the general condition of the patient permits. Posteroanterior, lateral, oblique and erect (or lateral decubitus if the state of the patient does not permit an erect film) films are taken, and examined for:

(1) the number and extent of rib fractures,
(2) widening of the mediastinum (due to ruptured aorta),
(3) loculated air in the mediastinum (due to perforated oesophagus),
(4) pneumothorax or haemothorax,
(5) lung parenchymal damage,
(6) traumatic diaphragmatic hernia.

INTERMITTENT POSITIVE PRESSURE VENTILATION (IPPV)
Artificial ventilation rarely needs to be resorted to as an emergency in patients with flail chest, and rapid deterioration is usually due to other factors, such as cardiac tamponade, hypovolaemia, pneumothorax or haemothorax. IPPV is usually used to prevent slow cardiac and respiratory deterioration consequent upon the inefficient flail segment.

The advantages of IPPV are:

(1) It does not require the integrity of the bony thorax, and during inspiration in IPPV all parts of the chest wall are subjected to the same pressure acting from within the chest; thus the flail segment moves with the rest of the chest wall, no paradoxical movement occurs, pain is reduced, and healing at the fracture sites is encouraged.
(2) Ventilation by IPPV means that the patient does not have to do the increased work required to maintain adequate gas exchange in the presence of the inefficient lung and chest mechanics.
(3) Removal of secretions is made much easier by the insertion of an endotracheal or tracheostomy tube.
(4) Adequate analgesia can be given without fear of respiratory depression.

CONSERVATIVE MANAGEMENT

Lesser degrees of flail chest can often be treated conservatively, if the patient can clear his secretions adequately and maintain reasonable PO_2 and PCO_2 levels without distress. This is frequently the case with a posterior flail segment, in which the flail segment may be adequately splinted by the surrounding muscles.

Oxygen is given by mask to maintain the arterial PO_2 level at about 80–100 mmHg (10–13 kPa). If the PO_2 is less than 60 mmHg (8 kPa) on 30–40% oxygen, ventilation is necessary.

Pain relief may produce a dramatic improvement in respiratory function and the ability to cough. Local analgesic techniques, such as intercostal, paravertebral or continuous thoracic epidural blocks, are particularly useful, although the latter two may produce hypotension.

The opinion of a thoracic surgeon may be urgently required for

(1) a widening mediastinum suggesting aortic rupture.
(2) loculated gas in the mediastinum suggesting oesophageal rupture
(3) a traumatic diaphragmatic hernia,
(4) rupture of a major bronchus causing a continuous broncho-pleural air leak.

Once the initial assessment and classification of the patient has been completed, and immediately life-threatening conditions have been treated, each patient is thoroughly examined in a systematic way to ensure that all injuries have been noted. It is often suitable to start at the patient's head, and work down, examining the head, eyes and face, neck and spinal column, the chest, abdomen, pelvis and limbs for injury.

The management of head injuries is described on p. 75.

Tension pneumothorax

The term 'tension pneumothorax' implies not only a major collapse of the lung on the side of the pneumothorax with a positive pressure within the pleural space relative to the atmosphere, but also a shift of the mediastinal structures to the opposite side, which may cause kinking of the great vessels and circulatory embarrassment.

AETIOLOGY

A tension pneumothorax usually develops either spontaneously following rupture of a subpleural bulla or following trauma. There is a valvular mechanism which enables air to enter the pleural space in inspiration, but prevents egress of the air in expiration, so the air in the pleural space increases in volume and in pressure with each breath, causing increasing respiratory distress and hypoxia. A simple pneumothorax may rapidly become a tension pneumothorax if the patient undergoes IPPV.

DIAGNOSIS
Diagnosis is made more easily in injured patients. Obvious trauma to the chest, with tenderness over fractured ribs, possibly with surgical emphysema, a tracheal shift to the opposite side, and the affected side of the chest hyperresonant to percussion leads to the diagnosis. Bronchospasm may be present.

In patients with spontaneous development of a tension pneumothorax, the presenting complaint is usually increasing short- ness of breath, associated as above with tracheal shift and hyper- resonance of the affected side. The patient will be distressed and often cyanosed, with his chest in the inspiratory position.

If the condition of the patient is not desperate, a chest X-ray should be taken in the semi-erect position to confirm the diagnosis.

MANAGEMENT
If the condition of the patient is critical, a large needle-through-can- nula device, as used for intravenous infusions, should be thrust through the chest wall, either in the 2nd intercostal space 30 mm lateral to the sternal edge, or in the anterior axillary or mid-axillary line in the 4th or 5th intercostal space. This will permit the release of the air under pressure and improve the general condition of the patient until an intercostal drain can be inserted into the pleural space and connected to an underwater seal. (Figure 12.4).

If the clinician is in doubt about the diagnosis, but is faced with a serious and deteriorating situation, he can insert a small needle (18 or 21 SWG) on a 20 ml syringe, through the chest wall on the side of the presumed pneumothorax, and attempt to aspirate. The diagnosis is correct if air is readily aspirated into the syringe, and rushes out of the needle when the syringe is removed. If a wrong diagnosis has been made, a minor pneumothorax of little significance is produced.

Insertion of intercostal drain
Following emergency decompression of the tension pneumothorax, an intercostal drain should be inserted into the pleural space under cond- itions of sterility and adequate analgesia. An erect or semi-erect chest

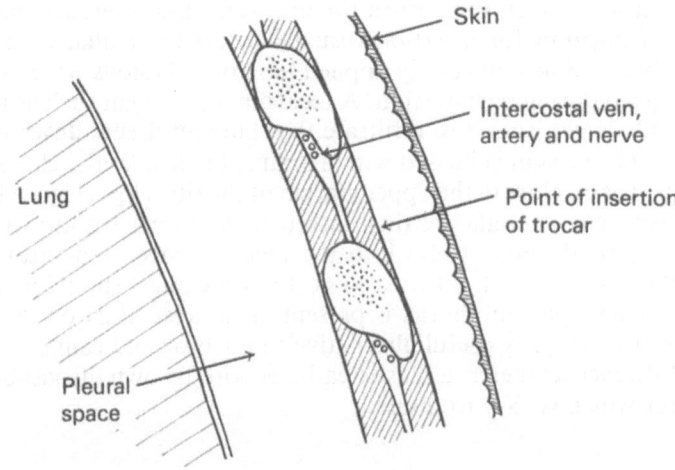

Figure 12.2 Insertion of intercostal drain

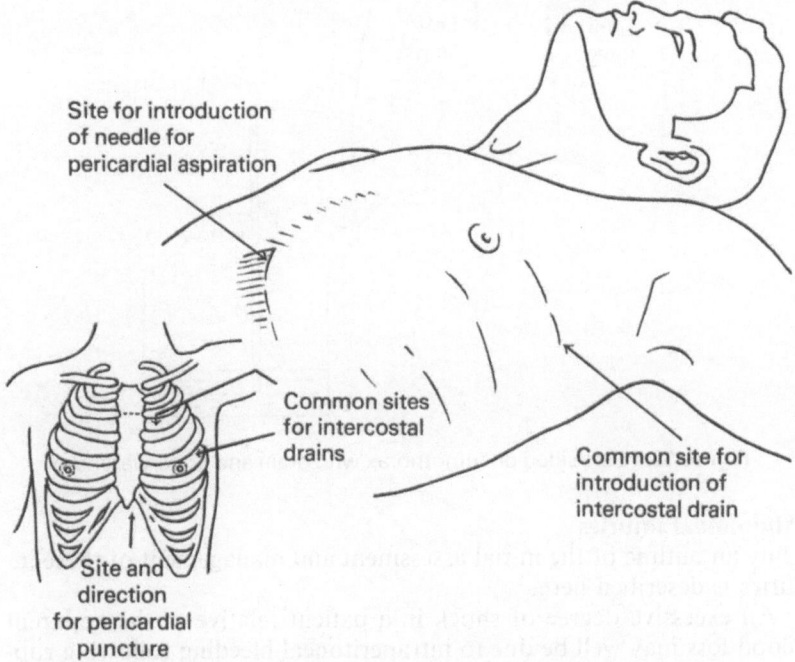

Figure 12.3 Sites for insertion of intercostal and pericardial drains

X-ray must be taken to confirm the diagnosis and to ensure that the intended position for insertion (usually below the axilla, as above) is suitable, and has no closely applied lung or adhesions which might be damaged during the insertion. A local analgesic agent such as ligno-caine (lidocaine) is used to infiltrate the skin and tissues down to the pleura, and the skin is incised with a scalpel blade over the chosen in-tercostal space, close to the upper margin of the rib below (Figure 12.2). The trocar and cannula are then inserted, the trocar withdrawn, the catheter passed about 10 cm into the pleural space, and sutured in position. A catheter of at least 18 FG (French Gauge) should be used, but if a haemopneumothorax is present, a catheter of 24 or 28 FG is more satisfactory. A useful alternative to a trocar and cannula is the Argyll thoracic catheter, a plastic catheter with its own disposable in-troducer which is easy to insert.

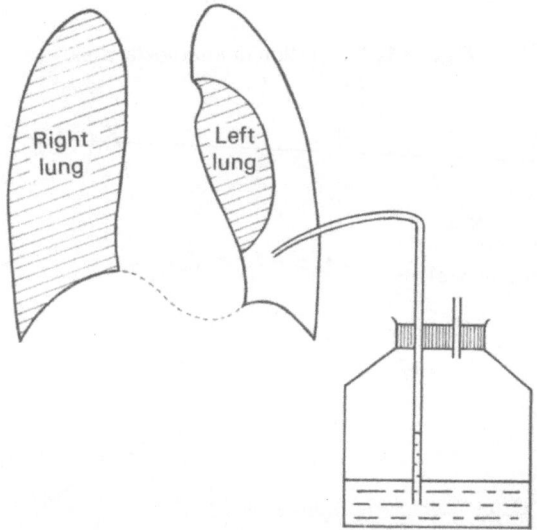

Figure 12.4 Left-sided pneumothorax with drain and underwater seal

Abdominal injuries
Only an outline of the initial assessment and management of these in-juries is described here.

An excessive degree of shock in a patient relative to the apparent blood loss may well be due to intraperitoneal bleeding following rup-ture of solid organs such as the liver, spleen or kidneys. Details of the type of trauma are helpful, but the history from the patient is often unavailable or unreliable if head injury or shock is present.

Examination of the abdomen will reveal obvious penetrating injuries and often 'pattern bruising' on the skin from overlying clothing, which implies a severe compression force and a high incidence of intra-abdominal injury. Tenderness of the abdomen and loin may be present, with or without abdominal distension.

Haematuria implies kidney or bladder damage, but inability to micturate or bleeding from the urethra suggests bladder or urethral rupture.

Radiography of the abdomen may show:

(1) loss or distortion of kidney or splenic outlines in renal or splenic rupture,
(2) fracture of the lower ribs, which may mean liver or splenic damage,
(3) rupture of the diaphragm.

Peritoneal lavage with a syringe of saline and a needle sometimes shows intraperitoneal bleeding, but other damage such as ruptured bowel which is not associated with intraperitoneal bleeding may still be present and remain undiagnosed.

Spinal injuries

These may be due to dislocation or fracture dislocation, of the vertebrae, or rupture of the posterior ligaments. In the latter injury radiographs of the spine may appear normal even in the presence of cord damage or instability.

Symptoms and signs depend on the spinal level and the neurological damage incurred. Further damage must be minimized by immobilization as soon as possible. Patients with cervical spinal injury should have a cervical collar until more definitive immobilization or traction can be undertaken, since besides the protection it affords, it is a constant reminder to medical and nursing staff that cervical instability may be present.

Other injuries

Fractures in general should be immobilized to reduce pain and fat embolization. Deformities or dislocations which cause arterial or venous obstruction or nerve entrapment must be quickly corrected. Soft tissue injury in a limb compartment may lead to pressure necrosis of tissue unless fasciotomy is undertaken.

13

Initial treatment in burns

Types of burn injuries
Three degrees of severity in burn injuries are recognized.

(1) *Superficial burns involving only the epidermis*
These heal without scarring and are characterized by erythema and blistering.

(2) *Partial thickness burns*
In these only the superficial dermis has been significantly damaged, and healing can take place from those deeper elements of the dermis which have survived such as hair follicles and sebaceous glands.

(3) *Whole thickness skin loss*
Where this occurs, spontaneous healing can only take place from the edges of the burn, and therefore skin grafting will eventually be required in such burns more than 2 to 3 cm across.

Areas with partial thickness burns are sensitive to pinprick. This permits areas with partial thickness burns, which should heal spontaneously, to be differentiated from areas of full thickness loss which are completely analgesic.

INITIAL MANAGEMENT
First, the adequacy of the airway and of ventilation must be checked, especially in patients who are unconscious, who have facial burns or who may have inhaled smoke. Laryngeal oedema can easily develop, and inhaled fumes, for example from burning plastics, can produce insidious deterioration of lung function. Intubation or even tracheostomy may be required. In acute upper airway obstruction due to laryngeal oedema, a large intravenous cannula (SWG 12) thrust

into the lumen of the trachea can be life-saving. The trachea should be immobilized by the index finger and thumb of one hand (Figure 13.1) while this is done. When aspiration of air confirms the position within the trachea, the cannula is connected to an oxygen supply and oxygen insufflated at a flow rate of 4 – 5 litres/min. This should enable the patient to be kept oxygenated while specialist assistance is obtained. An alternative procedure is puncture of the cricothyroid membrane with a scalpel.

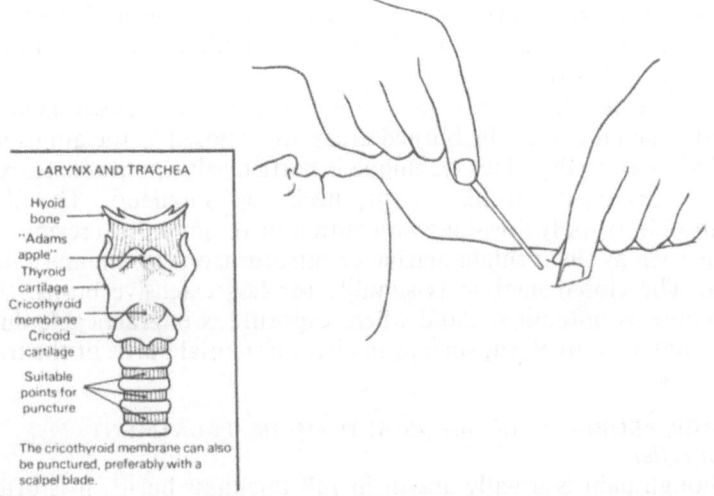

LARYNX AND TRACHEA

Hyoid bone
"Adams apple"
Thyroid cartilage
Cricothyroid membrane
Cricoid cartilage
Suitable points for puncture

The cricothyroid membrane can also be punctured, preferably with a scalpel blade.

Figure 13.1 Tracheal puncture

Second, the percentage area of burn involved is roughly estimated (p. 249). In children this is more difficult, as the surface areas of the head and trunk expressed as a percentage of the total body surface are greater in children than in adults, and this must be taken into account. If the area of partial or full thickness burn exceeds 20% in adults or 10% in children an intravenous infusion is set up.

Third, fluid replacement is commenced with plasma or a plasma substitute (p. 272) after blood samples for haemoglobin, haematocrit, urea and electrolytes and cross-matching have been taken. The formula on p. 250 is only a guide; improvement in the circulation is shown by increasing urinary output and falling haematocrit levels, as well as by improved pulse rate, blood pressure and filling of peripheral veins. Blood transfusion may be required (p. 250).

Fourth, the aims of local treatment for care of the burned surface are to:

(1) minimize infection,
(2) prevent further tissue damage and loss,
(3) provide optimal conditions for healing.

Particular care must be taken of the eyes and eyelids if these are involved. Instillation of fluorescein into the conjunctival sac makes diagnosis of corneal damage easier where there is doubt. If the cornea is exposed chloramphenicol ointment should be instilled and the advice of an ophthalmologist obtained without delay.

Circumferential burns on the limbs may have a tourniquet effect on the distal circulation, and incision of the coagulum may be required to prevent venous stasis.

Treatment of burned surfaces is by either open or closed methods. In the open method, the burned areas are exposed to the atmosphere and allowed to dry. This technique is particularly applicable to extensive burns of the trunk, groins, neck and shoulders. The closed method is to apply dressings with antibiotic or antiseptic creams or lotions such as silver sulphadiazine or nitrofurazone to minimize infection. The closed method is suitable for less extensive burns, those treatable as outpatients, and where exposure is impracticable due to the total area involved, such as in circumferential burns of the trunk.

OTHER PROBLEMS IN BURNS AND THEIR TREATMENT
Pain relief
Although pain is usually absent in full thickness burns, it is often a constant feature where there are large areas of partial thickness or superficial burns, and may require large and repeated doses of narcotic analgesics for many days. Entonox (premixed nitrous oxide 50% and oxygen 50%) inhalations are often useful to provide immediate analgesia.

Acute renal failure
Acute renal failure may develop.

Infection
Since burn wounds are avascular, systemic antibiotics are of little value in combating local infection at the burn site, and are not routinely given. Some specialized units, however, give prophylactic benzyl penicillin to reduce the risk of streptococcal infection. Care must be taken, however, to treat any infection which becomes systemic. Gram-negative septicaemia is particularly dangerous.

14

Patients requiring urgent pain relief

Pain is a very demanding symptom, and many varied conditions such as myocardial infarction, renal colic or childbirth may require urgent pain relief. When the best method of relieving a particular painful condition is being sought, the cause of the pain (perhaps smooth muscle spasm, distension of a viscus, or local pressure on a nerve trunk) and the type of pain (whether steady or intermittent, sharp, dull or boring) should be considered as well as the pharmacological effects and side-effects of a particular analgesic agent. Occasionally no analgesic may be required; if an anginal attack is precipitated by paroxysmal supraventricular tachycardia, the correct treatment is that of the cause – the arrhythmia – rather than the effect – the pain. Narcotic analgesics are best for dull steady boring pain, and less satisfactory for intermittent or colicky pain.

Agents given for pain relief
NARCOTIC ANALGESICS
Morphine
Morphine is still the drug of choice among powerful analgesics, and may be given intramuscularly, subcutaneously or intravenously.

Following subcutaneous or intramuscular administration, the analgesic effects of a dose of morphine are not maximal for 1–2 h, or considerably longer in states of poor peripheral perfusion as in shock; the only rapidly effective method of administration is to give a slow intravenous injection – 0.1 mg/kg morphine sulphate can be given slowly over 5 min, and a further dose of half the initial dose may be given after 15 min if required. If the patient is in severe pain, respiratory depression is rarely a problem at this dose level except in patients liable to CO_2 retention.

The subcutaneous or intramuscular dose is 10–15 mg for a 70 kg man, scaled down according to weight for children and women. For patients over 70 years old half that dose is frequently sufficient.

Sedation and euphoria are often produced, which can be of value in myocardial infarction and other conditions with marked mental distress. Peripheral vasodilatation occurs, reducing the right ventricular preload, and improving pulmonary oedema due to left ventricular failure.

The side-effects of morphine are:

(1) *Hypotension and bradycardia* are sometimes seen, especially if the intravenous route is used. As a consequence, in myocardial infarction, morphine is usually given intramuscularly or subcutaneously.

(2) *Nausea and vomiting* occur frequently.

(3) *Smooth muscle tone* is increased, so conditions causing pain due to smooth muscle spasm may be worsened; bronchospasm may increase.

(4) *The fetal brain* takes up morphine more readily than pethidine (meperidine) and so is not normally given to pregnant women who are expected to deliver within the following 12 h.

Other side-effects occasionally seen are dysphoria, dizziness, sweating and itching.

Pethidine (meperidine)

Pethidine can be given intravenously in 10 mg increments until adequate pain relief is obtained. A total dose of 1 mg/kg may be necessary, but a high incidence of vomiting is found if more than 0.5 mg/kg is given.

The incidences of respiratory depression and nausea and vomiting are similar to morphine, but pethidine does not cause smooth muscle spasm, and it is safer to use in obstetrics than morphine since fetal respiratory depression is less.

NITROUS OXIDE (ENTONOX)

A useful method of producing good pain relief which may be self-administered or administered by non-medically qualified personnel is by the use of the Entonox apparatus. This consists of a mixture of equal volumes of nitrous oxide and oxygen in a pressurized cylinder with a demand valve similar to that in self-contained underwater breathing apparatus (SCUBA). When inhaled, excellent analgesia of very rapid onset (and recovery) is obtained, which is extremely useful for short-term pain relief, for example when splinting fractures or transporting accident victims. Symptoms and signs of disease are easily elicited on discontinuing inhalation, which may not be the case following parenteral narcotic administration. An added benefit is the high concentration of oxygen inspired (50%).

The side-effects of Entonox are nausea and vomiting which occur in 30–40% of patients. Following prolonged administration over several days marrow depression can develop.

LOCAL ANALGESIC BLOCKS

Local analgesic blocks should not be forgotten where applicable; techniques such as epidural or intercostal blocks, or even local infiltration in fractures, are often more effective than narcotics and produce little cardiovascular or respiratory disturbance.

15

Complications of spinal and epidural analgesia requiring urgent treatment

During both extradural (epidural) and intradural (spinal) analgesia there is widespread sympathetic blockade which usually extends for one or two spinal segments beyond the limits of the sensory loss. Due to the consequent loss of vasomotor tone, there is arteriolar and venous dilatation in the affected segments, with an increase in the vascular capacity and in venous pooling, and a drop in the blood pressure. This fall in the blood pressure is not usually of great significance, but severe hypotension can occur in the presence of:

(1) Pre-existing hypovolaemia, where the blood pressure is being maintained only by maximal sympathetic activity.

(2) A reduction in venous return. The best example of this is the supine hypotensive syndrome of late pregnancy. If a woman in the last trimester of pregnancy lies supine, the weight of the uterus and its contents may completely obstruct the inferior vena cava, reducing venous return, and therefore the cardiac output and the blood pressure. In the presence of intact sympathetic reflexes, the woman is often able to compensate by an increase in vasoconstriction and venoconstriction, which produce an improved venous return, cardiac output and blood pressure. This physiological compensatory mechanism is prevented by the sympathetic blockade associated with extradural or intradural analgesia, and a profound drop in the blood pressure can result.

(3) A more extensive segmental blockade than was intended, due to:

    (a) an excessive dose of analgesic agent;
    (b) a dose of local analgesic intended for epidural injection being injected intradurally. A much higher volume of solution is required for extradural analgesia. If this volume is inadvertently injected intradurally a total spinal injection results, with potentially disastrous effects (see below);

(c) the patient being wrongly positioned by the anaesthetist, and the analgesic solution allowed to migrate cephalad, producing a more extensive sympathetic block.

The treatment of hypotension in extradural or intradural analgesia is that of the underlying condition. Any hypovolaemia should be urgently treated with plasma substitutes, while excessive sympathetic blockade can be treated with vasopressor drugs such as ephedrine (alpha and beta-adrenergic stimulant) or metaraminol (also alpha and beta-stimulant – p. 29). Apnoea may occur due to the analgesic agent passing cephalad in the cerebrospinal fluid blocking the intercostal and phrenic nerves or producing medullary ischaemia, and demands urgent artificial ventilation.

Special cases
THE SUPINE HYPOTENSIVE SYNDROME OF PREGNANCY
If a woman in labour with epidural (or spinal) analgesia has a sudden severe drop in blood pressure, the possibility of caval occlusion should be considered, especially if the drop follows a change in position from lateral to supine.

Management
(1) Turn the patient on to her left side. A head-down position should *not* be used.
(2) Infuse 500 – 1000 ml crystalloid solution, such as normal saline.
(3) Commence oxygen therapy to the mother with a mask; this should improve the oxygen delivery to the fetus, whose well-being is immediately compromised by any fall in maternal arterial pressure.
(4) If no immediate improvement results, give 5 mg ephedrine intravenously, repeated every 5 min until improvement occurs.
(5) If changing the position of the patient, infusing fluid, and giving ephedrine produces little benefit, consider other possible causes such as amniotic fluid embolism (p. 24).

ACCIDENTAL TOTAL SPINAL
When an accidental total spinal occurs, the local analgesic solution spreads widely in the cerebrospinal fluid, and apnoea and profound hypotension occur. If severe hypotension develops within 10 min of an epidural 'top-up', and is associated with apnoea, a total spinal is the most likely diagnosis, and may have resulted from the migration of the tip of the epidural catheter into the intradural space.

Management
  (1) Give artificial respiration by any means available. Intubation
      and ventilation should in any case be undertaken as soon as
      possible, since artificial ventilation will be required for about
      2 h.
  (2) Ephedrine is given in a dose of 5 mg intravenously, repeated
      three or four times if necessary. Plasma expanders may also be
      given in the acute situation, but there is a danger of circulatory
      overload when the block wears off if the circulation has been ex-
      cessively expanded.

MASSIVE EPIDURAL
This is a poorly understood condition in which the patient gradually
becomes apnoeic about 20 min after a dose of local analgesic is given
into the epidural space. No drop in the blood pressure occurs. Artificial ventilation is required for about 2 h. No obstetric patient has
been described with this condition.

TOXIC REACTIONS
Toxic reactions to local analgesics are rare, and are usually due to in-
advertent intravascular injection. Convulsions can occur, and are
treated in the same manner as epileptic fits (p. 54). Cardiac arrest has
been described following intravascular injection of solutions containing adrenaline (epinephrine).

16

Pre-eclampsia and eclampsia

Pre-eclampsia
Pre-eclampsia is acute hypertension of pregnancy occurring at any time after 24 weeks gestation, and is said to be present when the blood pressure reaches or exceeds 140/90 mmHg on two occasions 24 h apart, with or without proteinuria, and in the absence of any pre-existing cardiovascular or renal disease. In severe cases a triad of oedema, hypertension and proteinuria develops.

PATHOLOGY
Most organs, but particularly the kidneys and liver, suffer damage due to arteriolar fibrin deposition. A bleeding tendency may develop due to disseminated intravascular coagulation (DIC) while the utero-placental circulation and thus the fetus become increasingly compromised as placental function declines. Despite the raised blood pressure and the oedema, a patient with severe pre-eclampsia actually has a reduced circulating blood volume and may show signs of hypovolaemia.

In pre-eclampsia, the risks to the mother are:

(1) the development of eclampsia,
(2) renal failure,
(3) cardiac failure,
(4) intracerebral bleeding,
(5) disseminated intravascular coagulation.

The risks to the fetus are hypoxia, acidosis, and death. The precarious blood supply to the fetus via the placenta may be abruptly cut off by placental infarction or separation from the placental site.

Eclampsia
Eclampsia is characterized by epileptiform convulsions. It is usually preceded by pre-eclampsia, but can appear without hypertension, and

is then indistinguishable from grand mal convulsions. The fits have both tonic and clonic phases, and if treatment is not swiftly instituted they increase in frequency and duration until cardiorespiratory failure occurs with death of both the mother and the fetus.

Signs of impending eclampsia are:

(1) Cardiovascular signs – rapidly rising diastolic pressure (> 100 mmHg).
(2) Cerebral signs – photophobia, visual disturbances, headache and generalized twitching.
(3) Gastrointestinal signs – epigastric pain and vomiting.
(4) Renal signs – increasing proteinuria, oliguria or anuria.

MANAGEMENT

Management of eclampsia requires (1) antihypertensive drugs, (2) adequate analgesia, and (3) anticonvulsants with sedative properties.

The aims in the management of eclampsia are to:

(1) control the convulsions – diazepam is the drug of choice;
(2) maintain the airway and adequate oxygenation if the patient is unconscious;
(3) maintain or institute treatment for pre-eclampsia;
(4) monitor both mother and fetus – particularly maternal conscious level, blood pressure, urinary output and fetal heart rate;
(5) deliver the fetus either vaginally or by Caesarean section as soon as reasonably possible;
(6) continue to observe for recurrence of eclampsia up to 48 h after delivery.

The development of DIC may require fresh frozen plasma and heparin (p. 271). In severe cases the hypovolaemia and oedema may be reduced and tissue perfusion improved by infusion of salt-poor albumen.

Antihypertensive drugs

The blood pressure should be reduced gradually to prevent any precipitous falls in uterine blood flow which might further compromise the fetus.

In the United Kingdom the most commonly used agent is hydrallazine; it is given intravenously and has a rapid effect. The dose is titrated against the response, by giving 5 mg intravenously every

5 min until the diastolic blood pressure is less than 110 mmHg. If more than 20 mg is required, further doses should be given more slowly, 5 mg every 15 min intravenously until control is achieved. A maintenance dose of 2–20 mg/h preferably by infusion pump will be required.

An alternative is diazoxide (p. 58). The sudden drop in pressure associated with diazoxide therapy may be disadvantageous to the fetus, if placental blood flow is only just adequate.

Analgesia

Adequate pain relief is best achieved by the use of epidural analgesia. This not only removes the pain of labour, with its associated hyperventilation and rise in blood pressure which may predispose to convulsions, but also produces a sympathetic block which may improve uteroplacental and renal blood flow. Epidural analgesia should never be undertaken when a coagulation disorder is present.

Alternatively, pethidine (meperidine) must be given in adequate amounts with inhalational analgesia as required (nitrous oxide/oxygen mixture – Entonox – appears to be the safest).

Anticonvulsants

Diazepam is both a sedative and an excellent anticonvulsant, and is the drug of choice for the acute management of convulsions. The appropriate dose for any patient is fairly variable, and it is best given intravenously at a rate of 2.5 mg every 2–3 min until the patient is drowsy and relaxed. If the patient has convulsions, diazepam is given faster at a rate of 5 mg/min; usually 10–30 mg is enough to terminate the convulsions. Equipment for airway maintenance and resuscitation must be at hand. An intravenous infusion providing 2.5–5 mg/h is usually adequate to maintain the sedative and anticonvulsant actions until delivery.

Diazepam is associated with neonatal hypotonia and poor temperature regulation in the newborn if a total dose greater than 20 mg is given to the mother, but terminating the convulsions is of course the primary consideration.

Chlormethiazole is available in 0.8% solution and is an effective sedative and anticonvulsant. It is given initially at a rate of 4 ml/min until the patient is adequately sedated, then reduced to a suitable rate – usually about 1 ml/min – to maintain the effect. It can be used with diazepam. A drip counter or paediatric burette is useful to ensure that overdosage with maternal respiratory depression does not occur.

Thiopentone is an excellent anticonvulsant, but an overdose is easily given, and it is best administered by anaesthetists.

Magnesium sulphate is used more in the United States than in the United Kingdom. It is an anticonvulsant, and it is also said to have diuretic and antihypertensive activity.

An initial dose of 4 g magnesium sulphate in 20% solution is given intravenously over 4 min, then 1 g/h by infusion. The aim is to achieve serum magnesium levels of 3–4 mmol/l and the serum concentration of magnesium should be monitored if possible. A sign of overdosage is the disappearance of the tendon reflexes. Overdosage is treated with slow intravenous injection of calcium gluconate solution. As the excretion of magnesium ion is mainly by the kidneys, if the urine output falls to less than 30 ml/h the dose of magnesium sulphate should be reduced.

17

Neonatal resuscitation

Neonatal apnoea
About 15% of babies born in general maternity hospitals are apnoeic 2 min after birth. Apnoea, however, is often unpredictable – the art of obstetrics is in expecting the unexpected.

Predictability of the need for resuscitation
If the women whose babies are at risk could be accurately predicted during pregnancy or labour, neonatal resuscitation would cease to be a problem.

Some cases are predictable, for example:

(1) Women who have had repeated doses of narcotic analgesics and sedation.
(2) Breech presentation, twin pregnancies, and forceps delivery (except low forceps delivery with epidural analgesia).
(3) Women with prolonged labours (especially with prolonged second stage) or with fetal distress.
(4) Women with a history of pre-eclampsia, hypertension or antepartum haemorrhage.

Pathophysiology
An understanding of the survival mechanisms of the fetus is necessary for the application of logical treatment. Consider a fetus whose uneventful progress down the birth canal in the second stage of labour is rudely interrupted by the sudden loss of placental circulation by premature separation of the placenta or obstruction of its cord vessels. The sequence of events is shown in Figure 17.1.

First of all the fetus attempts to breathe. If this is unsuccessful (that is, if the fetus is still in the birth canal) the respiratory attempts stop after a short period, and the heart rate declines.

This period of apnoea is termed primary apnoea (or asphyxia livida

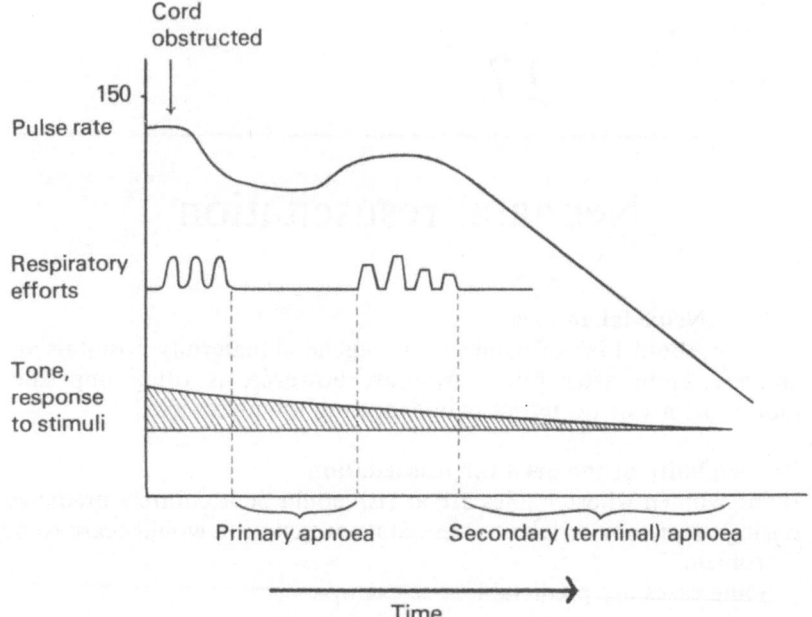

Figure 17.1 Events in fetal apnoea

in old textbooks). The muscle tone and the response to stimulation such as suction of the mouth and nostrils would be good in this period if they could be tested.

After a further period the heart rate rises again, and the fetus makes gasping attempts at respiration. If these do not rapidly result in oxygenation of the vital centres, the gasps cease, the heart rate slowly declines, and cardiac arrest occurs.

This second period of apnoea is termed secondary or terminal apnoea (asphyxia pallida in old texts) and is characterized by lack of response to stimulation, poor muscle tone, and a heart rate less than 100 beats/min (bpm). Only ventilation can retrieve this deteriorating situation.

Therefore, two groups of apnoeic infants can be described:

(1) A group with heart rate of usually 100 bpm or more, with good muscle tone and good response to stimuli. Treatment of these infants is less urgent and clearing the airways in an atmosphere of oxygen-enriched air may well induce inspiration. These are infants with primary apnoea.

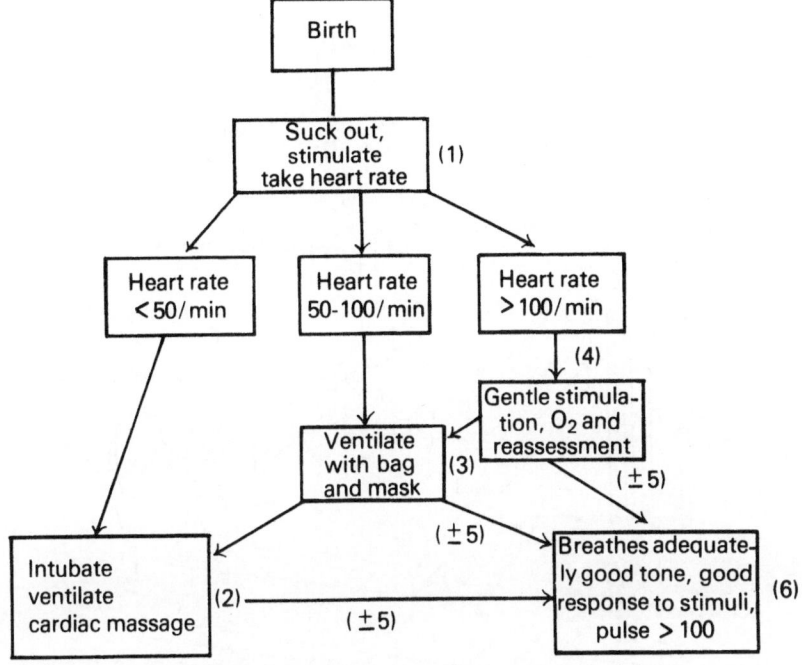

Figure 17.2 Management of fetal apnoea

(2) A second group with heart rate usually less than 100 bmp, pale in colour, with poor tone and no response to stimuli. These infants are in terminal apnoea and require ventilation and possibly external cardiac massage.

There are babies, however, who do not fit easily into either category. These may have respiratory depression following administration of narcotics such as pethidine or sedatives to the mother in labour, acidosis from prolonged hypoxia, or reflex apnoea and bradycardia from stimulation of the larynx by over-enthusiastic suction or a blob of mucus.

Technique of resuscitation
Many different approaches to neonatal resuscitation have been described. Figure 17.2 is a flow diagram which attempts to set out a simple yet clear approach. The numbers in brackets in the diagram refer to the numbered paragraphs below. The resuscitation apparatus

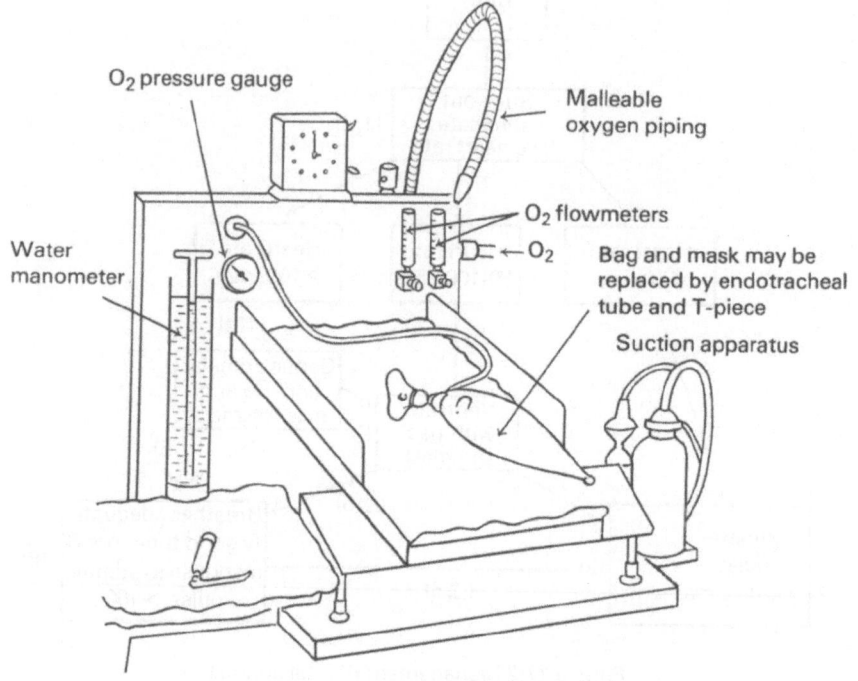

Figure 17.3 Typical resuscitation apparatus

should be checked before use, and anyone who may have to resuscitate newborn infants must be fully conversant with the equipment they will have to use.

(1) Immediately after the birth, the infant's mouth and nostrils are aspirated with a soft catheter or mucus extractor under direct vision. The tip of the catheter should never be passed blindly over the back of the tongue, as this can cause reflex apnoea and bradycardia. The child is then received into a prewarmed towel, which is used to dry and stimulate him. If apnoeic, the baby is transferred to the resuscitation apparatus. A stopclock is started, and the infant's heart rate measured over 10 s. This can be done with a stethoscope, but is often more conveniently done by feeling the pulse in the umbilical stump.

(2) If the heart rate is less than 50 bpm, immediate intervention is required, with intubation, ventilation, and external cardiac massage.

INTUBATION

The laryngoscope usually available is the straight-bladed type (Figure 17.4). People with limited experience in intubating neonates may well find the curved Macintosh blade easier to use.

Macintosh type blade

Magill type blade (see also Figure 17.6)

Flat bladed type

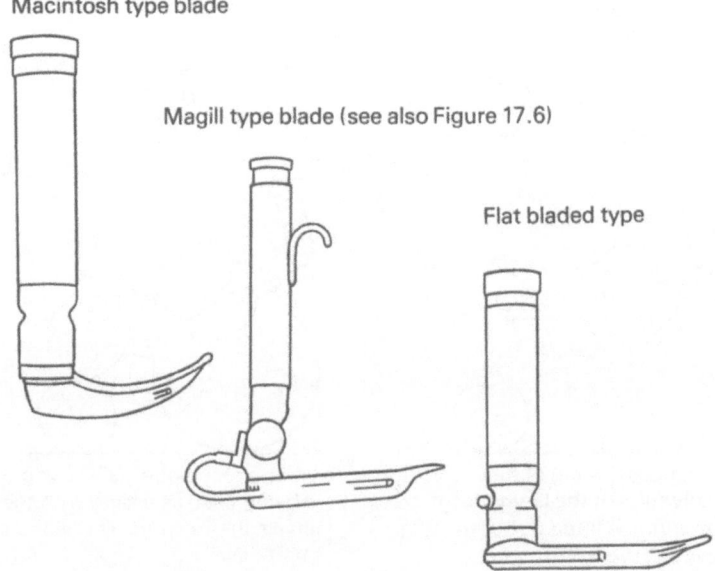

Figure 17.4 Laryngoscopes used in neonatal resuscitation

For ease of intubation, the baby should be placed on a level or slightly head-down surface with a rolled up towel under the shoulders. If the head is now extended, the mouth, larynx and trachea are in a straight line (Figure 17.5) and the only obstruction to a view of the larynx is the tongue. The laryngoscope merely lifts the tongue to expose the larynx.

With the child in the position described, the blade of the laryngoscope is inserted in the right side of the mouth and passed over the tongue, lifting it and pushing it to the left, until the epiglottis is visualized. The epiglottis is picked up with the tip of the blade, and the laryngoscope lifted in an upwards direction to expose the larynx. The most common mistake in intubation is to use the blade of the laryngoscope as a lever to prise up the tongue, with the upper gum margin as a fulcrum (Figure 17.5).

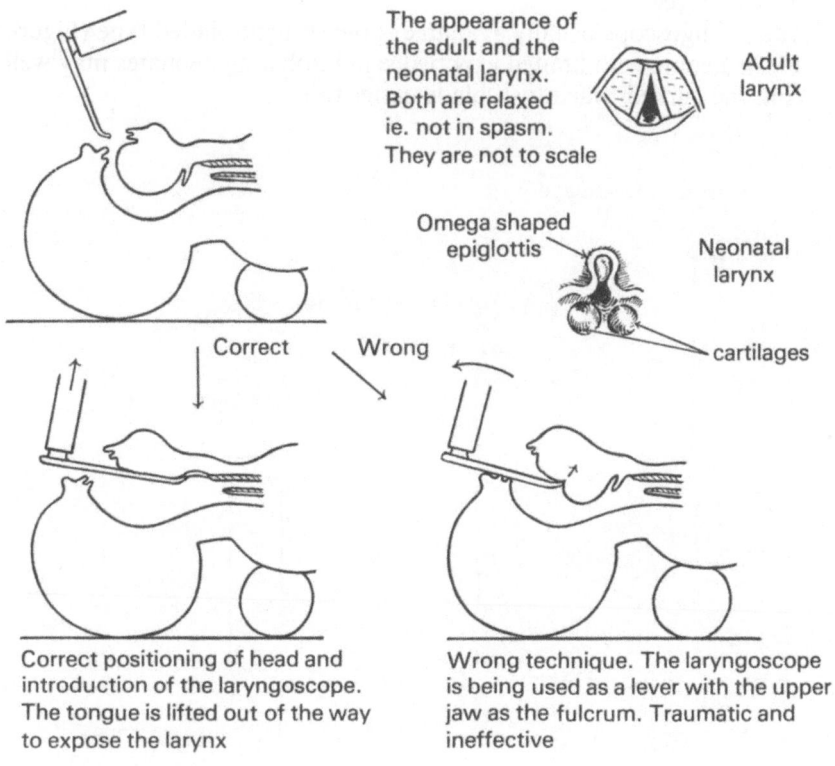

The appearance of the adult and the neonatal larynx. Both are relaxed ie. not in spasm. They are not to scale

Adult larynx

Omega shaped epiglottis

Neonatal larynx

cartilages

Correct   Wrong

Correct positioning of head and introduction of the laryngoscope. The tongue is lifted out of the way to expose the larynx

Wrong technique. The laryngoscope is being used as a lever with the upper jaw as the fulcrum. Traumatic and ineffective

Figure 17.5 Neonatal intubation, the adult and the neonatal larynxes

VENTILATION

A T-piece system is often used as in Figure 17.7, or a self-inflating bag may be used with an endotracheal connection. The former is simpler but requires an oxygen supply. When a finger occludes the end of the T-piece, as in A in Figure 17.7, the flow of fresh gas produces inspiration, and when the finger is lifted, expiration takes place. A fresh gas flow rate of 2 – 3 litres/min is adequate; higher flows can cause excessive intrapulmonary pressure and alveolar rupture. A respiratory rate of 15 bpm is adequate. A relatively high pressure of 30 cm water is often required initially to inflate the lungs, but this should be reduced to 20 – 25 cm water as soon as possible. Adequacy of ventilation is best assessed by chest movements and improvement in the pulse rate and general condition. Auscultation of the chest must be undertaken to exclude intubation of the oesophagus and to ensure that both lungs are being inflated.

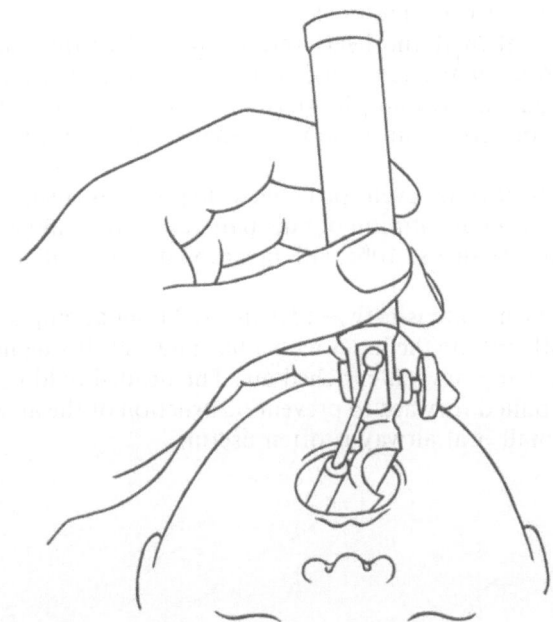

Figure 17.6 Method of holding a laryngoscope

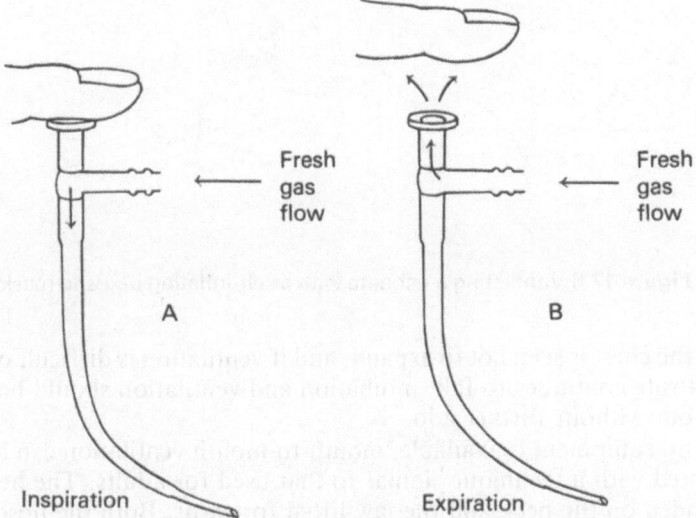

Fresh gas flow

Fresh gas flow

A

B

Inspiration

Expiration

Figure 17.7 Ventilating a neonate with a T-piece

EXTERNAL CARDIAC MASSAGE

This is undertaken if the heart rate drops to less than 50 bpm. In neonates cardiac massage is carried out by two fingers on the middle of the sternum, depressing the sternum about 0.75 cm/sec. As with adults, four or five compressions alternate with an inflation of the lungs.

Acidosis following even prolonged hypoxia is usually quickly reversed following institution of adequate respiration and circulation, and infusions of glucose 10% with bicarbonate solution are rarely required.

(3) If the heart rate is between 50 and 100 bpm attempts should be made to gently inflate the lungs with a bag and well-fitting mask, as in Figure 17.8, using oxygen-enriched air. The head should be extended and the jaw pulled forward to prevent obstruction of the airway by the tongue. A small oral airway is often useful.

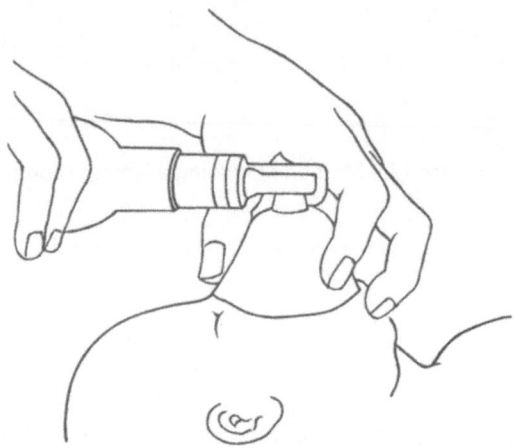

Figure 17.8 Ventilating a neonate with a self-inflating bag and mask

If the chest is seen not to expand, and if ventilation is difficult or the heart rate continues to fall, intubation and ventilation should be carried out without further ado.

If no equipment is available, mouth-to-mouth ventilation can be attempted with a technique similar to that used for adults. The head is extended on the neck and the jaw lifted forwards. Both the nose and the mouth of the child are covered by the mouth of the operator, but the child's lungs should be inflated using only the operator's cheeks as bellows rather than the expiratory muscles. This prevents excessive pressure being applied to the infant's airways.

(4) If the heart rate is 100 bpm or higher, then the general condition of the infant is good, and he is likely to be in primary apnoea. His heart rate should be monitored, and his feet flicked now and again as a stimulus to breathing, while his mouth and nose are maintained in an oxygen-enriched atmosphere, so that maximum advantage can be gained from any respiratory attempt. If the child is apnoeic after a minute, gentle inflation with a bag and mask can be carried out as above.

(5) If the mother has had several doses of narcotic analgesics such as pethidine (meperidine) during labour, fetal respiration may be depressed, but this is readily reversed by naloxone given to the infant as 0.01 mg/kg body weight, intravenously or intramuscularly. Naloxone has no effect on respiratory depression due to sedatives or acidosis.

(6) Successful resuscitation should produce a neonate with a heart rate of about 140 bpm, regular respirations, good tone and response to stimuli as in the traditional Apgar scoring system. The colour of the infant is often an unreliable guide to the effectiveness of therapy, and in spite of obvious wellbeing, he may take several hours to become pink.

SECTION II
PRACTICAL VENTILATION

18

Terminology

The ability to artificially ventilate the lungs by bag and mask (p. 133 or through an endotracheal tube (p. 171) is essential in all hospital departments. There is no doubt that many lives are saved without the resuscitator having detailed knowledge of his apparatus or of how to use it with the greatest benefit to the patient. However, the initial improvement in the condition of the patient is not always maintained, partly due to an insufficient understanding of the meaning and importance of such entities as tidal volume (p. 121), minute volume (p. 124), dead space (p. 124) and composition of alveolar air, all of which are readily influenced by the technique adopted by the resuscitator. It is therefore important that anyone involved in resuscitation should have a clear understanding of such terms.

For descriptive purposes it is convenient and conventional to define the quantities of gas involved in gaseous exchange within the respiratory tract, or different parts of a ventilation circuit, as specific static volumes. Obviously this is not strictly so because their definitions create non-existent anatomical or physiological barriers. Exchange of gas between adjacent sections of the respiratory tract is continuously taking place due to diffusion and to the rhythmical distortion of the lungs by the adjacent cardiac contractions. Nevertheless, provided this is appreciated, definitions of lung volumes can be very helpful in understanding the aims and principles of pulmonary resuscitation.

Tidal volume (V_T)

The tidal volume (V_T) of air is defined as the volume of air breathed in or out during a normal quiet respiration. The inexperienced resuscitator, when ventilating a patient, tends to push into the patient a quantity of air much greater than a normal tidal volume. Over-ventilation in this way can impede the venous return to the right side of the heart and cause hypotension (p. 152). The phrase 'normal quiet

121

respiration' is particularly important because in most resuscitative procedures involving artificial ventilation the aim is to imitate as closely as possible the normal movements of respiration.

Normal values in the adult vary from 400 to 500 ml. The full-sized normal baby has a V_T of 20 ml, and in the premature baby a V_T of 10 ml is usual.

V_T is measured by means of a Wright's respirometer (Figure 18.1) plugged into a face mask which is then applied carefully and firmly over the patient's nose and mouth in order to prevent leakage of expired air between the face and the mask. Provided again that no leak exists, it can also be plugged into the catheter mount (see Figures 19.1, 19.2) leading from the endotracheal tube. If the patient is breathing spontaneously it is immaterial whether the V_T is measured during inspiration or expiration.

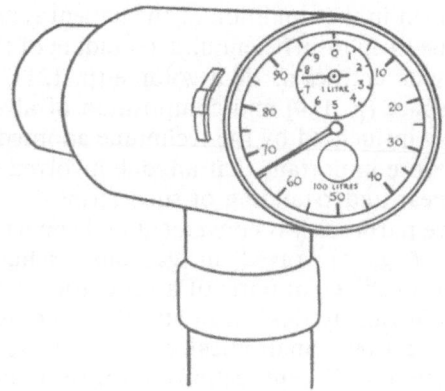

Figure 18.1 Wright's respirometer for measurement of tidal volume. The patient breathes into the respirometer and the amount of expired or inspired air is recorded on the dials

Another use of the respirometer is to measure the tidal volume of air leaving the patient and to compare it with the volume of gas that the ventilator is supposed to be delivering to the patient. For example, if the V_T leaving the patient on expiration is 300 ml and the V_T leaving the ventilator on inspiration is 800 ml, then 500 ml (800 − 300 ml) has been lost somewhere to the atmosphere. Leakage is due to insufficient inflation of the cuff surrounding the endotracheal tube, an incompletely closed valve, insecure connections between the various pieces of tubing and apparatus in the circuit, or a faulty gasket in the humidifier. Therefore, because of the possibility and likelihood of leaks it is essential to measure the V_T leaving the patient and not believe implicitly that its value is identical to the V_T leaving the ventilator.

Whenever long lengths of corrugated tubing constitute part of the circuit, even if the circuit is leakproof, there is no guarantee that a V_T of 500 ml delivered from a ventilator will cause 500 ml to enter the lungs. In fact the volume of gas entering the lungs is usually 100–150 ml less than that expelled from the ventilator. This discrepancy is due to the fact that distensible tubing is used to connect the patient to the ventilator. During the inspiratory phase (p. 155) some of the gas put out by the ventilator distends the tubing and is temporarily captured therein instead of passing into the lungs, so the actual measured V_T is less than the volume given out on inspiration by the ventilator. During the expiratory phase (p. 155) the positive pressure in the circuit falls and the rubber tubing in the circuit resumes its non-expanded state, simultaneously extruding its temporarily captured gas to the atmosphere without it ever entering the lungs; for example:

During inspiration

if volume of gas leaving ventilator = 500 ml
and volume of gas temporarily captured in expanding rubber tubing = 100 ml
the volume of gas entering lungs = 500 ml − 100 ml = 400 ml

During expiration

volume of gas leaving lungs = 400 ml
and volume of gas temporarily captured in previous expanded rubber tubing = 100 ml
total volume of gas leaving circuit = 400 + 100 ml = 500 ml

Consequently, if the required normal V_T of a patient during spontaneous ventilation is 500 ml, the V_T delivered by the ventilator should be set at 600–650 ml to allow for expansion of the corrugated tubing.

FACTORS REDUCING V_T

Common causes of diminished tidal volume are the failure to support the jaw in an anaesthetized or comatose patient, the presence of foreign material or sputum in the respiratory tract, head injury, and overdosage with alcohol, sedative or analgesic drugs.

Minute volume
Minute volume is defined as the total amount of air that is breathed in
or breathed out in 1 minute. If the tidal volume is 450 ml and every
breath is similar then a respiratory rate of 12 per minute would constitute a minute volume of 5400 ml.

∴ minute volume = tidal volume × respiratory rate per minute.

Minute volume can be measured using the standard Wright's
respirometer (Figure 18.1) but it is frequently displayed as a continuous readout on the electronic version. Normal minute volume in
an adult is 5−8 l/min.

Dead space volume (V_D)

ANATOMICAL
Anatomical dead space is that volume of air within the respiratory
tract which does not partake in respiratory exchange, and extends
from the mouth and nose down to but not including the alveoli. For
most purposes the dead space is regarded as being 2 ml for every 1 kg
(1 ml/lb) body weight. An average adult therefore has an anatomical
dead space of about 150 ml.

Alveolar air
This is the air in contact with the pulmonary capillaries. Its gaseous
composition is virtually the same as that in the lower part of the
trachea at the end of expiration. Therefore, at this stage, part of the
alveolar air ends up in the dead space and during the next inspiration it
returns to the lungs.

Air movements between atmosphere, dead space and alveoli
A clear understanding of air movements during spontaneous respiration is essential before and when using resuscitation apparatus.

EXPIRATION
On expiration (Figure 18.2) the deflating lungs squeeze some of the
stale alveolar air into the dead space. Fresh air already existing in the
dead space at the end of the previous inspiration is forced out of the
nose and mouth into the atmosphere without ever entering the lungs.
As expiration continues part of the stale air is then expelled into the atmosphere, but that part of the alveolar air which is last to leave the
lungs ends up in the dead space.

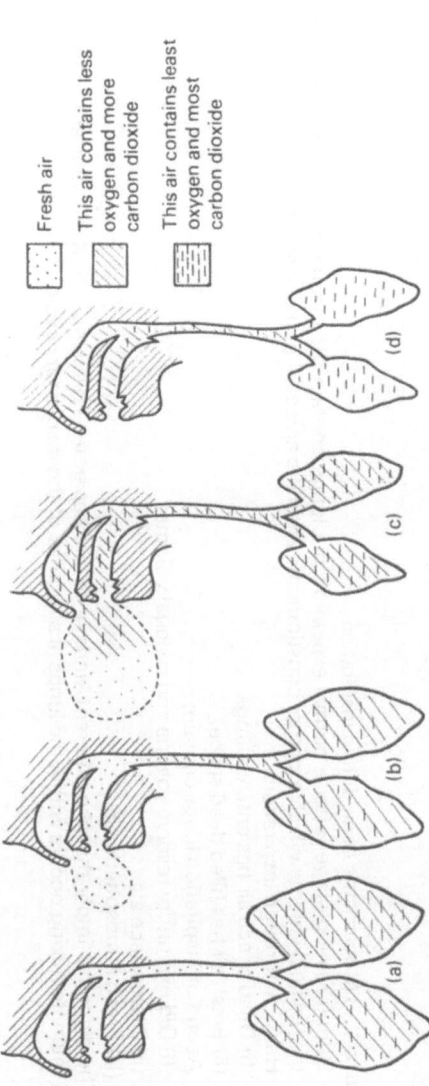

Figure 18.2 Movements of air during expiration

(a) At start of expiration lungs contain air which has given up part of its oxygen to the blood and in return has received carbon dioxide from the blood. It can be regarded as stale air.

(b) Halfway through expiration:
  (i) The unaltered fresh air in the dead space is breathed out without ever entering lung.
  (ii) Some of stale air has moved out into the dead space.

(c) At the end of expiration:
  (i) Some stale air is expelled from nose and mouth.
  (ii) Dead space contains stale air.
  (iii) Some stale air remains in lungs.

(d) (i) During expiratory pause (between end of expiration and start of next inspiration) gaseous exchange still occurs in lungs.
  (ii) Air remaining in alveoli (alveolar air) becomes more stale with a decreasing amount of oxygen and an increasing amount of carbon dioxide until another inspiration washes out the alveoli again (see Figure 18.3)

The diagrams imply that the different kinds of air are separate. This is not so. It is important to realize that intimate mixing occurs within the lungs at all stages of the respiratory cycle.

Legend (within figure):
Fresh air
This air contains less oxygen and more carbon dioxide
This air contains least oxygen and most carbon dioxide

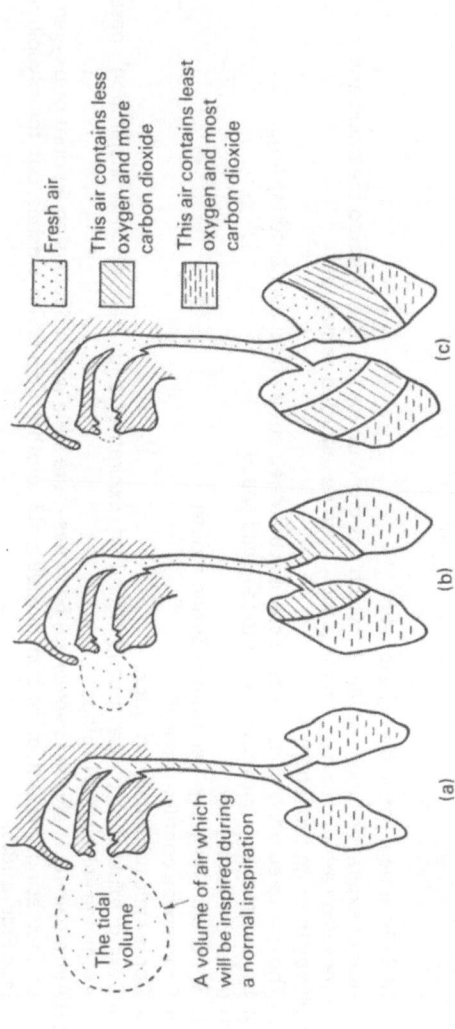

Figure 18.3 Movements of air during inspiration.

(a) During resting stage (after a normal expiration the lungs contain the expiratory reserve volume and the residual volume which together constitute the air in the alveoli, i.e. the alveolar air).

(b) Halfway through inspiration:
(i) Dead space air has entered lungs.
(ii) Fresh air has filled dead space.

(c) At end of inspiration lungs contain:
(i) Old expiratory reserve volume and residual volume.
(ii) Dead space air.
(iii) Fresh atmospheric air.

The diagrams imply that the different kinds of air are separate. This is not so. It is important to realize that intimate mixing occurs within the lungs at all stages of the respiratory cycle.

Therefore, at the end of expiration the dead space contains alveolar air which has a lower oxygen and higher carbon dioxide concentration than the fresh atmospheric air because it has already taken part in respiratory exchange with the pulmonary capillaries.

INSPIRATION

The presence of the dead space in the respiratory tract means that not all the inspired air that enters the mouth enters the lungs. On inspiration (Figure 18.3) the dead space air, consisting of alveolar air from the previous expiration, is first to enter the lungs and is followed by an in-flow of fresh air. The alveoli now contain 'old' alveolar air which was present in the alveoli at the start of inspiration, dead space air and fresh air. At the same time the remainder of the tidal volume of fresh air comes to reside in the dead space. Therefore, only part of the inspired air effectively ventilates the alveoli.

Effective tidal volume (V_A)

The above events explain the meaning of 'effective tidal volume' which is defined as that part of the tidal volume which enters the lungs and is able to take part in gaseous exchange with the blood. The effective tidal volume (V_A) (volume entering alveoli) is equal to the actual volume (V_T), minus the dead space volume (V_D).

In other words

Effective tidal volume = tidal volume − dead space volume
V_A = $V_T - V_D$
If tidal volume = 440 ml
and dead space = 140 ml
then effective tidal volume = 440 − 140 = 300 ml

Effective minute volume (alveolar ventilation − V_A)

The effective minute volume is derived by adding together all the effective tidal volumes breathed in 1 minute. If all the tidal volumes are approximately equal, a reasonable estimate of the effective minute volume is obtained by multiplying a typical effective tidal volume by the respiratory rate.

Effective minute volume = effective tidal volume × number of respirations per minute

If effective tidal volume   = 330 ml
and respiratory rate   = 12/min
then effective minute
volume   = 330 × 12
                              = 3960 ml

The effective minute volume is frequently referred to as the alveolar ventilation and is depicted $\dot{V}_A$. The dot over the V denotes measurement of volume over a period of time, usually 1 minute.

The significance of the above term is seen in disturbances of ventilation and is perhaps best illustrated by following the course of an imaginary, previously healthy patient who has had a chest operation (Tables 18.1 to 18.5).

Table 18.1 Before operation

Normal tidal volume V_T = 450 ml
Dead space volume V_D = 150 ml
Effective tidal volume V_A = 300 ml
Respiratory rate   = 10/min
Alveolar ventilation $\dot{V}_A$ = 300 × 10
                                                       = 3000 ml/min = 3 l/min

Respiratory exchange is normal

Table 18.2 Soon after operation. V_T is reduced due to the effects of pain and anaesthetic drugs. The tidal volume has fallen to two-thirds of its original value but the dead space remains the same

Tidal volume V_T = 300 ml
Dead space volume V_D = 150 ml
Effective tidal volume V_A = 150 ml
Alveolar ventilation $\dot{V}_A$ = 150 × 10
                                                       = 1500 ml/min = 1.5 l/min

Therefore, reducing the tidal volume by a third has reduced the alveolar ventilation to a half. Reducing the tidal volume produces a greater relative reduction in the effective tidal volume and alveolar ventilation

Table 18.3 After operation. The patient manages to obtain sufficient oxygen, but the build-up of carbon dioxide stimulates breathing and ventilation is soon increased by increasing the rate and depth of his respirations. If pain is severe he responds mostly by increasing his respiratory rate to 20/min

Effective tidal volume V_A = 150 ml
Respiratory rate   = 20/min
Alveolar ventilation $\dot{V}_A$ = 150 × 20 ml/min
                                                       = 3000 ml/min = 3.0 l/min

Alveolar ventilation has therefore reverted to normal

Table 18.4 Two days after operation. Accumulated sputum has caused part of the lung to collapse and reduced the tidal volume by another 50 ml to 250 ml

| Effective tidal volume V_A | = 250 − 150 ml |
| | = 100 ml |

Therefore reduction of tidal volume from 450 to 250 ml reduces the effective tidal volume by two-thirds from 300 ml to 100 ml. If the respiratory rate remains at 20/min alveolar ventilation $\dot{V}_A$ would be = 100 × 20 = 2.0 l/min

Table 18.5 Response to the respiratory centre increases the rate to 30/min in an attempt to maintain the PCO_2 at its normal value of 40 mmHg (5.3 kPa)

Effective tidal volume V_A	= 100 ml
Respiratory rate	= 30/min
Alveolar ventilation $\dot{V}_A$	= 100 × 30 ml/min
	= 3000 ml/min = 3.0 l/min

Therefore, a tidal volume of 250 ml has to be moved three times as often to provide the same ventilation as that normally produced when the tidal volume is 450 ml and the respiratory rate is 10/min (see Table 18.1)

It is apparent, therefore, that the patient who breathes rapidly and shallowly is ventilating inefficiently and perhaps inadequately to maintain a satisfactory respiratory exchange.

Furthermore, additional respiratory effort increases muscular work and causes fatigue unless the atelectasis is relieved either by coughing or by endobronchial suction.

Such patients should always be observed carefully because they are on the brink of respiratory failure (p. 223) and may need actual resuscitation. At this stage it is worth noting that the most effective way of improving alveolar ventilation is by increasing the depth of respiration (Table 18.6). However, increasing the tidal volume is not

Table 18.6

Tidal volume V_T	= 750 ml
Dead space V_D	= 150 ml
Effective tidal volume V_A	= 600 ml
Respiratory rate	= 4/min
Alveolar ventilation $\dot{V}_A$	= 600 × 4
	= 2400 ml/min = 2.4 l/min

Comparison between Tables 18.6 and 18.4 show that four deep breaths of 750 ml produce more ventilation than 20 breaths of 250 ml

always practicable because of the increased airway resistance and trapping found in some respiratory disorders.

Table 18.7 Further atelectasis reduces the tidal volume to 180 ml. Increasing fatigue prevents the patient increasing his rate of respiration, and alveolar ventilation becomes even less efficient so that asphyxia supervenes

Tidal volume V_T	= 180 ml
Dead space V_D	= 150 ml
Effective tidal volume V_A	= 30 ml
Respiratory rate	= 20/min
Alveolar ventilation $\dot V_A$	= 20 × 30 = 600 ml/min

Table 18.8 If the tidal volume decreases further to 150 ml to equal the dead space volume then the effective tidal volume is nil and exchange of gases between the atmosphere and the alveoli is nil

Tidal volume V_T	150
Dead space volume V_D (ml)	150
	———
Effective tidal volume V_A (ml)	0
Respiratory rate	10/min
Effective minute volume (ml)	10 × 0
	= 0
Alveolar ventilation $\dot V_A$	= 0

From the above it is seen that asphyxia gradually increases as the tidal volume falls and approaches the dead space volume, whereupon the respiratory movements are less and less effective and eventually serve only to move dead space air in and out of the lungs without any fresh air entering the respiratory tract.

Increasing the tidal exchange between atmospheric air and the alveoli is one of the main aims of resuscitation. One aid to improving alveolar ventilation is to decrease the dead space, which can be done by endotracheal intubation or tracheostomy.

Dead space
DECREASING DEAD SPACE

Reduction of dead space allows a higher proportion of inspired air to enter the lungs.

Tracheostomy bypasses the upper half of the respiratory tract so that air enters the trachea without passing through the nose, mouth, pharynx and larynx. The dead space following tracheostomy consists of the tracheostomy tube, the lower end of the trachea, and the bronchi and bronchioles. Tracheostomy has the effect of reducing the dead space to half of its original value (Table 18.9).

Table 18.9 Effect of tracheostomy or endotracheal intubation on dead space

	(a)	(b)	(c)	(d)
Tidal volume V_T (ml)	350	275	275	300
Dead space volume V_D (ml)	150	150	75	75
Effective tidal volume V_A (ml)	200	125	200	225
	before tracheostomy or endotracheal intubation	before tracheostomy or endotracheal intubation	after tracheostomy or endotracheal intubation the dead space is halved	after tracheostomy or endotracheal intubation the dead space is halved

Endotracheal intubation has a similar effect but after intubation the dead space consists of the endotracheal tube, the lower end of the trachea, and the bronchi and bronchioles. Because the endotracheal tube has a larger capacity than the tracheostomy tube, endotracheal intubation is almost, but not quite, as effective as tracheostomy in reducing the dead space. However, this small discrepancy between their effectiveness in reducing dead space can be ignored for most practical purposes.

Because endotracheal intubation is easier to perform and immediately reversible, in that the endotracheal tube can be withdrawn and reinserted more readily, attention in this chapter is directed mostly towards the effects on the dead space of endotracheal intubation.

Tables 18.9(a) and (b) show that if the dead space is 150 ml, any factor that decreases the tidal volume from 350 to 275 ml reduces the effective tidal volume from 200 ml to 125 ml. Endotracheal intubation, by reducing the dead space to 75 ml, restores the effective tidal volume to 200 ml (Table 18.9(c). The patient can then ventilate his lungs as effectively as the patient who is not intubated but whose tidal volume is 350 ml. Endotracheal intubation, therefore, helps to restore his respiratory exchange but at the expense of losing the ability to cough effectively and humidify his inspired gases.

A further look at Table 18.9 reveals that an intubated patient with a tidal volume of 300 ml (Table 18.9(d)) can ventilate his lungs more effectively than a non-intubated person whose tidal volume is 350 ml (Table 18.9(a)).

Apparatus dead space
The anatomical dead space extends from the bronchioles to the region where the expired air leaves the body, namely the nose and mouth. Any valveless piece of equipment such as a Schimmelbusch mask,

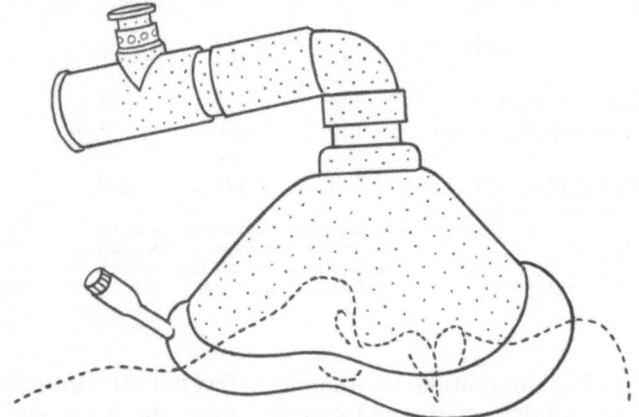

Figure 18.4 Apparatus dead space (stippled)

for giving open ether, when applied to the face increases the dead space by an amount equal to the internal volume of the applied equipment. Anatomical dead space and apparatus dead space together constitute the *total* dead space.

The face mask dead space reduces the effective tidal volume (V_A) and its value may become very significant if the patient's tidal volume (V_T) is restricted due to disease or drugs because it can cause the accumulation of carbon dioxide. Special care is necessary in choosing the size of face mask for a baby because too large a mask may have a volume far in excess of the baby's tidal volume so that little or no exchange of air occurs between the atmosphere and the baby's lungs.

Most anaesthetic circuits incorporate an expiratory valve, in which case the apparatus dead space is that volume of the apparatus which extends from the patient to the expiratory valve (Figure 18.4). Increasing the dead space is usually disadvantageous and precautions are taken to reduce it to a minimum. Usually this involves placing an expiratory valve close to the mouth and introducing a flow of fresh gas near the mouth so that any stale gas lingering there is flushed away. The rationale behind these precautions is clarified by an elementary knowledge of the various circuits used in resuscitation (Chapter 19).

19

Basic equipment – resuscitation bags and circuits

Effective resuscitation requires knowledge of the components and use of basic equipment. Essentially, effective ventilation needs a supply of air or oxygen and a rubber bag, usually referred to as a reservoir bag (p. 147), to squeeze the air or oxygen into the patient. A valve, the expiratory valve (one type of which is the 'non-return valve'), is necessary to allow the air or oxygen to escape into the atmosphere during expiration.

The non-return valve
The function of the non-return valve is to allow all the air or oxygen squeezed from within the reservoir bag to enter the lungs, and allow all the expired gases to vent into the atmosphere instead of passing back into the anaesthetic circuit and subsequently being reinhaled. This type of valve forms the basis of the portable resuscitation bag.

Portable resuscitation bags such as the Ambu or Air Viva incorporate bag and valve in one unit. If these are unavailable a suitable circuit can be built from standard anaesthetic equipment (p. 136). It is important to be familiar with all the components and connections, which must be immediately available otherwise valuable time is lost before resuscitation can start.

Portable resuscitation bag (Ambu, Air Viva etc.)
The portable resuscitation bag is robust, easy to handle, has a minimum of connections and can function effectively. Pressure on the bag forces air into the patient; release of the bag allows expiration through the non-return valve. Simultaneously the bag returns to its original shape and draws into itself, through a separate entrance, a further bagful of fresh air (Figure 19.1).

Oxygen can be introduced by connecting rubber tubing leading from a cylinder or piped oxygen supply to a protruding nipple situated near the tail of the resuscitation bag. It should be remembered that release of the bag causes it to fill so that it sucks in both fresh air and oxygen. If the oxygen flow rate is 6 l/min, that is 100 ml/s, and the volume in the bag is 300 ml, then if the bag fills over a period of 1 second it will suck in 100 ml of oxygen and 200 ml air, giving an oxygen : air ratio of 33 : 66% with a total oxygen percentage of 33 plus 66 × 21/100 = approximately 46%

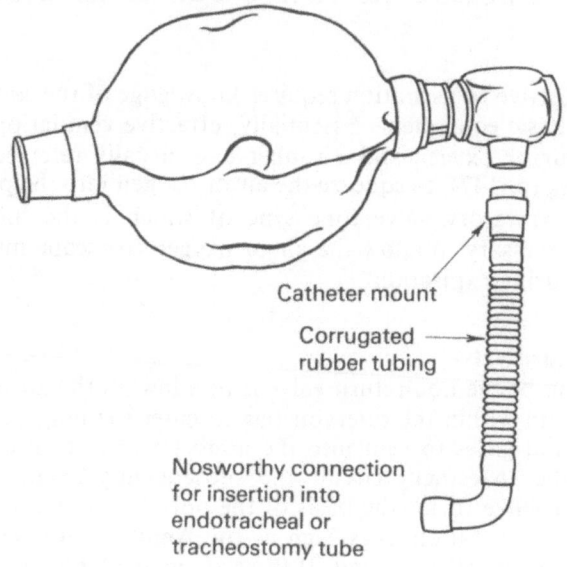

Catheter mount

Corrugated rubber tubing

Nosworthy connection for insertion into endotracheal or tracheostomy tube

Figure 19.1 'Ambu' portable resuscitation bag. The valve is the non-return type

In practice, the actual percentage of oxygen acquired within the bag depends on many factors such as the compliance of the bag, the flow rate of oxygen, rate of filling of air and rate of release of the bag by the hand of the resuscitator. However, one thing is sure, the connection of an oxygen supply to the standard portable resuscitation bag certainly raises the oxygen percentage that can be delivered to the patient but not up to 100%; therefore, if it is essential to deliver 100% oxygen to the patient, the standard portable resuscitation bag is unsatisfactory.

Recently the Ambu bag has been fitted with an additional plate-like attachment which blocks the air entry into the bag so that connection to an oxygen supply does ensure the administration of 100% oxygen.

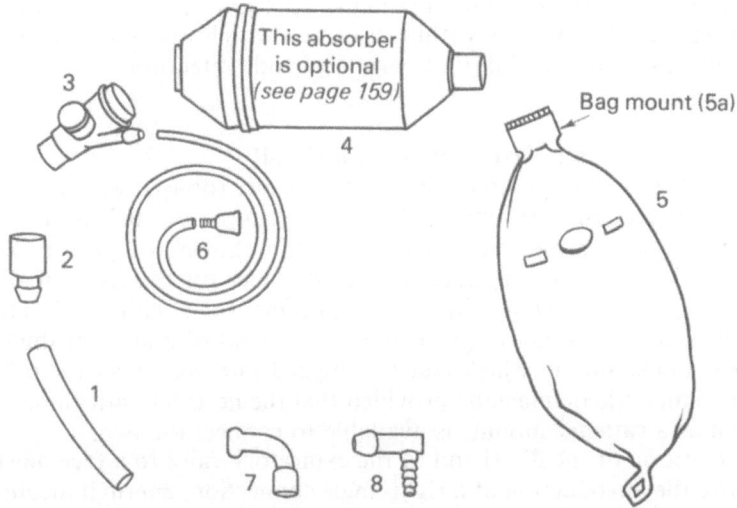

Figure 19.2 Circuit for performance of intermittent positive pressure
ventilation (IPPV). Key:
1   Rubber tube which connects with endotracheal tube via a Nosworthy
    connector (7) or Rowbotham oral connector (8)
2   Catheter mount
3   Expiratory valve with feed (attachment for oxygen supply line)
4   Water's carbon dioxide absorber (canister)
5   Reservoir bag with bag mount (5a)
6   Air or oxygen supply tube for connection to air or oxygen cylinder, pipe
    line or anaesthetic machine
7   Nosworthy connector
8   Rowbotham connector

The pop-off expiratory valve (for example, Heidbrink)
This type of valve is spring-loaded and is often seen on the circuit attached to the anaesthetic machines, usually positioned very close to
the face mask. Its function is to allow the escape of expired air and
surplus gas from the circuit without allowing entry of atmospheric air
from outside. However, during expiration only part of the expired
tidal volume (V_T) is discharged into the atmosphere. The remainder
passes back towards the reservoir bag and is returned to the lungs with
a supply of fresh gas when the bag is compressed during the next inspiratory phase (p. 144). This reinhalation of expired gas is known as
rebreathing, the extent of which depends on the fresh gas flow rate. If
the fresh gas, which is usually oxygen, is delivered to the circuit at
6 l/min there will be little carbon dioxide retention (p. 140). Fresh gas

flow rates of less than 6 l/min should incorporate a carbon dioxide absorber (p. 159) because rebreathing is greater with lower flow rates and thus increases the possibility of carbon dioxide retention.

How to build an effective resuscitation circuit
The ideal resuscitation circuit should be simple, robust, versatile and easy to understand and manipulate. An example of such a circuit (known as the Mapleson C circuit, p. 138) is shown in Figure 19.2). This particular expiratory valve carries the inlet for the entry of the fresh gas, the two being called the 'expiratory valve with feed'. The feed is connected to an oxygen cylinder by means of a piece of thick-walled rubber tubing which can be plugged into the oxygen supply from an anaesthetic machine provided that the necessary attachment, known as a catheter mount, is available to connect the two.

Connection of the distal end of the expiratory valve to a face mask requires the introduction of a right-angle connection, a term indicated by its shape. On the other hand connection of the wide exit part of the expiratory valve to the narrower endotracheal connection of an endotracheal tube needs a catheter mount and a small piece (12 cm) of rubber tubing. Attachment of the reservoir bag with its bag mount to the expiratory valve completes the circuit. If a carbon dioxide absorber is indicated it is introduced between the valve and the bag (p. 159).

Resuscitation with the anaesthetic machine
As a piece of resuscitation apparatus the anaesthetic machine has many advantages. Usually it is well-serviced, robust, stable and fairly mobile. Its shelves carry basic resuscitation equipment such as oral airways, face masks, laryngoscopes, endotracheal tubes and Magill's intubating forceps (see Figure 22.5), and often a selection of drugs for use in a wide variety of emergency conditions.

Many different varieties of circuit are available for attachment to an anaesthetic machine, some complex and best restricted to use by anaesthetists. The non-anaesthetist practitioner is advised to restrict his use to the Mapleson A (p. 137), C (p. 138) and E (T-piece, p. 140), and the 'to and fro' circuit (p. 159).

To achieve adequate ventilation of the lungs it is essential for the resuscitator to understand what happens to the composition of the gases in the tubing connecting the patient to the machine during the various stages of respiration. As mentioned above (p. 121) the reader should realize that adjacent volumes of gases mix with one another and are not delineated as shown in Figures 19.3 to 19.16, although

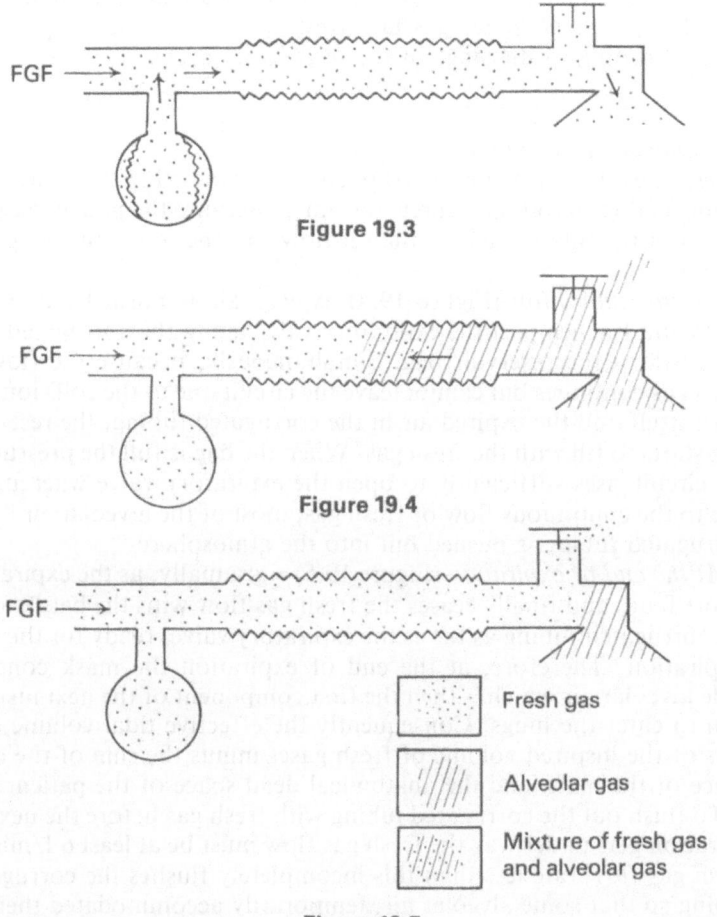

Figure 19.3

Figure 19.4

Fresh gas

Alveolar gas

Mixture of fresh gas and alveolar gas

Figure 19.5

Figures 19.3 – 19.5 Composition of gas flow in Mapleson A circuit during spontaneous ventilation. **Figure 19.3** Inspiration; **Figure 19.4** Midway through expiration; **Figure 19.5** End of expiration

they do serve a purpose in explaining why the flow of fresh gas (FGF—fresh gas flow) should not fall below certain values.

MAPLESON TYPE A CIRCUIT
This circuit is found connected up and ready for use in most casualty departments.

It is advisable to divide the gases in the patient and circuit into alveolar gas, dead space gas and fresh gas. Their relative positions vary according to the stage of the respiratory cycle.

Spontaneous respiration
During inspiration (Figure 19.3) fresh gas, from within the anaesthetic tubing and reservoir bag, enters the lungs. Because the patient extracts gas from the tubing quicker than it flows in, the reservoir bag partly empties.

During expiration (Figure 19.4) expired air is pushed out of the lungs and trachea past the expiratory valve along the corrugated tubing towards the reservoir bag. Simultaneously, because the flow of fresh gas continues but cannot leave the circuit due to the collision between itself and the expired air in the corrugated tubing, the reservoir bag starts to fill with the fresh gas. When the bag is full the pressure in the circuit rises sufficiently to open the expiratory valve whereupon, due to the continuous flow of fresh gas, most of the alveolar air in the corrugated tubing is pushed out into the atmosphere.

At the end of expiration (Figure 19.5) – gradually, as the expiratory effort fades and finally ceases the fresh gas flow wins the battle to fill the corrugated tubing as far as the expiratory valve, ready for the next inspiration. Therefore, at the end of expiration the mask contains stale alveolar air which is then the first component of the next inspiration to enter the lungs. Consequently the effective tidal volume consists of the inspired volume of fresh gases minus the sum of the dead space of the mask and the anatomical dead space of the patient.

To flush out the corrugated tubing with fresh gas before the next inspiration gets under way the fresh gas flow must be at least 6 l/min. A fresh gas flow rate less than this incompletely flushes the corrugated tubing so that some alveolar air, temporarily accommodated therein, is reinhaled during the next inspiration. If this reinhalation is marked and prolonged it eventually leads to carbon dioxide retention. On the other hand, fresh gas flows greater than 6 l/min are wasteful.

MAPLESON TYPE C CIRCUIT (FIGURES 19.6 to 19.8)
Spontaneous ventilation
During inspiration (Figure 19.6) fresh gas enters the lungs from the anaesthetic tubing and the reservoir bag. However, a greater volume of fresh gas is taken by the patient from the reservoir bag than is being added to it from the fresh gas source, and therefore the bag partly empties.

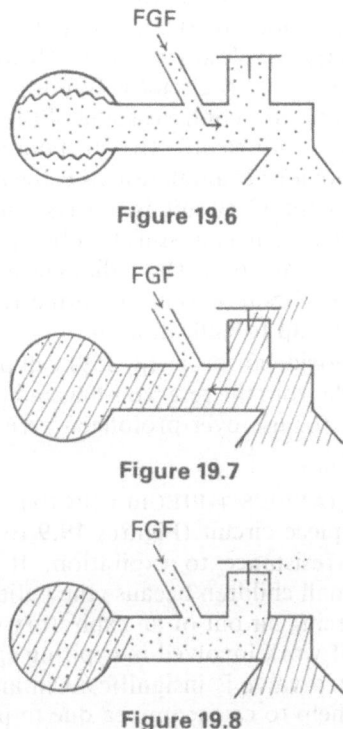

Figure 19.6

Figure 19.7

Figure 19.8

Figures 19.6 – 19.8 Composition of gas flow in Mapleson C circuit during spontaneous ventilation. **Figure 19.6** Inspiration; **Figure 19.7** Midway through expiration; **Figure 19.8** End of expiration. Key as in Figures **19.3 – 19.5**

During expiration (Figures 19.7) expired air has a choice of two destinies; some of it leaves through the expiratory valve and the remainder enters the reservoir bag. Likewise, the fresh gas has a similar choice: some is vented into the atmosphere and wasted. The rest of the fresh gas enters the reservoir bag which now contains a mixture of fresh gas, dead space gas and alveolar gas, and gradually reinflates.

At the end of expiration (Figure 19.8), as the expiratory effort fades, more and more fresh gas enters the reservoir bag, thereby diluting that part of the alveolar air which has not been ejected through the expiratory valve. When the bag is full the continuing flow of fresh gas passes through the valve into the surrounding atmosphere.

The last part of the alveolar air to leave the lungs comes to rest in the trachea and mask, so this is the first component to enter the lungs during the next inspiration. In this respect this Mapleson C circuit does not differ from the Mapleson A circuit. However, during inspiration, the reservoir bag in the A circuit is full of fresh gas, but in the C circuit the reservoir bag also contains some of the alveolar air. Consequently, the C circuit is not as effective in spontaneous respiration in preventing carbon dioxide accumulation as is the A circuit because the inspiratory gas from the C circuit is always contaminated by stale alveolar air; nevertheless, it is a useful, robust, easy-to-manage circuit, and because the rate of carbon dioxide build-up is slow, the resuscitator should not hesitate to use it with a fresh gas flow rate of 6 l/min for periods of up to half an hour.

Use of a carbon dioxide absorber (p. 159) can prevent the reinhalation of carbon dioxide from the reservoir bag and thereby render the C circuit perfectly safe for use over prolonged periods.

MAPLESON TYPE E (AYRE'S T-PIECE) CIRCUIT

The Mapleson E T-piece circuit (Figures 19.9 to 19.12) is valveless, so cause negligible resistance to expiration. It is, therefore, very suitable for use in small children because the patient does not have to use any energy in forcing air out of an expiratory valve. Although the additional amount of work involved in expiring against the resistance of a correctly adjusted valve is insignificant in an adult, it can soon tire an ill baby and help to cause apnoea due to physical exhaustion.

Its lack of resistance to expiration makes it useful for patients of all ages with head injuries because it does not raise the central venous pressure with the concurrent increase in pressure in the jugular and intracranial veins.

Its drawbacks are: first, that it has no reservoir bag and so is less adaptable for IPPV in the adult, and second, it is more wasteful because the fresh gas flow needs to be higher than in the Mapleson A and C circuits, in the region of 9–12 l/min for the adult patient.

Spontaneous ventilation
During expiration (Figures 19.11 and 19.12) expired air leaves the lungs and enters the corrugated tubing. Throughout expiration the fresh gas flow also enters the corrugated tubing and pushes the expired air further and further along until eventually some or all of the stale air is thrust out of the distal end into the atmosphere.

At the end of expiration (Figure 19.12) – as expiration finishes the proximal end of the corrugated tubing fills with fresh gas. Any stale alveolar air remaining in the tubing is positioned at the distal end.

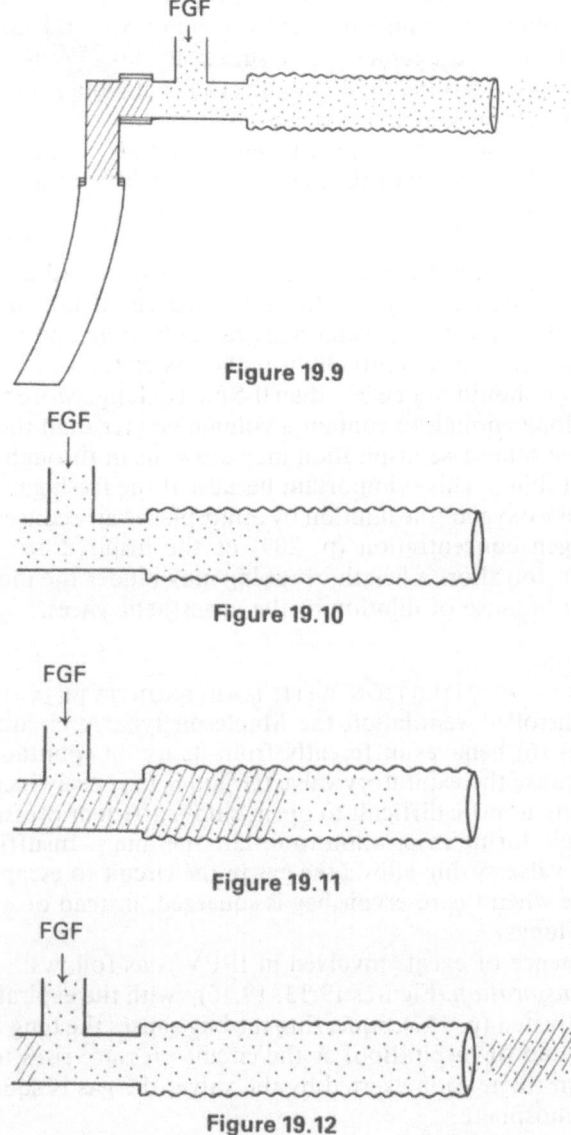

Figures 19.9 – 19.12 Composition of gas flow in Mapleson E circuit during spontaneous ventilation. **Figure 19.9** Start of inspiration; **Figure 19.10** End of inspiration; **Figure 19.11** Midway through expiration; **Figure 19.12** End of expiration. Key as in **Figures 19.3 – 19.5**

On inspiration (Figures 19.9 and 19.10) fresh gas is first drawn into the lungs from the proximal part of the tubing. Any stale alveolar gas in the distal part of the tubing is also sucked towards but never reaches the patient, provided the tidal volume (V_T) is less than the volume of fresh gas in the proximal part of the tubing.

If the fresh gas flow is insufficient and fails to push the stale alveolar air out of reach of the next inspiratory effort then some stale air is reinhaled.

Length of corrugated tubing – The tubing can be either 1, 2 or 3 metres long because every breath of expired air, if not immediately thrust into the atmosphere, is pushed gradually more and more distally down the tube until eventually it makes its exit.

The tubing should not be less than 0.5 metres long. More precisely it should be long enough to contain a volume greater than the patient's tidal volume otherwise inspiration may draw air in through the distal end of the tubing. This is important because if the fresh gas flow consists of 100% oxygen, the dilution by atmospheric air reduces the fractional oxygen concentration (p. 209) of the inspired fresh gas. In anaesthesia, too short a length of tubing may hinder the induction of anaesthesia because of dilution of the anaesthetic gases.

CONTROLLED VENTILATION WITH MAPLESON TYPE A CIRCUIT
During controlled ventilation the Mapleson type A circuit (Figures 19.13 to 19.16) behaves differently from its use in spontaneous ventilation because the expiratory valve tension is purposely increased (p. 156), making it more difficult to open, since sufficient pressure has to be generated during inspiration to inflate the lungs. Insufficient tension in the valve spring allows the gas in the circuit to escape into the atmosphere when the reservoir bag is squeezed, instead of working to inflate the lungs.

The sequence of events involved in IPPV is as follows:

During inspiration (Figures 19.13, 19.16), with the expiratory valve suitably adjusted (p. 157), squeezing the bag causes the lung to inflate, and at the end of inspiration, as the circuit pressure rises to become greater than the tension exerted by the valve, the gas is squeezed out into the atmosphere.

During expiration (Figures 19.14, 19.15) release of the reservoir bag causes the pressure in the circuit to drop. The patient breathes out and into the corrugated tubing. This alveolar gas causes the fresh gas to flow into and fill the reservoir bag. When the bag fills, and the pressure rises in the circuit, gas begins to force its way through the ex-

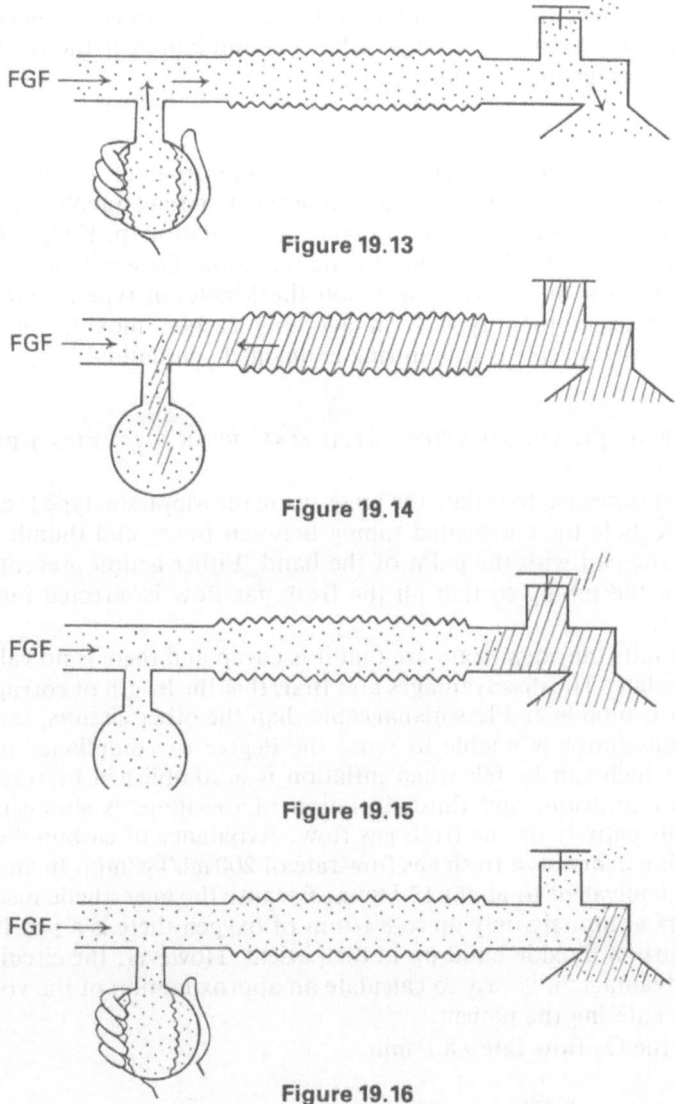

Figure 19.13

Figure 19.14

Figure 19.15

Figure 19.16

Figures 19.13 – 19.16 Composition of gas flow in Mapleson A circuit during controlled ventilation. **Figure 19.13** End of first inspiration; **Figure 19.14** Midway through expiration; **Figure 19.15** End of expiration; **Figure 19.16** Further inspirations. Key as in **Figures 19.3 – 19.5**

piratory valve. If all the alveolar air is not ejected it is the first component of the corrugated tubing to be reinhaled with consequent carbon dioxide retention. This possibility is minimized if the fresh gas flow is greater than 6 l/min.

CONTROLLED VENTILATION WITH MAPLESON TYPE C CIRCUIT
Controlled ventilation with the Mapleson C circuit involves similar gaseous interchange as with spontaneous ventilation (p. 138); 6 l/min fresh gas flow avoids carbon dioxide retention. Generally it is stated that during spontaneous ventilation the Mapleson type A circuit is more efficient than type C in avoiding carbon dioxide retention whereas the reverse is true during controlled ventilation.

CONTROLLED VENTILATION WITH MAPLESON E (AYRE'S T-PIECE) CIRCUIT
All that is needed to inflate the lungs using the Mapleson type E circuit is to occlude the corrugated tubing between finger and thumb or to block the end with the palm of the hand. Either action prevents gas leaving the tubing so that all the fresh gas flow is directed into the patient.

In adults the advantages are that it is cheap and there is no valve to manipulate. The disadvantages are: first, that the length of corrugated tubing is mobile and less manageable than the other circuits; second, the resuscitator is unable to sense the degree of compliance of the lungs which can be felt when inflation is accomplished by reservoir bag compression, and third, inflation of the lungs is slow since it depends entirely on the fresh gas flow. Avoidance of carbon dioxide retention demands a fresh gas flow rate of 200 ml/kg/min. In an adult this is equivalent to about 12 l/min. Because the anaesthetic machine delivers accurately only up to 8 l/min of oxygen there is a possibility of a carbon dioxide build-up in the patient. However, the circuit has one advantage: it is easy to calculate an approximation of the volume of gas entering the patient.

Let the O_2 flow rate = 8 l/min

$$= \frac{8000}{60} \text{ ml} = 130 \text{ ml/s}$$

Then obstruction of the corrugated tubing for 3 seconds will force 130 × 3 = 390 ml into the patient.

The timing of the technique is as follows:

Time	Action	Result
At the count 1	Occlude the corrugated tubing	Inspiration starts
At the count 2, 3	Maintain the occlusion	Inspiration continues
At the count 4	Release the corrugated tubing	Expiration starts
At the count 5, 6	Nil	Expiration ends

A 6 second respiratory phase with equal duration of the inspiratory and expiratory components is not physiological. Nevertheless, as a temporary circuit it is a useful addition to other resuscitation circuits. If the fresh gas flow can be increased to 12 l/min which is equivalent to 200 ml/s, the inspiratory phase, in delivering 400 ml tidal volume, can be reduced to 2 seconds which makes it more acceptable physiologically.

As in the use of other circuits it is important to observe the extent of chest movements that occur whenever the corrugated expiratory tube is occluded.

In children and especially babies (p. 114) this circuit is excellent. A child aged 10 years requires a gas flow of about 6 l/min. For example,

Let the tidal volume V_T = 200 ml
Respiratory rate   = 15/min
Then the minute volume   = 200 × 15 = 3 l/min
Required O_2 flow rate from
  machine   = 6 l/min

∴ Occlusion of expiratory limb for 2 seconds delivers 2 × 100 = 200 ml which is the demanded tidal volume.

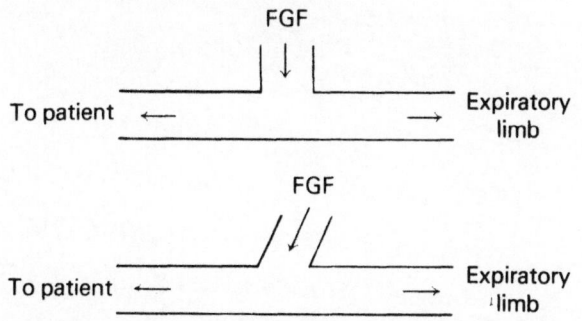

Figure 19.17 Variation in shape of Ayre's T piece

The Mapleson type E or Ayre's T-piece circuit is the basis of many expensive neonatal resuscitation machines. Sometimes apparently different circuits vary only in the shape or direction of the expiratory limb of the T, or in the direction of entry of fresh gas flow (Figure 19.17). All that has happened is that the T has been bent. For resuscitation the behaviour of the gas flows and the technique of their use can be regarded as identical. Use of the T-piece in neonatal resuscitation is discussed in Chapter 17.

Although it is true that one circuit is superior to another according to whether spontaneous or artificial ventilation is desirable this fact should not deter the employment of *any* of these circuits in an emergency situation. The immediate primary aim in resuscitation is to restore the airway and re-establish adequate pulmonary gaseous exchange. Only if resuscitation is prolonged is there any need to ensure that the most appropriate circuit is used. Usually the circuit can be altered accordingly at a later stage in the resuscitation procedure.

20

The reservoir bag – its use in spontaneous and controlled ventilation

Functions of the reservoir bag during spontaneous ventilation

'Squeeze the bag' or 'watch the bag' are expressions frequently heard in the operating theatre or casualty department. The 'bag' refers to the reservoir bag which forms an important part of an anaesthetic or resuscitation circuit.

To understand the functions of the reservoir bag two considerations are necessary:

(1) The anaesthetic machine is usually set to deliver a fresh gas flow of 6 l/min.
(2) During a normal spontaneous respiration the patient inspires a tidal volume of 450 ml in 1.5 seconds. If the inspiratory flow of gas were constant during this time the flow rate would be $450/1.5 = 300$ ml/s, which is equivalent to 18 l/min. But the flow rate of air entering the lungs during inspiration is not constant and at some stage reaches $30-40$ l/min.

Therefore, when the patient inspires, the machine cannot cope with the immediate demands. It cannot provide sufficient fresh gas flow to satisfy the sudden inspiratory requirements of the lungs. This problem is overcome by inserting a reservoir bag between the anaesthetic machine and the patient. As the patient inspires, any gas that cannot be supplied immediately by the machine is sucked out of the bag which actually acts as a reservoir; the bag therefore, diminishes in volume during inspiration. An immediate question is 'why restrict the fresh gas flow to 6 l/min when the demand of the patient is greater'? The answer is that there is no reason why a higher gas flow cannot be used but it leads to an expensive waste of fresh gas, most of which is vented out of the expiratory valve during the other stages of respiration. Furthermore, the oxygen flowmeters read accurately only to 8 l/min. A greater flow of oxygen causes the rotating bobbin to rise and stick at

147

the top of the flowmeter tube and it is then no longer capable of indicating what flow of oxygen is being delivered; 6 l/min is adequate to avoid carbon dioxide retention in an adult in the Mapleson type circuits A (Figure 19.3) and C (Figure 19.6).

SIZE OF RESERVOIR BAG

The adult-sized reservoir bag is the 2 litre, which means that its capacity is 2 litres when it is fully but not forcibly distended. The smaller version for the younger patient has a capacity of 1 litre. The bag may be provided with a loop at the bottom so that the bag can be folded over and the loop hooked onto a knob on the top of the bag mount. This procedure reduces the bag's functional capacity to half if a smaller bag is desired but unavailable.

Much mystique surrounds the choice of size of reservoir bag, but the size chosen is immaterial provided that the bag can cope with a sudden demand on its contents. It must not collapse completely during inspiration, so its capacity should be greater than the patient's tidal volume.

In the case of a child the smaller bag is more suitable because his small tidal volume causes greater fluctuations than if the 2 litre one is used, and the child's respirations can be more easily and accurately assessed; a 2 litre reservoir bag can nevertheless be used in the young patient if necessary.

Squeezing the bag by hand is termed manual ventilation. It is a procedure often performed by the anaesthetist, and to the onlooker appears to require little special skill. But, as in all types of artificial ventilation, the purpose is to ensure an adequate tidal exchange without upsetting the circulatory dynamics of the venous return to the heart. To accomplish these aims the resuscitator needs to be familiar with his resuscitation apparatus and to understand what he is trying to accomplish without doing harm to the patient.

LUNG CHARACTERISTICS – HOW TO SQUEEZE THE BAG

Because some lungs are larger than others they require the introduction of a larger volume of air to satisfy their tidal volumes. To ensure inflation the stiff lung needs generation of higher pressure in the bag than does the more compliant lung. The asthmatic, with bronchospasm, requires the inflation and expiration periods to be extended because of the narrowing of the air passages with consequent resistance to air flow. The emphysematous lung has lost its elasticity, and deflation needs a longer expiratory time than does the normal lung. It is immediately obvious that the characteristics of the lung and air passages influence the volume, pressure and rate of flow of the gas passing into the patient. Many varieties of ventilator are on the market with special specifications, invented to cope with the different characteristics found in different lungs. It is, however, true to say that no ventilator has yet been invented that is universally adaptable to deal with all eventualities. Fortunately all resuscitation procedures requiring IPPV can effectively be performed manually, but constant attention is essential, and the practitioner must 'see, feel and listen'.

What to see

Much can be learned by watching a person relaxing or asleep, and noting how little the chest and abdomen move with respiration. In fact, the observer would worry were the respiratory movements too pronounced. Nevertheless, manual ventilation by the inexperienced usually produces heaving chest and abdominal movements more conducive to those of a patient who has just completed a 100 metres sprint. The resuscitator, therefore, should squeeze the bag sufficiently to produce respiratory movements similar in extent to those anticipated in normal quiet respiration.

What to feel

With experience it is possible to feel the extent of lung inflation during inspiration, but until this skill is developed there is need to correlate the 'feel' of the bag while watching the patient's respiratory movements.

WHY THE BAG IS NOT EMPTIED DURING INFLATION

The reason is as follows:

Let the fresh gas flow rate from the machine   =   6 l/min
   or cylinder   = 100 ml/s
Let the patient's required tidal volume (V_T)   = '400 ml

Then, if the entrance to the bag is occluded, by nipping between finger and thumb or (what amounts to the same thing) if the bag is prevented from filling by being grasped firmly by the hand, none of the fresh gas flow enters the reservoir bag. As a result, 100 ml/s of fresh gas flows into the corrugated tubing towards the patient. Therefore, by simply grasping the bag and preventing its filling, 100 ml of the required 400 ml tidal volume (V_T) is directed towards the patient; a grasp of 2 s deflects 200 ml of fresh gas towards him.

From the above it is seen that the actual volume which needs to be squeezed out of the bag is equal to the tidal volume (V_T) minus that delivered by the machine or cylinder whilst the bag is being squeezed.

For example, a 1 s squeeze delivers 100 ml

∴ Amount needed to be squeezed out of the bag to satisfy the tidal volume (V_T) requirement = 400 ml − 100 ml = 300 ml

This 300 ml is approximately only a third the volume of a 1 litre bag and one-seventh the volume of a 2 litre bag. Therefore, it is unnecessary and *can be harmful* to empty the bag completely during inflation. The bag should be squeezed gently with one hand, preferably between the thumb and the outer three fingers, a technique which restricts the strength of the grasp and thus the amount of gas discharged from the bag. The use of both hands for bag compression is unnecessary and unwise; it is remarkable that patients survive when an aggressive two-handed technique is adopted because it can seriously impede the venous return and cause hypotension. The reservoir bag should therefore be approached firmly but handled gently like a peach, and not squeezed hard like a lemon.

DURATION OF SQUEEZE DURING INFLATION

Keeping the bag squeezed directs all the fresh gas into the corrugated tubing in addition to that which has been expelled from the bag during compression.

Let the bag compression expel 300 ml
The additional fresh gas entering the corrugated tubing
= 100 ml/s

∴ Compression for 1 s directs 300 ml + (100 × 1) ml = 400 ml towards the patient

Compression for 2 s directs 300 ml + (100 × 2) ml = 500 ml towards the patient

Compression for 3 s directs 300 ml + (100 × 3) ml = 600 ml towards the patient

If the whole 600 ml enters the lungs it is too much to satisfy the 400 ml requirement of that particular patient, and will result in hyperventilation, a fall in P_ACO_2 and P_aCO_2, and a respiratory alkalosis.

Lowering of the carbon dioxide level in the blood may prevent spontaneous ventilation starting when the decision is taken that IPPV is no longer necessary. Furthermore, maintenance of a high pressure in the lungs during inflation can cause hypotension. The reason for this is described below.

Central venous pressure changes during spontaneous ventilation
During inspiration
The chest wall moves outwards and the diaphragm downwards causing the intrapleural pressure to become more subatmospheric and the lungs to expand. This fall in pressure imparts a traction effect on the walls of the great veins in the chest and sucks blood towards the heart. Inspiration is thereby a major factor in increasing the cardiac venous return.

During expiration
The collapse of the chest wall and elevation of the diaphragm increases the intrapleural pressure and as a result the great veins are compressed so that venous return to the heart is impaired. This effect is most noticeable during the Valsalva manoeuvre in which a forced expiratory effort with a closed glottis increases the pressure exerted on the great veins and prevents blood returning to the heart.

At this point it can be recalled that in normal circumstances the cardiac output = venous return, and peripheral resistance × cardiac output = blood pressure. Therefore, a fall in venous return causes a fall in both cardiac output and blood pressure. IPPV can have similar effects on the blood pressure as described below.

Central venous pressure changes during controlled ventilation
Contrary to what occurs during inspiration in spontaneous ventilation, when chest cage expansion precedes lung inflation, in controlled ventilation the lungs expand first followed by expansion of the chest wall and descent of the diaphragm.

During inflation
The pressure is applied to the reservoir bag and gas is forced into the lungs. The intrapulmonary pressure rises and the lungs inflate.

Inflation of the lungs pushes the thoracic cage outwards so that it too expands. As a result the intrapleural space is trapped between lung and cage, and being squeezed between them its pressure rises so that its value becomes positive. Simultaneously the great veins are similarly subjected to the rise in pressure and their blood flow is diminished or prevented. Both cardiac output and blood pressure fall.

During expiration
Release of the reservoir bag allows the pressure to fall in the circuit. The elasticity of the lungs and chest wall initiate expiration, and the intrapulmonary pressure returns to normal atmospheric pressure. Also, the intrapleural pressure diminishes, so removing the obstruction to the central venous return. Cardiac output increases and the blood pressure returns to normal.

EFFECTS OF PROLONGED INTRATHORACIC PRESSURE
Prolonged interference with the venous return to the heart causes hypotension and can occur during IPPV if the inflation pressure generated in the lungs is too high, is maintained for too long, or if the intrapulmonary pressure is not allowed to fall to atmospheric pressure at the end of expiration. Therefore, during IPPV, attention is paid to the extent and duration of both inflation and expiration.

EXTENT AND DURATION OF INFLATION
The immediate aim of IPPV during inflation is to introduce a tidal volume of gas into the lungs. Immediately pressure is applied to the bag, the pressure in the lungs begins to rise continuing until the pressure on the bag is released. Therefore, at every fraction of a second during inflation a different intrapulmonary pressure is present. The sum of all these pressures, taken at intervals of fractions of a second, divided by the sum of all these times during which the pressure is recorded gives the average pressure exerted over the total time taken by inflation. This average pressure is more often called the mean pressure.

$$\therefore \text{Mean pressure} = \frac{\text{sum of all pressures recorded at intervals of fraction of a second}}{\text{sum of all the times during which the pressure is recorded}}$$
(= inflation time in seconds)

In physiology books this expression is recorded with the use of symbols

Σ = sum of

d = a little bit of something

dP = a little bit of the total pressure

dT	$=$	a little bit of the total time
$\bar{P}$	$=$	mean pressure

Then $\bar{P} \quad = \dfrac{\Sigma dP}{\Sigma dt}$

This equation reads 'the mean pressure is equal to the sum of all the pressure readings divided by the sum of all the time intervals over which the pressures were recorded'. Such information is obtainable by computer, and is recorded graphically in Figure 20.1 where mean pressure = the sum of all the hundreds of values of P, that is at Y_1, Y_2 etc. between $Y_0 \rightarrow Y_e$ divided by the sum of the time intervals from $X_0 \rightarrow X_e$

If all the values of Y are added together they constitute the area under the graph. If all the time intervals are added together they give the total time. Therefore, the mean pressure equals the

$$\frac{\text{area under the graph}}{\text{time from start to end of inflation}}$$

Figure 20.1 shows the intrapulmonary pressure generated during inflation; Figure 20.2 shows the same pressure recorded during deflation. Combining Figures 20.1 and 20.2 gives Figure 20.3, where expiration or deflation starts at e.

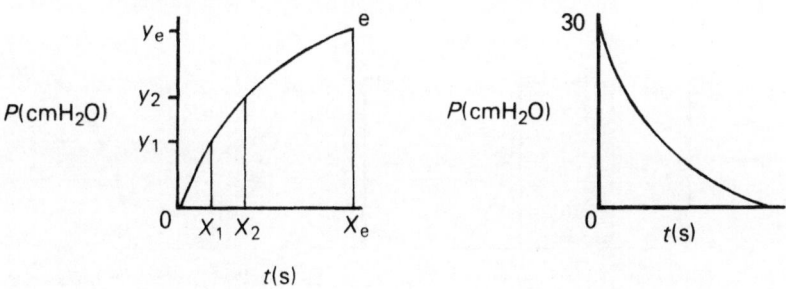

Figure 20.1   **Figure 20.2**

Figures 20.1, 20.2, and 20.3 show that the intrapulmonary pressure remains above atmospheric until expiration ends. Therefore, at all times during inflation and deflation there is some interference with venous return.

Significance of Figure 20.3
Using the same criteria as before, the mean pressure during the whole inflation–deflation cycle is equal to the area under the graph (shaded) divided by the time taken for the cycle. Figure 20.3 yields important information in that because $\bar{P}$ =

$$\frac{\Sigma dP}{\Sigma dt} \text{ and } \Sigma dP \text{ is equal to the area,}$$

an increase of the area (vertically lined) will therefore increase the mean pressure $\bar{P}$.

In Figure 20.4, the area enclosed by the graph, and therefore the mean pressure, is increased by elevating the maximum inflation pressure from 30 cm to 40 cm water (horizontally lined).

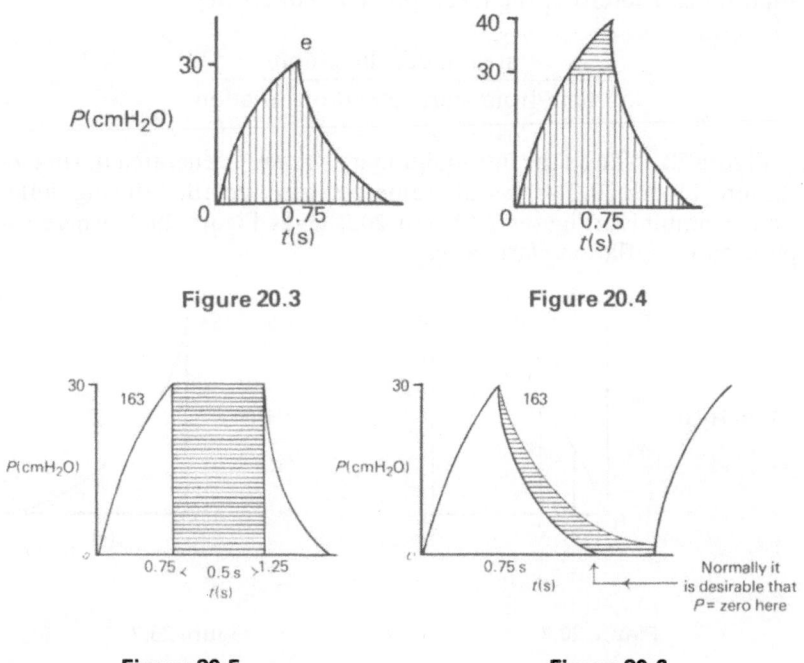

Figure 20.3   Figure 20.4

Figure 20.5   Figure 20.6

$\bar{P}$ is also increased in Figure 20.5 where the maximum inflation pressure is maintained for an extra 0.5 s, that is from 0.75 s to 1.25 s.

$\bar{P}$ is also increased in Figure 20.6 where the intrapulmonary pressure is not allowed to fall to zero before the next inflation starts.

Conclusion

From Figures 20.1 to 20.6 above and from other information it is recognized that to provide a satisfactory tidal exchange with minimal impairment of the venous return, various conditions are required:

(1) The appropriate tidal volume is introduced into the lungs.
(2) The mean pressure is kept as low as possible by
    (a) restricting the maximal pressure generated in the lungs during inflation,
    (b) restricting the duration over which the maximal inflation pressure is applied,
    (c) allowing free exit of air from the lungs,
    (d) allowing a pause of about 1 s between the end of expiration and the beginning of the next inspiration.

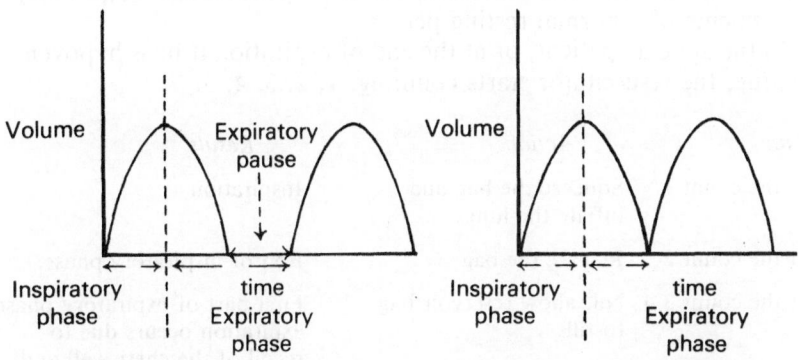

Figure 20.7 Respiratory cycle – normal breathing

Figure 20.8 Respiratory cycle – rapid breathing (tachypnoea)

RESPIRATORY CYCLE

A normal adult breathing quietly breathes in, immediately breathes out, and then has a brief rest before the next inspiration starts. The normal respiratory cycle is divided into two phases: the inspiratory phase and the expiratory phase (Figure 20.7). The inspiratory phase lasts from the beginning of inspiration to the end of inspiration. The expiratory phase extends from the end of the previous inspiration to the beginning of the next inspiration. The first part of the expiratory phase extends from the end of inspiration to the end of expiration. The second part of the expiratory phase is called the respiratory pause, and is that part of the cycle between the end of expiration and the beginning of the next inspiration. During tachypnoea the respiratory pause is absent (Figure 20.8).

The respiratory pause is important, especially during IPPV, because it is at this point where the intrathoracic pressure is normally lowest, allowing the free flow of venous blood back to the heart.

Practical points on resuscitation
The resuscitator needs to appreciate the effects that artificial inflation of the lungs has on the blood pressure, otherwise he may find the blood pressure soon becomes unrecordable. He should develop a suitable rhythmic technique as described below.

Technique of applying IPPV with resuscitation bag
Rhythmical compression and relaxation of the reservoir bag are performed in such a way that the chest and abdominal movements are similar in extent and duration to the spontaneous respiratory movements of a normal resting person.

In the apnoeic patient, or at the end of expiration if he is hypoventilating, the resuscitator starts counting, 1, 2, 3, 4, 5.

Time	Action	Result
At the count 1	Squeeze the bag and inflate the lungs	Inspiration
At the count 2	Release the bag	End of inspiratory phase.
At the count 3,4	Nil, allow reservoir bag to fill	First part of expiratory phase; expiration occurs due to recoil of the chest wall and lungs
At the count 5	Nil, bag is full, ready for start of next cycle	Second part of expiratory phase, that is, expiratory pause; lungs are immobile

Technique of performing manual IPPV with expiratory valve and anaesthetic circuit
The following instructions are suitable for performing IPPV with the Mapleson A and C type circuits (p. 142–144).

Valve adjustment 1
Let the anaesthetic machine or oxygen cylinder deliver a flow rate of 6 l/min oxygen, then screw the valve in an anticlockwise direction until it is completely open. Squeeze the reservoir bag. The gas forced out has the choice of effortlessly leaving the circuit through the fully

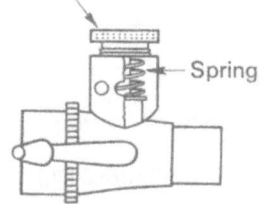

Circular disc – when turned clockwise closes valve. When turned anti-clockwise opens valve

Spring

Figure 20.9 Expiratory valve

opened expiratory valve or working hard by entering the lungs and lifting the overlying ribs and chest wall; naturally the gas chooses to pass through the valve into the atmosphere. Consequently it is stated that the resistance of the lungs and chest walls to inflation is greater than the resistance of the valve. No gas enters the patient.

Valve adjustment 2
Screw down the valve by half a turn in a clockwise direction to increase the tension of the valve spring and make it more difficult for the gas, squeezed from the bag, to escape into the atmosphere. Compression of the bag at this stage forces some air into the lungs but most still leaks into the atmosphere.

Valve adjustment 3
Continue to screw the valve clockwise in quarter turns until the resistance of the valve spring approximates to that attributed to the elasticity of the lungs and the weight of the chest wall. Gas can now enter the lungs or leave the valve with equal ease. Movements of the chest wall should now resemble those of normal quiet spontaneous inspiration.

Valve adjustment 4
Unscrew the valve a quarter turn anticlockwise. Next, release the reservoir bag to allow expiration to start. The natural elastic recoil of the lungs and chest wall forces the expired air into the corrugated tubing and then out into the atmosphere.

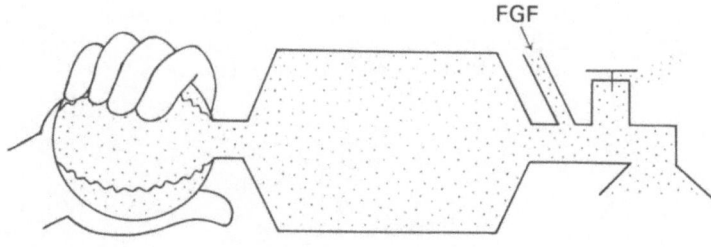

Figure 20.10

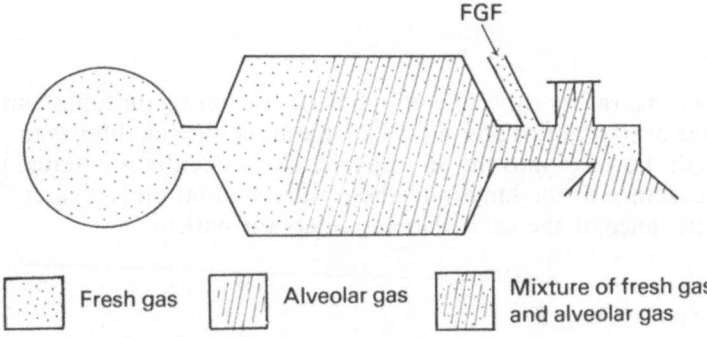

Figure 20.11

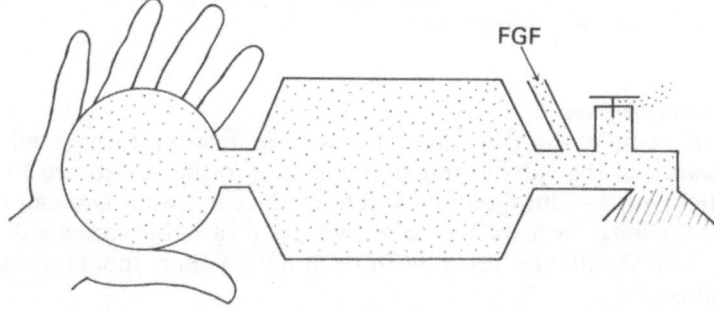

Figure 20.12

Figures 20.10 – 20.12 Composition of gas flow in Mapleson C circuit and
absorber, i.e. 'to-and-fro' circuit during controlled ventilation
Figure 20.10 First inspiration; **Figure 20.11** Midway through expiration
alveolar gas has its CO_2 removed; **Figure 20.12** Start of subsequent
inspiration

As when using the portable resuscitation bag the procedure is to

Count 1,   squeeze the bag
Count 2,   release the bag
Count 3, 4, 5   allow the lungs to empty

Finding the correct tension in the spring to ensure proper ventilation is not easy and readjustments are often necessary. It is important to observe the movements produced by resuscitation efforts, and not to rely on the hiss from the valve as gas passes through into the atmosphere. The hiss denotes one thing only, that gas is escaping into the atmosphere; it does not indicate gas is entering the lungs. Lung expansion is only indicated when the chest is *seen* to expand.

IPPV with Mapleson circuit C and carbon dioxide absorber

Allow the anaesthetic machine or oxygen cylinder to deliver a supply of oxygen at the rate of 2 l/min. The technique of ventilation is identical to that described above with the Mapleson type A and C circuits.

When the expiratory valve is appropriately adjusted, an oxygen flow rate of 2 l/min produces adequate oxygenation and ventilation provided that the carbon dioxide canister clears the carbon dioxide from the expired air on its way to and from the reservoir bag before re-entering the lungs. Because the expired air goes to and from the absorber during expiration and inflation respectively, the circuit used in this way is known as a 'to and fro' circuit or system (Figures 20.10 to 20.12).

FUNCTIONS OF THE CARBON DIOXIDE ABSORBER

The function of the carbon dioxide absorber is first to clear the expired air by absorbing its carbon dioxide, and second to economize on the flow rate of fresh gas.

The carbon dioxide absorbing agent is soda-lime in the form of granules which are artificially coloured, usually pink. Reaction with carbon dioxide turns the soda-lime white. Although patchy changes from pink to white occur within a few minutes on the outside of the granules this is not an indication for their renewal; only when the granules are uniformly white is there need to renew the soda-lime. Usually fresh soda-lime is needed after $\frac{1}{2} - 1$ h in a person who is being hyperventilated to correct carbon dioxide retention because of the increased amount of carbon dioxide flowing through the absorber. With a normal or low PCO_2 the soda-lime remains effective for $6 - 8$ h.

Precautions when using absorber
Carbon dioxide absorbers must never be used with trichloroethylene because it reacts with the soda-lime to form dichloracetylene which can cause cranial nerve palsies.

Efficient ventilation demands that the absorber is leakproof. Loss of gas during manual IPPV is usually due to soda-lime dust fouling the rubber seal between the body of the absorber and its screw-on lid. Leakage is avoided by ensuring that the rubber seal is dust-free. The absorber should be filled completely with soda-lime granules and its sides gently tapped to allow them to settle otherwise the gas passing through the absorber chooses the path of least resistance and flows over the granules, between them and the inner wall of the cylinder, rather than taking the intergranular path. This diminishes the efficiency of the absorber.

Heat evolved during use
Chemical reaction between carbon dioxide, soda-lime and expired water vapour produces heat so that the canister becomes very warm. This is a normal event and is noticeable within a few minutes of use. The canister never becomes sufficiently hot to burn the patient. However, in a hyperpyrexial patient it is unwise to reintroduce hot air into the patient, and frequent change of canister is advisable. To prevent wastage it is better to have two canisters and change them over every 10 min, allowing the spare one to cool whilst the other is in use. Change of soda-lime in necessary every 2 − 3 hours.

In hypothermia it is advisable to retain heat, and the return of hot air into the patient helps to achieve this aim (this is the basis of mountain and cave rescue apparatus). A small amount of water is added to the soda-lime to help the generation of heat which is then directed by means of a resuscitation bag into the patient and thereby adds to his body heat. Some rescuers add a little carbon dioxide from a tiny sparklet bulb to the soda-lime, again to produce heat and warm the inspired air, yet avoiding burning the victim's respiratory mucosa. Rescuers consider that the apparatus is portable and robust.

Positioning the canister
Those working in hospitals regard the canister as a heavy unwieldy object which is difficult to position. It is usually placed so that it rests on the pillow besides the patient's head; care must be taken to ensure that it does not rest directly on his forehead. The unpadded canister rim, pressing on the supraorbital and supratrochlear nerves can cause troublesome residual analgesia of the same side of the forehead.

Protective padding
Protection of the eye from overlying metal or rubber circuit components is essential if corneal abrasions are to be avoided. Usually the 'protective' padding consists of sorboplastic material, but basically, this too is dangerous because it is very abrasive and any movement of it on the exposed cornea acts like sandpaper. It is essential to first close the eyes carefully and maintain closure by sticky tape.

21

Ventilators

A ventilator is a piece of equipment whose function is to move gas in and out of the lungs. The intermittent positive pressure ventilation (IPPV) that its use entails is non-physiological and can disturb normal circulatory dynamics, the main disturbance being a decrease in venous return to the heart during inspiration (p. 152). Table 21.1 illustrates the differences in intrapleural pressure associated with both normal spontaneous and artificial ventilation.

Table 21.1

	Ventilation	
	Normal spontaneous	*Artificial*
During inspiration	intrapleural pressure ↓	intrapleural pressure ↑
	∴ venous return ↑	∴ venous return ↓
During expiration	intrapleural pressure ↑	intrapleural pressure ↓
	∴ venous return ↓	∴ venous return ↑

In spite of these pressure derangements, ventilators have revolutionized the treatment of poliomyelitis, tetanus, head injuries and many other conditions in which prolonged artificial ventilation is needed until normal function returns. A ventilator must only be used if the patient is intubated or has a tracheostomy.

Types of ventilators

Hundreds of different types of ventilators have been invented, from the relatively simple to the extremely sophisticated, all claiming, in some way or another, to possess certain characteristics which produce a pattern of respiratory exchange in the patient resembling his normal ventilation.

In this chapter it is possible to mention briefly only the basic facts involved in ventilator use. However, a little knowledge and familiarity, achieved by repeated practical use, will enable the practitioner to employ a valuable and reliable piece of resuscitation equipment.

CLASSIFICATION
Many different and complex classifications are available. The simplest way is to divide them into three main groups, the pressure-cycled, the volume-cycled and the time-cycled.

PRESSURE-CYCLED VENTILATOR
The pressure-cycled ventilator inflates the patient's lungs until a predetermined intrapulmonary pressure is achieved. When this pressure is reached the machine stops its inflating action and allows the lungs to deflate before starting off another respiratory cycle. Because the cycling of the machine relies on the build-up of a previously selected pressure or 'preselected' pressure, it is said to be pressure-cycled.

Intrapulmonary pressure (airway pressure)
It is important to realize that the actual pressure sensed by the ventilator and recorded on its gauge is the pressure in the upper airway. However, in this chapter airway pressure is replaced by 'pressure within the lungs' or 'intrapulmonary pressure' in an attempt to provide an elementary knowledge of ventilator mechanisms.

Because the child's lung can hold less than the adult, less gas needs to be pushed into the younger patient to produce the same intrapulmonary pressure. For example, if the preselected pressure reaches 25 cmH$_2$O (2.5 kPa) the 400 ml may be needed in the adult, but to obtain the same pressure in a 12-year-old child may require the introduction of only 200 ml.

Effects of respiratory obstruction
If the flow of gas into the patient is obstructed, the pressure selected for the end of the inspiratory phase is reached earlier in the cycle and so inflation of the lungs is automatically arrested by the machine. Expiration follows and after the expiratory pause there is another shortened inspiratory phase. The result is that the machine gallops along instead of maintaining its natural leisurely trot. Consequently,

if the machine increases its rate there is need to aspirate accumulated secretions or remove some other cause of respiratory obstruction.

Effects of leaks on the ventilator

Any leak in the circuit causes the ventilator to take longer to build up the preset intrapulmonary pressure because extra gas needs to be pumped into the circuit to compensate for the leakage. As a result the inspiratory phase is prolonged. If the leak is very marked the ventilator may be incapable of compensating fully and be unable to fill the lungs and complete its cycle. As it cannot start a new cycle it stops its pumping action. Massive leaks result from accidental disconnection between the rubber tubing and ventilator or patient, or due to deflation or rupture of the cuff around an endotracheal or tracheostomy tube.

VOLUME-CYCLED VENTILATOR

Preselection of the volume that the machine delivers to the patient determines the extent of lung inflation. When it has pumped this preselected volume of gas into the patient it stops its inflating action and allows the lungs to deflate before it starts off another respiratory cycle. Because the rhythm, or cycling, of the machine depends on delivery of this certain selected volume, the machine is said to be volume-cycled.

The time taken for the inspiratory phase is again variable and varies with the ease or difficulty with which air can be pumped into the lungs.

Effect of respiratory obstruction

Even if respiratory obstruction occurs the ventilator still tries to deliver its preselected volume of gas. If, therefore, the ventilator is set to deliver 600 ml of gas and one lung suddenly collapses due to a blocked bronchus, then it tries to force the entire 600 ml into the remaining patent lung. As a result there is too much air in the uncollapsed lung to be accommodated comfortably and the pressure rises above the desired level. This rise in intrapulmonary pressure is immediately transmitted to the pleural cavity, thus raising the intrapleural pressure and impeding the return of blood by the great veins to the heart. Cardiac output falls and hypotension occurs.

Inflation pressures should not be too high and should be maintained only long enough to inflate the lung adequately. In most normal lungs the pressure reached at the end of inspiration should be

25–30 cmH$_2$O. A sudden rise in pressure or a gradual creeping up of pressure readings demands instant investigation and removal of the obstruction which is usually in the form of secretions or due to kinking of a piece of connecting tubing.

Effect of leakage

If leakage occurs, as it does when the cuff of an endotracheal tube is inadequately inflated, the inflating gas takes the path of least resistance and escapes into the atmosphere. Therefore, only part of the ventilator's output enters the lungs. Also, the ventilator disposes of its preselected volume earlier than if the circuit were fully intact. This reduces the duration of the inspiratory phase, and the ventilator increases its rate of cycling. Usually there is a hissing or swishing sound, depending on the extent of the leak and there is diminished movements of the patient's chest. He shows gradual or immediate signs of asphyxia according to whether the leak is slight or massive.

TIME-CYCLED VENTILATOR

Whereas the pressure-cycled ventilator cycles when a preselected pressure is reached in the lungs, and a volume-cycled ventilator cycles when a preselected volume is delivered, the time-cycled ventilator cycles when it has inflated the lungs for a preselected period of time. It then allows expiration for a fixed period of time after which starts the inspiratory part of the next cycle. For example, if 1.5 seconds is the time selected for the duration of inspiration and 4.5 seconds for the duration of expiration, then the time-cycled ventilator inflates for 1.5 seconds, allows 4.5 seconds for expiration and then starts another cycle.

The timing mechanism is not influenced by the characteristics of the patient's lungs or the presence of secretions.

Effects of respiratory obstruction

Because the ventilator is set to inflate for 1.5 s it tries to accomplish its task even if some obstruction is present. In consequence a high pressure may build up in the lungs, indicated by the gauge on the machine, and may impede the venous return and cause profound hypotension. Pressure build-up beyond a certain level causes a safety valve to blow off thus preventing damage to lung tissue.

Effects of leakage

Leakage in the circuit does not alter the ventilator's rhythm. Even if all the air is pushed out past a ruptured cuff of an endotracheal tube, so that little gas enters the patient, the machine still spends 1.5 seconds trying to inflate the lungs and allows 4.5 seconds for them to deflate.

VENTILATOR PRECAUTIONS

Ventilators are robots; many of them, and especially the time-cycled, continue remorselessly, irrespective of what they are doing to the patient. The regular clicking of the ventilator every time it cycles is no guarantee that all is well. However, the time-cycled ventilator is no more and no less dangerous than any other type. As in all apparatus the resuscitator needs to get to know the ventilator. He should respect its usefulness, realize its limitations but never trust it. It can go wrong, and it often will go wrong, usually as a result of misuse or neglect.

Consequently, the patient on a ventilator should never be left alone. Constant vigilance of the ventilator is necessary but this should be accompanied by similar attention to the patient, ensuring that the ventilator is providing the necessary ventilatory requirements.

In case there is a mechanical or electrical failure, the person in charge of ventilation must ensure that the doctor and nurse can work the ventilator by hand, as is achieved by turning the appropriate lever to 'manual ventilation'. Furthermore, they should learn how to disconnect the patient from the ventilator and maintain an adequate respiratory exchange by using a portable resuscitation bag (p. 133) or a reservoir bag and valve (p. 136).

Indications for ventilator treatment

It is not always easy to decide if and when a patient needs to be put on a ventilator but basically he can usually be placed in one of two categories. Category 1 consists of those who cannot breathe spontaneously. This group of patients needs immediate ventilation by some form of mechanical means. Category 2 consists of those patients who can breathe spontaneously but inadequately.

CATEGORY 1

Inability to make respiratory movements can be caused by severe depression of the respiratory centre or by failure of the muscles of respiration to contract. Familiar causative factors are overdosage of drugs, such as narcotics, hypnotics and anaesthetics; trauma; and infections such as encephalitis, all of which frequently produce profound depression of the respiratory centre.

Paralysis of the muscles of respiration may be due to muscle disease or occur when the impulses from the respiratory centre are prevented from reaching the muscle fibres as in poliomyelitis, or following the injection of a muscle relaxant.

In the category 1 patient the ventilator takes complete control of the ventilation since its mechanism is unimpeded by the patient because he himself is unable to produce any voluntary respiratory movements.

CATEGORY 2

When spontaneous respiratory movements are present but inadequate to produce effective ventilation it is advisable to ventilate the patient manually. Often, after 1 or 2 min, the resuscitator finds he is able to ventilate the patient without resistance. It is then obvious that the patient can be connected to the ventilator without help from muscle relaxants or narcotics (see below).

If, however, the patient's spontaneous respiratory movements persist against the attempts at artificial ventilation by means of a portable resuscitation bag, anaesthetic machine or ventilator, then it is necessary to deliberately produce either paralysis of the muscles of respiration or depression of the respiratory centre, thereby converting the patient into category 1 above. Popular muscle relaxant drugs used to produce respiratory paralysis are suxamethonium (succinylcholine), d-tubocurarine chloride, and pancuronium bromide; their mode of action and management are discussed on pp. 194–8. Great care and experience is needed for the safe usage of these drugs; they should not be given unless the user has had some anaesthetic training.

A popular choice is to use intravenous analgesic drugs such as morphine 5 – 10 mg, pethidine (meperidine) 50 – 100 mg, fentanyl 0.05–0.01 mg, and phenoperidine 1–2 mg, to sedate the patient sufficiently, and to depress the normal inborn rhythmical respiratory movements dictated by his respiratory centre, so that they are overpowered and taken over by the ventilator.

Another technique is to allow the patient and ventilator to breathe together, but they must quickly get into phase or rhythm with each other. As the patient actually inspires, the ventilator must simultaneously pump air into him. As he expires, the ventilator must allow gas to escape from the lungs. If the respiratory movements of the patient and the ventilator are out of phase, such as occurs if he starts to expire as the machine tries to inflate the lungs, he is said to be 'fighting the ventilator'. Clashing of patient and ventilator in this way prevents expiration taking place and increases the respiratory embarrassment. The conscious patient feels he is suffocating and becomes very distressed.

The problem of fighting the ventilator is solved by using a 'trigger mechanism' on the ventilator which stirs the machine into immediate action to produce one respiratory cycle. To set off the trigger mechanism requires an appropriate stimulus – which is any spontaneous inspiratory movement made by the patient.

THE TRIGGER MECHANISM

Consider a typical sequence of events. The patient is able to make voluntary respiratory movements but they are of insufficient magnitude to produce adequate ventilation, his spontaneous inspiration producing a tidal volume of only 100 ml instead of the requisite 400 ml. He is therefore connected to the ventilator and the 'trigger' switched to the 'on' position, so that when he tries to inspire spontaneously, he sucks gas from the ventilator. The suction or negative pressure he produces within the ventilator sets off the trigger mechanism. So as soon as the patient starts to take a spontaneous breath, that is, immediately he starts to inspire his 100 ml, the trigger is activated and makes the ventilator pump a preselected tidal volume of gas into his lungs at almost exactly the same time as he spontaneously inspires; he feels that he himself is responsible for the adequate chest movement. When the preselected volume has entered the lungs the ventilator permits expiration. The next spontaneous respiration again stimulates the trigger mechanism and the whole sequence is repeated.

The question arises as to what happens if the respiratory depression becomes so profound that complete apnoea supervenes or the efforts at spontaneous respiration are too weak to activate the trigger mechanism. In this event a safety mechanism incorporated in the ventilator then comes into play, as follows: if the trigger is not activated within 10 seconds after the previous inspiration the ventilator pumps gas into the patient without waiting for the message from the trigger mechanism itself; should the patient remain apnoeic the ventilator pumps a further tidal volume into the patient 10 seconds later. Although 5 or 6 breaths per minute are inadequate to maintain a normal respiratory exchange over long periods, they will keep the patient alive until adjustments have been made to the ventilator. If the observer is insufficiently acquainted with all the ventilator controls, the patient should be ventilated by hand, either by converting the ventilator to 'manual' or by disconnection from the machine and reconnection to a portable resuscitation bag.

VENTILATOR CONTROLS

The behaviour of the ventilator and its effects on the patient are controlled by a series of switches, knobs and dials, usually situated in the ventilator's front panel; many of these are self-explanatory. The ones listed below are common to most ventilators.

Inspiratory phase
This is the time between the start of inspiration and the end of the same inspiration (p. 155). The dial is graduated in seconds or fractions of seconds.

Expiratory phase
This is the time between the end of one inspiration and the beginning of the next inspiration (p. 155). The dial is graduated in seconds or fractions of seconds.

Expiratory pause
This is the time between the end of one expiration and the beginning of the next inspiration (p. 155). The dial is graduated in seconds or fractions of seconds.

Expired tidal volume
This is the volume of air leaving the patient, and is measured on a respirometer (p. 122 and Figure 18.1).

Airway pressure
Airway pressure is recorded on a dial with values usually ranging from -50 cmH$_2$O to $+50$ cmH$_2$O (-5 kPa to $+5$ kPa).

The sensor actually measures the pressure in the circuit close to the patient's mouth. If the ventilator is set correctly and there is no respiratory obstruction, the airway pressure is then similar to that in the lungs, and often loosely referred to as the intrapulmonary pressure (p. 163). If, however, obstructive airway disease is present, a longer time must be allowed for the airway pressure and the intrapulmonary pressures to approximate (p. 148).

All ventilators have a safety blowoff valve set at between 30 cmH$_2$O (3 kPa) and 80 cmH$_2$O (8 kPa) according to the individual model. This mechanism protects the patient if the pressure generated in the airway rises to undesirable levels.

Negative pressure control
When the ventilator is constructed to suck gas out of the lungs during expiration it has a negative pressure control. This, as the name im-

plies, produces a negative pressure in the respiratory tract during the expiratory phase. It is recorded on the airway pressure dial as -0 to $-50 \, cmH_2O \, (5 \, kPa)$. However, in spite of the wide range of negative pressure recordable, it is unusual to have the ventilator deliberately produce a negative pressure of more than $3-5 \, cmH_2O \, (0.3-0.5 \, kPa)$.

22

Endotracheal intubation

Endotracheal tubes

Endotracheal tubes are made of rubber or plastic. They may be plain or cuffed, and may also be armoured. They are further classified into oral and nasal types according to whether their principal use is intended for introduction through the mouth or nose (Figure 22.1).

Great care must be taken in selecting an endotracheal tube. Correct selection and management are life-saving; incorrect choice and mismanagement can be disastrous.

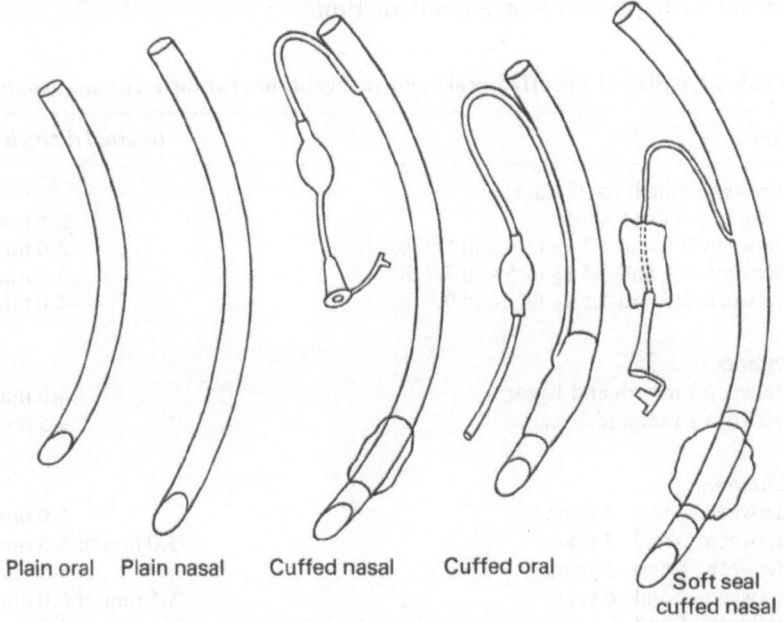

Plain oral Plain nasal Cuffed nasal Cuffed oral Soft seal cuffed nasal

Figure 22.1 Types of endotracheal tube

171

DIMENSIONS: WIDTH

Endotracheal intubation reduces the dead space (p. 131). Consequently, it may be argued that introduction of a narrow endotracheal tube is more efficient in dead space reduction. This is true but unfortunately decreasing the bore of the endotracheal tube increases the resistance to the passage of air through its lumen. Besides causing extra muscular work, if the patient is breathing spontaneously, and thereby increasing oxygen consumption, resistance to air flow may be so pronounced as to prolong inspiration and expiration sufficiently to impair adequate respiratory exchange. The choice of too narrow an endotracheal tube, therefore, causes insidious respiratory obstruction, eventual coma and death.

The resuscitator should choose the widest endotracheal tube that can be inserted without causing trauma to the vocal cords.

Table 22.1 gives an indication of suitable sizes according to the age of the patient; the appropriate size can be learned only by experience. The anaesthetist selects the tube he thinks will be most suitable but he must always have close by a tube of similar length one size smaller. If an organic obstruction is suspected he will also have ready several smaller sizes and may even resort to a plastic catheter as a temporary means of bypassing a severe obstruction.

Table 22.1 Size of uncuffed oral endotracheal tubes for different age groups

Age	*Internal diameter*
Neonates (birth to 28 days)	
up to 2.0 kg (4.4 lb)	2.5 mm
Between 2.0 and 2.5 kg (4.4 and 5.5 lb)	3.0 mm
Between 2.5 and 3.5 kg (5.5 and 7.7 lb)	3.5 mm
Between 3.5 and 4.5 kg (7.7 and 9.9 lb)	4.0 mm
Infants	
Between 1 month and 1 year	4.0 mm
Between 1 year and 2 years	4.5 mm
Children	
Between 2 and 3 years	5.0 mm
Between 3 and 4 years	5.0 mm or 5.5 mm
Between 4 and 5 years	5.5 mm
Between 5 and 6 years	5.5 mm or 6.0 mm
Between 6 and 7 years	6.0 mm
Between 7 and 8 years	6.0 mm or 6.5 mm
Between 8 and 10 years	6.5 mm

Table 22.1 (Continued)

Age	Internal diameter
Between 10 and 12 years	6.5 mm or 7.0 mm
Between 12 and 14 years	7.0 mm
Between 14 and 16 years	7.0 mm or 7.5 mm
Between 16 and 18 years	8.0 mm
Above 18 (female)	8.0 mm, 8.5 mm or 9 mm
Above 18 (male)	8.5 mm, 9 mm or 9.5 mm

Note: Another endotracheal tube, one size smaller than that anticipated, should be to hand before intubation is attempted.

The size stamped on the side of the endotracheal tube denotes the internal diameter of the lumen which increases in measurements of 0.5 mm. For males a 9.0 mm or an 8.5 mm is generally used, and for females an 8.5 mm or an 8.0 mm. The inexperienced resuscitator often finds it hard to believe that an 0.5 mm difference in diameter will be of any significance to the successful insertion of an endotracheal tube. Nevertheless it does matter; the tube should slide smoothly between the cords if laryngeal oedema is to be avoided.

DIMENSION: LENGTH

Various formulas are available for choosing the correct length of endotracheal tube but the easiest and most reliable method is to choose an oral endotracheal tube equal in length to 1 ½ times the distance between the corner of the mouth and the lobe of the ear on the same side. Nasal intubation requires a longer tube, of a length twice the distance between the corner of the mouth and the lobe of the ipsilateral ear. Too short a tube allows the tube to slip out of the larynx. Too long a tube allows the distal end to slip into the right bronchus, thereby causing collapse of the left lung (the signs and symptoms of this are described on p. 181).

INSPECTION

Before insertion, routine inspection of an endotracheal tube should always include examination of its lumen. The tube is held up towards a light and looked through as if it were a telescope. Examination in this way excludes the presence of any old blood, mucus and unwanted residents such as cockroaches.

ENDOTRACHEAL CONNECTORS

After introduction of the endotracheal tube there is usually need to connect it to the tubing of some resuscitation apparatus, by means of a metal or plastic endotracheal connector. These are made in many different sizes and shapes (see Figure 19.2). Correct choice of size is essential; four sizes are available (1, 2, 3 and 4), the bore of the distal end becoming wider as the number increases in magnitude. Two facts, however, are obvious. First, the proximal end of the endotracheal connection has to be of uniform bore in all sizes to fit into the corrugated rubber catheter tubing (see Figure 19.2). Second, the distal end has to be of a bore that fits snugly into the appropriate size of endotracheal tube. A third less well-known fact is that a small endotracheal connector can be held firmly by an endotracheal tube which is capable of housing an endotracheal connector one or even two sizes bigger. Introduction of too small an endotracheal connector causes resistance to respiration, and possible asphyxia.

It is essential to insert the largest endotracheal connector possible into the selected endotracheal tube, and to do this the connector must be lubricated with a few drops of water, spirit or non-irritant antiseptic solution. Lubricating jelly or cream is not recommended because it renders the tube too slippery to handle and may later cause the connector and tube to become separated from each other. Before any endotracheal tube is inserted into a larynx the upper 2 cm should be inspected to ensure that it is not split, and also to confirm that the attached connector is of large enough size.

The cuff

A cuffed endotracheal tube with its cuff deflated can be regarded as a plain endotracheal tube apart from the fact that the deflated cuff takes up space when being passed through the vocal cords. Also, laryngeal space is occupied by the rigid pilot tubing. This tubing is only 1 mm in diameter but in a child it is housed in the relatively narrow larynx at considerable expense of the tube's conducting airway. It therefore reduces the size of the bore than can be accommodated, and because of its rigidity it can produce laryngeal oedema. For these reasons the authors feel that cuffed endotracheal tubes should not be used in children under 8 years of age.

FUNCTIONS OF THE CUFF

Correct cuff inflation obliterates the space between the endotracheal tube and the tracheal wall, thus preventing regurgitated stomach contents or blood and saliva entering the trachea from the upper

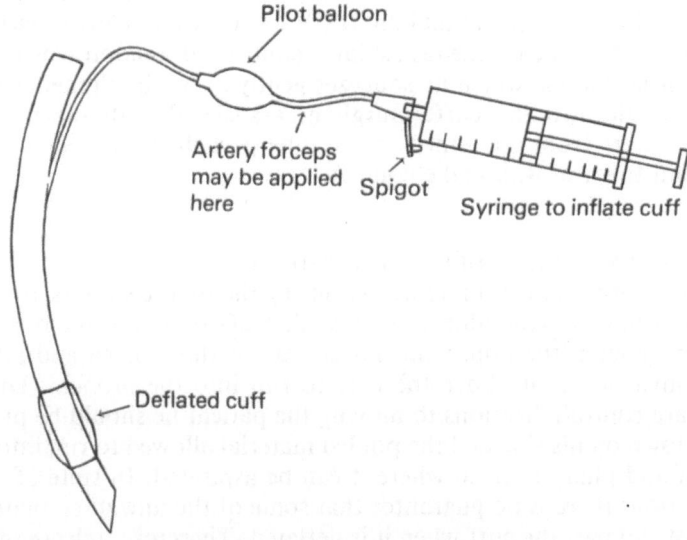

Figure 22.2 Cuffed endotracheal tube

respiratory tract. Also, an airtight seal is necessary for using controlled ventilation in adults (Figure 22.2).

TESTING FOR LEAKS
Before a cuffed tube is used the cuff should be tested to see if it is leakproof, so 2 ml or 3 ml of air are introduced into the balloon which should remain inflated. Larger volumes should not be injected because they only serve to stretch and weaken the cuff so that it may rupture later inside the patient. It should inflate normally. Bleb formation calls for the tube to be discarded.

PILOT BALLOON
A frequent question is 'how much air do you put into the cuff when the endotracheal tube is in the trachea?' The answer is that a 10 ml syringe is used to introduce enough air to inflate the cuff so it just produces an airtight seal between itself and the adjacent tracheal wall. The usual volume required is 2–5 ml.

Excessive cuff inflation creates the danger of tracheal mucosal necrosis but such a condition is unlikely to occur unless the excessive inflation is maintained for several hours. Insufficient cuff inflation allows foreign material and gas to slip past the cuff thereby increasing the risk of atelectasis and making IPPV less efficient. Correct cuff inflation is established if the resuscitator connects the endotracheal tube to an inflation bag which he squeezes gently as he simultaneously introduces air into the cuff. Gurgling, associated with the upward escape of air from the lumen of the tube past the cuff, ceases when cuff and tracheal wall make contact.

PRECAUTIONS WHEN DEFLATING THE CUFF
Deflation of the cuff is unnecessary during the first few hours after intubation unless extubation is indicated. Cuff deflation removes the barrier between the upper and lower part of the trachea and allows any saliva or vomit above the cuff to run into the bronchi. Unless there are contraindications to moving the patient he should be placed head down on his side and the pooled material allowed to run into the mouth and pharynx from where it can be aspirated. In spite of such precautions there is no guarantee that some of the unwanted material will not slip past the cuff when it is deflated. Therefore, release of the cuff should be followed immediately by suction of the lower trachea and bronchi by suction catheter.

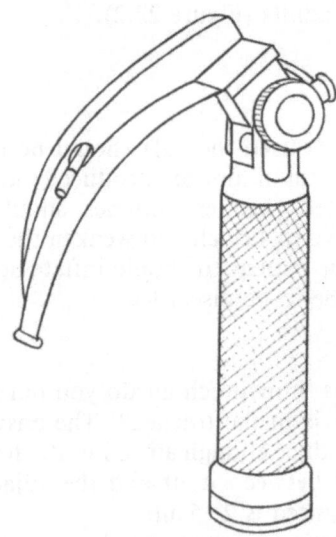

Figure 22.3 Macintosh laryngoscope (curved blade)

Oral endotracheal intubation

Insertion of an oral endotracheal tube is usually easy provided that the operator is able to get a clear view of the vocal cords. This depends on choosing the correct size and type of laryngoscope and on using it correctly.

TYPES OF LARYNGOSCOPE BLADE
Two main types of laryngoscope blade are available: the Macintosh with a curved blade (Figure 22.3), and the Magill with a straight blade (Figure 22.4).

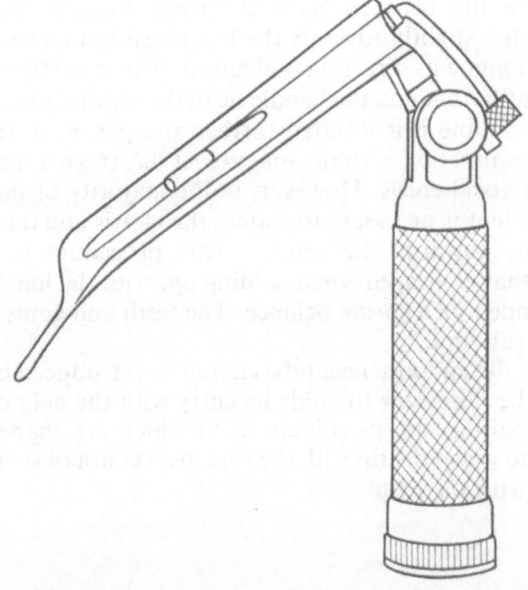

Figure 22.4 Macintosh laryngoscope (Magill blade)

The Macintosh laryngoscope blade has a groove along its entire length to accommodate the tongue, whereas the Magill blade has no groove for the tongue and is more difficult to use.

Size of blade
Blades are available in three sizes. The smallest blade is used in children up to the age of 18 months – 2 years. The next size is used in children

up to the age of 5-7 years. The blade must be long enough to reach the close vicinity of the glottis, and if there is doubt as to which of two different-sized blades to choose it is usually wise to start with the larger of the two. A skilled anaesthetist can often use the largest blade for all patients from 2 years of age to a full-grown adult.

Introduction of Macintosh curved blade

The head of the patient is placed midway between flexion and extension. The shoulders must not be on the pillow otherwise visualization of the glottis is made more difficult, especially in children (but see neonates, p. 113).

The blade is introduced into the right side of the mouth taking care not to trap the lips between blade and teeth. Initially the tip of the blade is directed slightly towards the left tonsil but as soon as it has captured the tongue its direction is changed, lifting the tongue as it advances, so that both it and the handle lie in the sagittal plane. With the blade in the midline it is inserted further and passed in front of the epiglottis to its junction with the tongue. At this stage it may be possible to see the vocal cords. However, in the majority of patients, one further movement is necessary to expose the glottis and this is a lifting of the tongue towards the ceiling. This procedure is sometimes described as that envisaged when holding up, with the hand, a sack of onions suspended on a spring balance. The teeth and gums should not be used as a fulcrum.

If the tip of the endotracheal tube cannot be introduced between the cords it may be necessary to guide its entry with the help of a pair of Magill's intubating forceps (Figure 22.5) which are shaped to allow the operator to grasp the tip with the forceps, yet not obstruct the view of the cords with his hand.

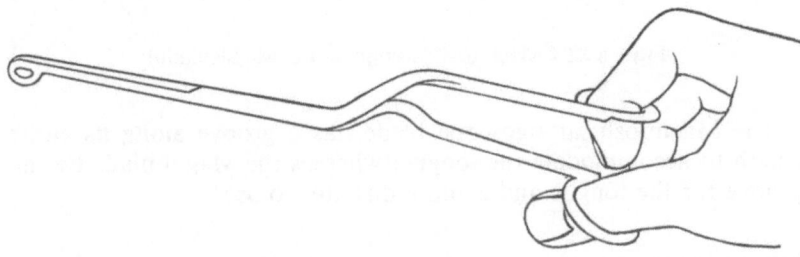

Figure 22.5 Magill's intubating forceps

Insertion of Magill straight blade

The introduction technique for the Magill blade is identical to that used with the Macintosh blade except that the tip of the blade is manoeuvred behind the epiglottis (beneath the epiglottis when the patient is supine) which is lifted to uncover the vocal cords. It is important not to advance the blade too far otherwise its contact with the vocal cords sends them into spasm. Further details are described in resuscitation of the newborn (p. 113).

Choice of oral or nasal tube

NASAL TUBE INTRODUCED ORALLY

To the inexperienced eye the nasal tube may appear identical to the oral type. However, the nasal endotracheal tube is thinner walled and so more flexible and more easily kinked; its curve is not so pronounced. In an emergency it can be introduced orally but the resuscitator should remember that the nasal tube is longer than its oral counterpart and may inadvertently slip into the right bronchus. This can be avoided by leaving the proximal 5 cm protruding from between the lips, but there is a danger of kinking occurring and asphyxiating the patient; so a nasal tube, when introduced through the mouth, should be replaced by an oral one at the earliest opportunity.

ORAL TUBE INTRODUCED NASALLY

The more pronounced curve in the oral tube makes it more difficult to pass through the nose than a nasal one, especially if the tube is of the cuffed variety. However a cuffed nasal or oral tube, passed through the nose, offers several advantages over the plain nasal variety. First the cuff can be inflated to prevent the inhalation of secretions and vomit and also allow IPPV. Second, it is more comfortable and it cannot be bitten or chewed, so that the danger of self-asphyxiation is less. However, the resuscitator should remember that the length needs to be greater when an oral tube is passed nasally than when the tube is inserted through the mouth, otherwise the tip slips out of the larynx.

Techniques of introduction

Manoeuvring the cuffed tube through the nose into the larynx is sometimes difficult and a few practical points are worthy of mention.

The lubricated tube should be held like a dart ready for throwing at the dartboard. The head is slightly extended beyond the neutral position and the tip inserted into the nostril in a backward (not an upward) direction. Gentle but firm pressure is needed to advance the tube into the nasopharynx where its position is noted by means of the laryngoscope. Magill's intubating forceps then grasp the end of the tube 2-5 cm behind the tip and guide it with the help of an assistant who pushes it gently further through the nose towards the larynx. With the tip 1 cm proximal to the laryngeal aperture the manoeuvre is stopped to assess the movement and position of the cords. At the opportune movement, as the cords are abducted, the tip of the tube is thrust quickly but gently through the glottis.

Difficulties of nasal intubation

Nasal intubation is generally much more difficult than oral intubation. Even expert anaesthetists sometimes find difficulty in manoeuvring the tip of the tube past the nasopharynx because it frequently becomes stuck behind a posterior pillar of the fauces. Rotation of the proximal end of the tube may free the distal end but if this fails the resuscitator should insert his finger and hook the tip of the tube out from behind the fauces.

Slight bleeding from the delicate mucous membranes is frequent, but clumsy manipulation of the tube can strip the mucosa from the pharyngeal wall.

Although individual circumstances demand which route is selected, in general oral intubation is usually chosen for the acute emergency. Replacement by nasal tube is performed later if there is danger of the patient biting the tube or if the period of intubation is likely to be prolonged.

The soft seal tube

This type of tube is prepacked and bears a large cuff made of very thin plastic which is reputed to produce minimal damage to the tracheal mucosa. Considerable care is needed when grasping the tip with the Magill's intubation forceps otherwise they tear the delicate cuff. Incorporated in the main tube, extending along its length is a radio-opaque linear marker which is useful in locating the tip of the tube and its proximity to the carina.

Such a tube, with its low pressure, high volume cuff, should be used in any patient who it is anticipated will require IPPV for more than 12 h. This is because the traditional tube causes chemical irritation to the tracheal mucosa, and its low volume, high pressure cuff is more liable to produce mucosal ulceration, particularly if hypotension is present. It is equally important to inflate the cuff of the soft seal tube with the minimum amount of air required to produce an airtight seal. This kind of cuff need not be periodically deflated. The soft seal tube is, however, more difficult to insert than the rubber tube which remains the tube of choice for emergency intubation. A recognized disadvantage is that the soft cuff puts up little resistance to any nasogastric tube mistakenly passed through the glottis. The consequences are obvious.

Complications of intubation

INTUBATION OF THE RIGHT BRONCHUS

Selection of too long an endotracheal tube usually results in its tip entering the right bronchus so that proper ventilation is only accomplished in the right lung. This results in carbon dioxide accumulation in the non-ventilated lung with a rise in PCO_2 and a fall in PO_2. Cyanosis may be present but is frequently absent or slight; sweating is often pronounced. Such events may extend over a period of 10–15 min but may also take several hours to develop. Diagnosis is made by noting the diminished movement of the left side of the chest associated with diminished or absent air entry in the left lung. If the patient is ventilated by hand there is usually an obvious increase in resistance to inflation. Withdrawal of the tip of the tube from the bronchus into the trachea restores full movement and air entry to the lungs. Chest X-ray may also be useful in establishing a diagnosis especially if the endotracheal tube contains a radio-opaque linear marker (p. 180).

INTUBATION OF OESOPHAGUS

Attempts at endotracheal intubation frequently result in the tube entering the oesophagus. This occasionally happens to the skilled anaesthetist, but it is a very frequent event with the trainee. It is usually avoided by correct use of the laryngoscope which lifts the tongue to provide a clear exposure of the vocal cords. Sometimes the tube slips from the larynx into the oesophagus due to the tube being too short, because of defective anchorage of the tube, or through head movements.

After endo-oesophageal intubation, various things happen according to whether the patient breathes spontaneously or with the help of IPPV.

Spontaneous ventilation

The introduction of the tube into the oesophagus of a spontaneously breathing patient may not affect him and if he continues to breathe spontaneously it does no harm and produces no symptoms, but if its position is in doubt its relationship to the vocal cords must be checked by laryngoscopy. If it is attached to a reservoir bag of the anaesthetic machine, some movements of the bag may take place but their magnitude will be less than those anticipated had the tube been correctly placed in the trachea. Often, however, its presence in the oesophagus is more obvious, producing belching of varying ferocity, sometimes accompanied by gastric contents passing up the endotracheal tube or alongside it into the mouth.

IPPV

Accidental endo-oesophageal intubation is often performed in the apnoeic comatose patient or one who has previously been rendered apnoeic by the injection of suxamethonium (p. 194). Insufflation of air through the tube from a resuscitation bag usually 'feels wrong' – there is a slightly increased resistance when inflating the stomach than there is when expanding the lungs. Also, the stomach usually returns the inflated gas to the bag slightly slower than do the lungs.

Sometimes during inflation or deflation, or both, a belching or bubbling noise is heard within the rubber tubing. Usually all the gas pushed into the stomach is returned to the bag, but at times the air enters the stomach and stays there. A bulge appears in the epigastrium and gradually abdominal distension increases markedly, eventually causing elevation of the diaphragm and interfering with lung movements. A further possibility is stomach rupture. During these events the apnoeic or almost apnoeic patient is unable to ventilate his lungs adequately and he becomes cyanosed.

From the above it may seem impossible not to immediately diagnose endo-oesophageal intubation. Nothing is further from the truth. Diagnosis can be very difficult in those patients who do not demonstrate increased resistance during inflation and who return all the gases to the resuscitator bag without producing adventitious sounds. The reason is that inflation of the stomach pushes up the diaphragm, squeezes the lungs and ejects some of their contents through the cords. Deflation of the stomach allows the diaphragm to fall, the lungs to expand to their original volume, and to suck air through the larynx. Sometimes air entry is audible in the lungs through a stethoscope. Therefore, a regular inflation–deflation sequence of the stomach constitutes a type of artificial ventilation which produces some degree of respiratory exchange and prevents the immediate onset of cyanosis. Ventilation produced is partly effective but insufficient, and gradually, perhaps over a period of 5 to 10 minutes or even longer, the patient deteriorates, his colour becomes bluish or pale, his pulse rate rises then becomes irregular, and death ensues.

Great care, therefore, is needed when performing intubation. The resuscitator should connect a reservoir bag to the endotracheal tube if the patient is breathing spontaneously and the movements should be commensurate with the respiratory movements.

If IPPV is used the resuscitator should make sure that the bag 'feels right', observe the abdomen to ensure that it is not increasing in size and listen to the chest carefully by stethoscope. The volume and characistics of air entry into the lungs should be noted carefully.

USE OF TOPICAL ANALGESIA

The extent and duration of laryngeal tolerance to the presence of an endotracheal tube are greatly increased by spraying the cords with 4% lignocaine (lidocaine). Initial contact with the local analgesic may cause temporary laryngeal spasm but this abates within 10–20 s. Nevertheless it is advisable to preoxygenate the patient before the lignocaine is used. Even better tolerance is established if the endotracheal tube is smeared with a local analgesic cream or gel. It is surprising how well the patient accepts an endotracheal tube provided that analgesia is satisfactory especially if he is very ill. Furthermore, it is recognized that after an hour or two the larynx appears to become insensitive to the presence of the tube. Provided the head or tube are not moved quickly or markedly it is sometimes possible to leave the tube in position for days without much discomfort, especially if it is introduced through the nose.

EXTUBATION AND THE INSENSITIVE LARYNX

Extubation combined with insensitivity of the larynx due to recent application of a topical analgesic, or to prolonged intubation as described above, exposes the patient to the dangers of regurgitation and inhalation of food.

Regurgitation

Regurgitation in the strong conscious patient is followed by swallowing or spitting out the gastric contents. Any gastric juice which does touch the cords causes immediate closure of the larynx until it is ejected. If, however, the patient is unconscious or weak, or the larynx is insensitive, it allows the gastric juice to flow into the bronchi. This results in infection or asphyxia. Deaths occur after anaesthesia as a result of regurgitation especially in the old, the very ill or the weak. It is sometimes remarked that aspiration has taken place during induction or maintenance of anaesthesia, when in fact it has occurred after return to the ward; for these reasons it is essential after extubation to

place the patient in the lateral position until he can cope adequately
with his reflexes.

Oral feeding should not be allowed for $2-3$ h after extubation.

Suction
Skilled suction through the endotracheal tube can remove obstructing
secretions and thereby enable a lobe to re-aerate. Faulty suction
technique can cause lung collapse and even heart failure.

CHOICE OF CATHETER
Sterility
The catheter should be sterile; a new disposable catheter should
preferably be used for every bout of suction. Should the cost prove
prohibitive or the prepacked type be unavailable the catheter can be
kept for $12-24$ h in a non-irritant antibacterial solution such as 0.1%
chlorhexidine and washed through with sterile water before insertion
into the trachea. Formalin vapour or irritant chemical solutions
should not be used for sterilization purposes because they may irritate
and damage the mucosa.

Before taking hold of the catheter the resuscitator should wash his
hands and put on a disposable glove. The ungloved hand is used for
unclean activities such as connecting the catheter to the suction apparatus.

Length
Catheter length should be adequate to reach as far down the
respiratory tract as is possible, and therefore should be sufficiently
long for its passage to be gently arrested as its tip lodges in one of the
smaller bronchi.

Lubrication
A fine covering of sterile lubricating jelly, saline, or water helps the
catheter slide down the trachea and minimizes the risk of mucosal
damage. Too much jelly introduced into a small bronchus may produce the atelectasis which the catheter is trying to relieve. For the same
reason the catheter should be empty of saline or water before entering
the trachea.

Shape
Some designs have a beak which is supposed to aid introduction of the
catheter into a specific main bronchus. It is the authors' opinion that

some types of prepacked catheter with an angulated tip are useless for this aim because the tip is too floppy and cannot be directed with any degree of accuracy; often this type of catheter is too short. By far the best type is the longer rubber Pinkerton catheter with its firm angulated tip which can be manipulated more successfully into a specific main brochus. However, it is more expensive than the others, is not disposable, and should be re-sterilized.

Size
The catheter diameter should be sufficient to allow aspiration of thick mucus, but should not be greater than half the width of the endotracheal tube otherwise atelectasis occurs if prolonged suction is inadvertently applied.

TECHNIQUE OF SUCTION
To avoid atelectasis and cardiac complications, suction should be applied only when withdrawing the catheter. Three different techniques are used. If a plain catheter is used it should not be connected to the sucker until the tip has been advanced into the bronchus. Another method uses a catheter which has an additional hole situated close to its proximal end (Figure 22.6). Connection of this type of catheter to the suction machine draws some air through the catheter tip but most

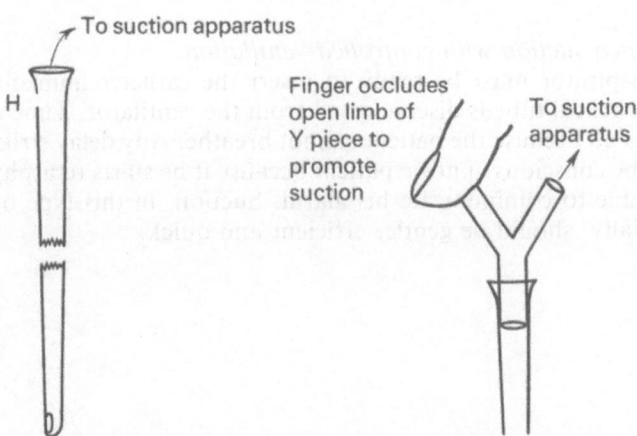

Figure 22.6 Straight catheter with hole (H) at proximal end

Figure 22.7 Y piece with catheter attached

through the hole (H). Suction is therefore not applied to the lungs until the hole (H) is occluded. The same principle applies if a Y piece of glass or plastic is inserted into a plain catheter (Figure 22.7); the bore of the Y piece should approximate to that of the catheter to enable air and mucus to pass freely through both stem and limbs. The stem of the Y is connected to the catheter, one of the limbs is joined to the suction apparatus, and the other left open to the atmosphere whereby it acts like the hole (H) in the catheter. Secretions can only be aspirated on occlusion of the open limb of the Y piece.

Introduction of catheter

After lubrication, and drainage if it has been kept in solution, the catheter is inserted quickly but gently down the trachea until it will go no further. Suction is applied by connecting the catheter to the suction apparatus or by occluding the side hole in the catheter or the open limb of the Y piece. Aspiration should not exceed 4–5 s.

Repeated suction with spontaneous respiration

Endotracheal suction is unpleasant and often frightening, and can cause profound fatigue if it produces a prolonged bout of coughing. It is advisable, therefore, to warn the patient before suction starts, allow him to rest and let his respirations return to normal before further suction is performed.

Repeated suction with controlled ventilation

The aspirator must be ready to insert the catheter immediately the endotracheal tube is disconnected from the ventilator. Time must not be wasted because the patient cannot breathe. Any delay strikes terror into the conscious apnoeic patient because if he starts to asphyxiate he is unable to communicate his alarm. Suction, in this type of patient especially, should be gentle, efficient and quick.

23

Intravenous anaesthetics

Resuscitation is often needed for the patient who has taken an overdose of barbiturates. On first glance, therefore, it may appear paradoxical that intravenous barbiturates, or similar drugs, have a useful role to play in resuscitative procedures. However, they are used in the conscious or semiconscious patient to induce sleep and render him oblivious to anaesthetic or surgical procedures. For example, in the casualty department, light anaesthesia is indicated prior to the administration of a muscle relaxant drug such as suxamethonium (p. 194) which is used to facilitate endotracheal intubation as the initial treatment of a stove-in chest. The induction of sleep prior to defibrillation attempts with a defibrillator is desirable because the procedure is distressing (p. 14).

Choice of intravenous anaesthetic
An assortment of drugs is available for the intravenous induction of anaesthesia. Popular ones are thiopentone (thiopental), methohexitone (methohexital) and alphaxalone with alphadolone, all capable of inducing anaesthesia within a few seconds of injection. Recovery time from anaesthesia is very similar for each, although slightly longer after thiopentone.

All intravenous agents are invaluable in resuscitation but must be treated with great respect. The precautions necessary before administration, the technique of their injection, and the constant surveillance necessary until recovery is complete, are common to all. Thiopentone has stood the test of time and is the drug with which the resuscitator should become familiar. For this reason the intravenous induction of anaesthesia for resuscitation procedures is in this chapter essentially restricted to the use of thiopentone.

Thiopentone (thiopental)
PHARMACOLOGY
Thiopentone is a quick-acting intravenous barbiturate. It induces sleep, but it is not an analgesic so it should not be given alone if the

pain caused by the original condition or by any surgical procedure performed is severe or prolonged. Such patients need analgesia too, either in the form of inhalational anaesthesia or as drugs such as morphine or fentanyl.

CONCENTRATION

Boxes of thiopentone contain two types of ampoule, one storing the drug in the form of a yellow powder, the other containing water. Both solute and solvent are obtainable in different quantities but the combination in popular use is thiopentone 0.5 g and water 20 ml. Thiopentone 0.5 g in 20 ml water is equivalent to thiopentone 2.5 g in 100 ml water. Therefore, mixing thiopentone 0.5 g in 20 ml water gives a 2.5% solution containing thiopentone 25 mg/ml. This strength of solution is least likely to cause either tissue necrosis or even gangrene (p. 189). Stronger solutions (such as thiopentone 1 g in 20 ml of water, giving a 5% solution) should *not* be used.

Mixing of solute and solvent

Addition of the water to the thiopentone is best accomplished by means of a 20 ml syringe and wide-bore needle or plastic cannula. Thorough mixing is obtained by repeatedly filling and emptying the syringe of thiopentone solution. If this is not done the top part of the thiopentone solution consists almost entirely of water, and the lower part of concentrated thiopentone – injection of the top solution will fail to put the patient to sleep whereas introduction of the lower solution may put him to sleep for ever!

DANGERS OF THIOPENTONE (THIOPENTAL)

Respiratory arrest

Depression of the respiratory system, sufficient to cause respiratory arrest, is almost instantaneous and universal. Provided that an overdose has not been given, the respiratory arrest lasts for 20–30 seconds after which spontaneous respirations reappear rapidly and ventilation quickly becomes adequate. If respiratory arrest continues beyond 20–30 seconds, or if the patient becomes slightly cyanosed or develops cardiac irregularities, then artificial ventilation is necessary by bag and mask until respiratory recovery has taken place.

Thiopentone must *never* be given unless the administrator has means of resuscitation immediately available.

Cardiovascular depression

Temporary hypotension frequently follows injection of thiopentone, because the drug depresses the vasomotor centre, the cardiac musculature and the muscular tissue in the arterioles. The extent of the cardiovascular depression depends on the dose given and the speed with which it is injected. Hypotension is usually of short duration, but frequent or preferably constant palpation of the pulse is necessary for 2−3 minutes after injection. Beyond this time hypotension, noted by sphygmomanometer reading or fall in pulse volume, calls for immediate lowering of the head end of the carrier. If this manoeuvre fails, a vasoconstrictor drug, such as metaraminol 5 mg intravenously, is indicated.

Thiopentone should. not be given where it is difficult or impossible to lower the patient's head. A theatre table or tilting carrier is much safer than a bed.

Extravenous injection

A 2.5% solution of thiopentone injected subcutaneously causes the appearance of a tender, hot, painful, erythematous swelling which usually subsides without treatment. A 5% solution causes abscess formation, and eventual necrotic ulceration which usually requires application of a skin graft; this solution should therefore be avoided. Extravenous thiopentone is treated by injecting into the spillage area 2 ml water or normal saline with hyaluronidase 1500 units; the latter lessens the possibility of permanent tissue damage by diluting the thiopentone and spreading it over a wider area.

Intra-arterial injection

An intra-arterial injection of thiopentone causes vascular spasm. Injection into the brachial artery causes severe pain in the fingers and/or the sensation of icicles running down the arm. Thiopentone 5% causes gangrene of the fingers (and possibly of the forearm) whereas thiopentone 2.5% intra-arterially is less likely to have such disastrous results.

After intra-arterial injection of thiopentone the needle should be left in the artery and through it injected procaine hydrochloride 20 ml of 0.5% solution followed by papaverine 40−80 mg in 10−20 ml saline. Some authorities recommend tolazoline 5 ml of 1% solution as an alphablocker. Others suggest brachial or stellate ganglion block or the administration of halothane (fluothane) to induce vasodilation. Heparin 7500−10000 units intravenously followed by 5000 units 6 hourly intravenously is also advocated. The limb is elevated and kept warm.

Avoid injecting thiopentone near to arteries. Injection should be into areas where arteries are usually absent, such as the lateral aspect of the antecubital fossa and particularly the dorsum of the hand. Nevertheless, aberrant arteries can run in these regions and trap the unwary.

DOSAGE
Adult dosage depends on many factors such as age, body weight, illness and the influence of other previously given medication (Figure 23.1).

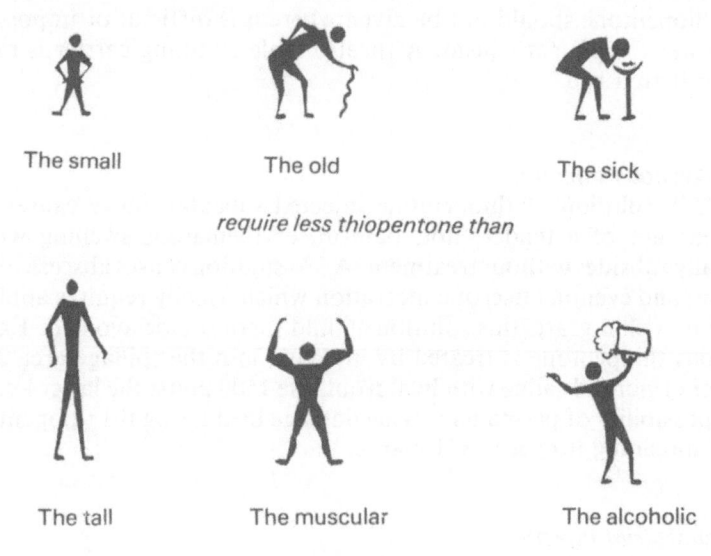

The small   The old   The sick

require less thiopentone than

The tall   The muscular   The alcoholic

Figure 23.1

The dose in fit children and adults is 4 mg/kg. Therefore, the fit adult weighing 70 kg (150 lb) needs 0.25 g, that is 10 ml of 2.5% solution.

The sick adult requires a quarter to a half of the fit adult dose according to body weight. An ill 80-year-old patient may need only 50−100 mg (2−4 ml of 2.5% solution) to put him to sleep.

RATE OF INJECTION
Rapid injection, within 3 seconds, of 5 ml 2.5% thiopentone solution (125 mg) usually causes sleep and respiratory arrest in a healthy 70 kg man. Slower injection of twice the dose over 20 seconds may just make him very drowsy, and spontaneous ventilation may persist.

Prolonged circulation time occurs in the elderly and the shocked, so the thiopentone takes longer to act, sometimes twice or three times as long as in the fitter patient. If this is not appreciated, the doctor, seeing the patient has not gone to sleep, may give a further dose which could cause profound hypotension.

Slow introduction of thiopentone is safer than rapid injection. The recommended rate for the healthy patient is 1 ml 2.5% solution (25 mg) per second. In the sick and the old, the rate of injection should be decreased to a half or a quarter.

TECHNIQUE OF INJECTION

Resuscitative equipment must be to hand. A suitable vein is selected on the dorsum of the hand, or in the lateral side of the antecubital fossa. Veins close to or overlying arteries are avoided.

The vein is observed and palpated to ensure that it is not pulsating, remembering that an artery too will not pulsate if the patient is hypotensive or if the grip on the arm, to make the veins prominent, is too tight and causes arterial occlusion.

Entry into the vein is followed by the injection of 1 ml thiopentone. The patient is asked 'Do you have any pain in your fingers?' A positive answer indicates an intra-arterial injection and further thiopentone must not be introduced, otherwise gangrene may result (p. 189). If pain is absent the injection is continued according to the state, weight and age of the patient (p. 190). The conscious patient should be encouraged to count out loud as the thiopentone injection continues. When he stops counting respiration usually stops, restarting within a few seconds. A further dose of thiopentone equal to half of that already given ensures that the patient is asleep.

If the patient cannot count out loud, thiopentone is injected until the eyelash reflex is lost. To elicit this reflex, the eyelash is touched gently; the conscious patient blinks. There is no need to touch the cornea and risk corneal damage.

24

Neuromuscular blocking drugs

Basic pharmacology

Figure 24.1 shows that Na^+ is the most prominent cation in the interstitial fluid; K^+ is the most abundant cation inside the cell.

Because there are more Na^+ ions outside than K^+ ions inside, the outside of the fibre is more positive than the inside, which is therefore relatively negative to the outside. Figure 24.1 can be simplified to Figure 24.2 and further simplified to Figure 24.3. As there is a difference in charge between the inside and the outside of the membrane, it is said that a potential difference exists or that the membrane has a potential. When the membrane is at rest the value of its potential, that is the potential difference between the inside and the outside, is known as the resting membrane potential and has a value around 70 mV.

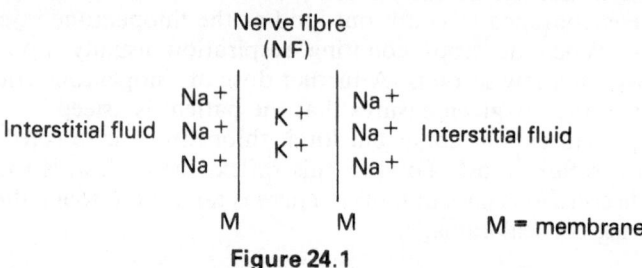

Figure 24.1

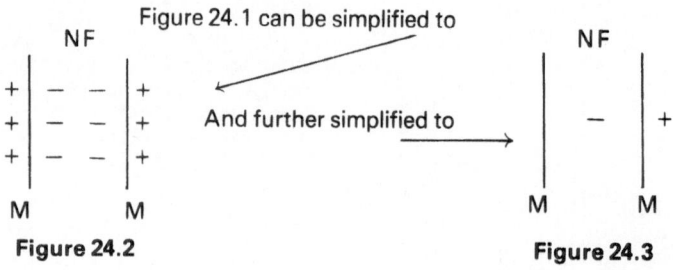

To maintain this potential the Na$^+$ ions are maintained outside the nerve fibre by an active process known as the sodium potassium pump or just the sodium pump.

When an impulse comes down the nerve fibre (Figure 24.4) the sodium pump mechanism is temporarily overwhelmed so that the Na$^+$ ions flow in and K$^+$ ions flow out of the fibres, but the Na$^+$ ions enter quicker than the K$^+$ ions move out (Figure 24.5). As a result the inside of the fibre becomes more positive until eventually there is no difference in charge, that is there is no difference in potential between the inside and the outside of the fibre. The membrane is no longer polarized, it is depolarized (Figure 24.6).

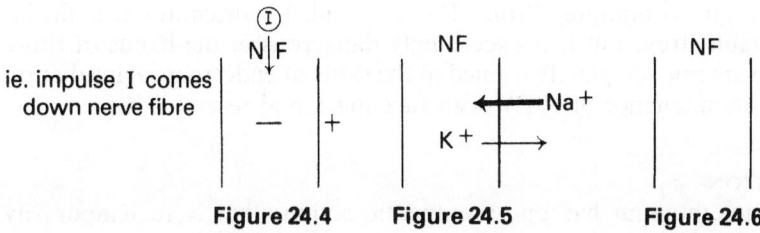

ie. impulse I comes down nerve fibre

Figure 24.4   Figure 24.5   Figure 24.6

Depolarization liberates the chemical transmitter acetyl choline at the neuromuscular junction (Figure 24.7), and this transmitter occupies receptors on the neuromuscular endplate (Figure 24.8) whose membrane likewise becomes depolarized. This depolarization spreads along the muscle membrane and the muscle contracts. After contraction the muscle relaxes and cannot contract again until the membrane repolarizes. The acetyl choline is destroyed by cholinesterase.

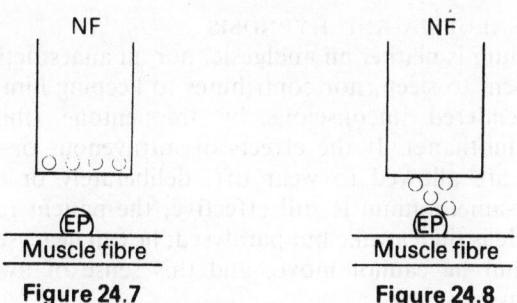

Figure 24.7   Figure 24.8

How muscle relaxants work
Basically they work in two different ways.

(1) By occupying the receptors on the neuromuscular endplate; thus they prevent the acetyl choline producing the depolarization necessary for muscular contraction. Drugs in this group are known as competitive blockers or *non*-depolarizing relaxants, and examples are d-tubocurarine chloride and pancuronium.
(2) By prolonging the depolarization so that further incoming quantities of acetyl choline are ineffective. Such drugs are known as depolarizers, the one most frequently used being suxamethonium (succinylcholine).

Suxamethonium
Suxamethonium is a depolarizing relaxant supplied in 2 ml ampoules, each 1 ml containing 50 mg. For the skilled resuscitator it is an invaluable drug, but it is exceedingly dangerous in the hands of those who are not adequately trained in the skills of endotracheal intubation and maintenance of IPPV with face mask and reservoir bag.

ACTION
Suxamethonium has one therapeutic action, that is to temporarily paralyse the voluntary muscles, and this it does without exception. Onset of paralysis is sudden, within 10−30 seconds, and is complete a few seconds later. Therefore, if it is injected to relax the muscles of the vocal cords and facilitate intubation, it simultaneously paralyses the muscles of respiration. Unless respiratory exchange is maintained for 2−5 minutes following its administration, by which time its activity has usually disappeared and spontaneous respiration has returned, the patient will die. Thus, after injection, it is vital to start and then maintain artificial ventilation while any sign of muscular paralysis persists.

LACK OF ANALGESIA AND HYPNOSIS
Suxamethonium is neither an analgesic, nor an anaesthetic. It neither puts the patient to sleep, nor contributes to keeping him asleep if he has been rendered unconscious by thiopentone (thiopental) or halothane (fluothane). If the effects of intravenous or inhalational anaesthetics are allowed to wear off, deliberately or accidentally, while the suxamethonium is still effective, the patient recovers consciousness. He is then awake but paralysed; he can hear, see, feel pain, and think, but he cannot move, and this sense of awareness can naturally cause distress.

Suxamethonium, therefore, must *never be given to a conscious patient*. Apart from the terror of being rendered paralysed whilst still conscious the widespread twitching that occurs on depolarization is

painful. According to circumstances a sleep dose of thiopentone
(p. 190) or similar acting drug is given immediately prior to the injection of suxamethonium. Sleep must be maintained during paralysis
with incremental doses of thiopentone 25 mg, or equivalent drug, or
by means of an inhalational anaesthetic.

Suxamethonium should not be mixed with thiopentone, and the two
given together, because the suxamethonium acts quicker than the
thiopentone so the patient twitches and becomes paralysed a few
seconds before the thiopentone has time to act.

MODE OF ADMINISTRATION
Administration is usually by intravenous injection in a dosage of
1 mg/kg (body weight). However, accurate assessment of the patient's
weight is not essential and suggested dosage is indicated in Table 24.1
below.

Table 24.1 Recommended dosage of suxamethonium

Patient	Dose
Adults (male)	100 mg (2 ml)
(female)	50 mg (1 ml)
Children (10 yrs old and above)	50 mg (1 ml)
(5–10 yrs old)	30 mg (0.6 ml)
(few weeks–5 yrs)	10–20 mg (0.2–0.4 ml)
Incremental doses – ¼ of above doses	

Smaller doses than those listed above usually paralyse the patient
completely but not for as long as the normal dose. It must be
understood that as little as 10–20 mg suxamethonium can cause
apnoea in the adult.

EXTRAVENOUS INJECTION
Extravenous injection can be either intramuscular or subcutaneous.

Intramuscular injection
Intramuscular suxamethonium is used when it is impossible to give it
intravenously due to difficult venepuncture. The dose is 2 mg/kg, or
twice as much as is given intravenously. Onset of muscular paralysis is
more gradual than intravenous injection, starting in about 1 min and
becoming complete in 2–3 minutes; duration of action is longer in
that it lasts for 10–20 minutes. Until muscular relaxation becomes

complete the administrator has to assist the gradually failing spontaneous respirations which is more difficult to accomplish than the controlled ventilation performed on the completely apnoeic patient. It should be appreciated, therefore, that ventilating the patient after intramuscular suxamethonium is often much more difficult than when it is given intravenously.

Subcutaneous injection
Absorption of suxamethonium after subcutaneous injection is almost as rapid as is intramuscular administration. This route is not recommended but it is mentioned because the drug is sometimes inadvertently injected perivenously when the needle slips out of the vein. When such an accident occurs the patient must not be left and must be observed carefully for the next 10 minutes in case his respirations begin to fail.

Complete apnoea can occur whilst attempts are made to re-enter a vein. To avoid a catastrophe it is essential that the doctor does not devote all his attention to the venepuncture, but assesses the colour of the patient's face and his respirations every 10 seconds.

DANGERS OF SUXAMETHONIUM
Lack of resuscitative skill
Unfamiliarity with the resuscitative bag and mask is an absolute contraindication to the use of suxamethonium. If the administrator is unable to achieve an adequate respiratory exchange by IPPV then in all probability the patient will die.

Prevention – A resuscitative circuit must be to hand and the attendant must be capable of using it effectively. Experience can be gained only under the direction of a doctor who has had some anaesthetic training.

Regurgitation
Regurgitation can and does occur after the injection of suxamethonium. Often the first indication that regurgitation has occurred is when the mouth is opened, prior to intubation, and a pool of gastric contents is found shimmering in the pharynx. The incidence of regurgitation is higher in less skilled hands than in those of the professional anaesthetist, partly due to the fact that the latter is more trained to ventilate the patient's lungs without simultaneously distending the stomach. Usually, however, the anaesthetist takes the additional precaution of applying cricoid pressure which is described below.

Prevention by applying cricoid pressure – Ideally the stomach should be emptied of its contents but this may be impracticable because of the urgent need for intubation. In such circumstances the cricoid cartilage is grasped between the fingers and thumb of an assistant. Counterpressure under the patient's neck is applied by the palm of the assistant's other hand. The cricoid cartilage is then pushed directly backwards. In this way it compresses and obliterates the lumen of the upper part of the oesophagus and prevents regurgitant fluid from entering the pharynx. Pressure is exerted 5 seconds after the start of the suxamethonium injection and is maintained until a cuffed endotracheal tube has been introduced into the trachea and the cuff suitably inflated. Release of the cricoid pressure may then allow gastric contents to extrude from the oesophagus into the pharynx, but they can then be removed by suction catheter without danger of them being inhaled.

In the above manoeuvre the anaesthetist takes a further precaution and saves valuable seconds if he takes a 10 ml syringe before he starts, withdraws the plunger to the 5 ml mark and inserts its nozzle into the pilot tubing. Also, close by he has a suitable pair of forceps so that once the endotracheal tube is in the trachea, he can inject the 5 ml of air immediately into the cuff, clip off the pilot tubing and thereby instantly secure the airway.

Bradycardia

Bradycardia, or rarely cardiac arrest, may occur within seconds of injecting suxamethonium. Injection of atropine, 500 μg intravenously, 1–2 minutes prior to administration of the suxamethonium, prevents this particular action. Some anaesthetists, however, do not always use atropine especially if the patient already has a tachycardia, with no untoward results. Atropine, therefore, is usually desirable but time must not be wasted in looking for it or giving it if the indication for the suxamethonium is urgent.

Increased salivation and bronchial secretions

Another parasympathomimetic side-effect of suxamethonium is excessive salivation and the outpouring of bronchial secretions, which does not occur in all patients, but can be so severe as to almost drown the patient unless they are removed by endobronchial suction catheter.

These salivary and bronchial secretions are inhibited by the prior injection of atropine, 500 μg injected intravenously 5–10 minutes before the introduction of suxamethonium. Again, atropine can be omitted if the administration of suxamethonium is urgent.

Incomplete recovery from suxamethonium
A patient, awakening from an anaesthetic which did not include a muscle relaxant, demonstrates slow and gentle movements of his voluntary muscles. A similar picture is portrayed if he has received a muscle relaxant provided the effects of the latter have completely worn off. If, however, the patient awakens whilst the suxamethonium is still active, then a characteristic picture appears. He partially opens his eyes, jerks his hands and feet but with minimal movement. His grip is weak, his tidal volume is diminished, he begins to go off-colour and if he is not ventilated he eventually becomes unconscious due to gradual asphyxiation. Visual examination shows that his vocal cords never completely shut and he is very easy to intubate. In such circumstances he must be ventilated until his muscle power recovers.

Prolonged apnoea
Suxamethonium is destroyed by an enzyme in the blood called serum cholinesterase or pseudocholinesterase. Low levels of this enzyme are sometimes found in liver disease, so suxamethonium is hydrolysed slower than usual and the return of normal ventilation is delayed.

More often prolonged apnoea is due to the presence of an abnormal gene, the patient having an abnormal pseudocholinesterase. The incidence of suxamethonium apnoea is believed to be one in every 3000 patients who receive the drug.

Apnoea due to suxamethonium can last for 9 – 12 hours. Shorter periods of apnoea (about half an hour) are not infrequent but usually the respiratory depression is due to an accumulation of factors such as the prior administration of narcotics or thiopentone followed by unintentional hyperventilation. In these circumstances application of a peripheral nerve stimulator demonstrates that neuromuscular transmission is normal. Usually all that is needed is to 'allow the patient to breathe'. The technique is as follows. Because excessive ventilation washes out the carbon dioxide from the lungs the blood PCO_2 falls, so the main stimulus of the respiratory centre is removed. The basis of treatment, therefore, is to allow the PCO_2 to rise so it can once more coax the respiratory centre into action. Raising the PCO_2 is accomplished by stopping the IPPV for 30 – 45 seconds. Oxygenation continues by diffusion through the endotracheal tube but the carbon dioxide gradually builds up in the lungs and blood. It is essential to watch both pulse and colour. Marked bradycardia, tachycardia or appearance of irregularities, or cyanosis or pallor demands the immediate restarting of the IPPV. If spontaneous ventilation does not return in 30 – 45 seconds, the lungs are ventilated gently once with the normal tidal volume (400 ml in an adult), and the whole cycle is repeated again. Unless the apnoea is due to an abnormal response to suxamethonium the above technique allows spontaneous ventilation to restart within 10 minutes.

Prolonged suxamethonium apnoea needs the help of an anaesthetist because IPPV must be maintained for several hours and he has to decide when the patient is able to breathe spontaneously and adequately. These patients need careful watching and a great deal of patience, but if properly looked after their recovery rate should be 100%.

A peripheral nerve stimulator can give considerable help as to the cause of the apnoea and the progress of treatment. There is no place for the injection of respiratory stimulants.

Composition of gas used in IPPV
The composition of the gas used in ventilating the apnoeic patient depends on his level of consciousness and the extent of his pain. Essentially the patient who is given suxamethonium falls into one of the following categories.

Unconscious and unresponsive to pain – This type of patient is ventilated with oxygen.

Conscious without pain – Because suxamethonium is non-anaesthetic, in that it does not cause or maintain narcosis, discontinuing a gaseous anaesthetic such as nitrous oxide and/or halothane allows consciousness to return. The patient soon is awake and paralysed. IPPV in this type of patient must be continued with oxygen 50 – 60% and nitrous oxide 50 – 40%; halothane 0.5% is added if the patient is fit and strong but is unnecessary if he is old and ill.

Conscious with pain – The presence of pain demands analgesia. Oxygen with nitrous oxide and perhaps halothane in the concentrations stated in above may suffice. If, however, pain is suspected of being severe or the patient is obviously restless, indicated by sweating or trying to move, then an analgesic such as fentanyl 0.05 – 0.1 mg, every ½ to 1 hour, is given intravenously.

SUMMARY OF PRECAUTIONS BEFORE ADMINISTERING
SUXAMETHONIUM
The following are necessary before suxamethonium is used.

(1) Skill to ventilate unconscious patient
(2) Skill to intubate
(3) Apparatus
  (a) Means of resuscitation, such as portable resuscitation bag and mask or anaesthetic circuit
  (b) Two laryngoscopes
  (c) Endotracheal tube
  (d) Airway
  (e) Suction apparatus (tested and working)
  (f) Knowledge of cricoid pressure
  (g) Tilting carrier
(4) Drugs
  (a) Thiopentone or similar drug if patient is conscious, followed by halothane or similar agent if pain is severe
  (b) Atropine.

25

Respiratory obstruction

Respiratory obstruction is a common cause of death. Fatalities occur sometimes because the condition is not recognized or because it is not suitably treated.

Signs of respiratory obstruction
Recognition of respiratory obstruction depends on the onlooker appreciating the normal respiratory movements of the chest and abdomen. Normally, as the chest expands so the diaphragm contracts; chest and abdomen move outwards together. Obstruction to respiration stimulates the respiratory muscles to greater effort to maintain an adequate pulmonary exchange. However, the diaphragm is more powerful than those muscles which surround and pull out the chest. As a result, on inspiration, the diaphragm moves down pushing out the abdomen but due to its superior strength it draws the chest inwards giving typical seesaw respiration attempts. During expiration the diaphragm moves upwards and the abdomen inwards. The chest wall, already pulled in to a position of expiration, moves little unless the respiratory obstruction is very severe when it may be forced outwards by the superior force of the diaphragm.

Contraction of the accessory muscles of respiration may be obvious and the nostrils may dilate. The patient may become pale or cyanosed, but it is wise to remember that cyanosis depends on the amount of reduced haemoglobin present in the blood. The anaemic patient may have insufficient haemoglobin to become cyanosed.

Behaviour disorders may become apparent. The patient may become irrational, restless and then becomes drowsy and stuporose.

The pulse rate usually increases but as hypoxia becomes more marked the tachycardia is replaced by bradycardia and irregularities. Blood pressure may rise at first due to carbon dioxide retention but eventually falls.

A rising temperature, especially in the already pyrexial patient, may

201

be apparent due to the increased work involved in trying to overcome the obstruction. Hyperpyrexia, especially in children, may lead to convulsions which themselves increase the rate of oxygen consumption and heat production thereby starting the vicious circle of hypoxia −convulsions−hypoxia (p. 43).

BREATH SOUNDS

The presence of respiratory obstruction is often missed because the attendant does not listen to the patient's breathing. Surrounded by a battery of electronic equipment it is thought perhaps too mundane to put an ear close to the patient's mouth to listen to what is going on; but this important, simple manoeuvre gives valuable information. Normal breathing is almost inaudible but the ear detects, with a fair degree of accuracy, the unobstructed outward flow of air during expiration. Normal breathing through an airway is more audible. The resuscitator can remind himself of its characteristics by keeping his own mouth open during inspiration and expiration. He will also notice that expiration takes twice as long to complete as does inspiration.

SLIGHT OBSTRUCTION

Slight obstruction leads to a diminution of the current of air detected by the ear but usually expiration, and sometimes inspiration, is more noisy, being accompanied by slight grunting, snoring or the crowing of laryngeal spasm.

Because the free passage of air is restricted, inspiration and expiration times are more prolonged. Prolonged expiration is usually most noticeable and its tone frequently becomes higher pitched.

SEVERE OBSTRUCTION

All the above signs are aggravated. Respiratory sounds become more noisy and the crowing of laryngeal spasm may be loud. Complete obstruction may be soundless but is accompanied by the seesaw type of respiration or complete respiratory arrest.

Relief of respiratory obstruction

Respiratory obstruction can be caused by flaccidity of the tongue, the presence of foreign material, laryngeal spasm, inflammation or tumour, or by a combination of all these. Treatment consists of removal of the cause where possible.

FLACCIDITY OF THE TONGUE

Fortunately the tongue is attached to the mandible, and elevation of the chin or pulling the jaw forward is usually sufficient to drag the tongue away from the posterior pharyngeal wall and restore the airway. This procedure almost appears unworthy of description yet correct support for the chin in some patients is a manoeuvre which is difficult to perform correctly even by skilled anaesthetists. The degree of neck extension and jaw protrusion differ markedly in different patients and they should be varied while listening to the air entry until eventually the jaw is positioned to guarantee maximum air entry.

Chin elevation, although usually desirable, can itself exacerbate respiratory obstruction especially in the edentulous because it approximates the lips. If, therefore, the nose is blocked by secretions, a deviated septum or by gauze packs, elevation of the chin may cause complete respiratory obstruction. Usually this problem is overcome by insertion of an airway but if this is not possible then the lips must be separated by the fingers.

Oral airway insertion

The flaccid tongue is bypassed by the insertion of a rubber or plastic airway, graded 00, 0, 1, 2, 3 and 4, the latter being the largest.

SIZE OF AIRWAY NEEDED

Babies up to 1 year of age require size 00 or 0.

Children from 1–5 years of age require size 0 or 1.

Children from 5 years to adults require size 1 or 2.

Adults require size 2, 3 or 4.

Correct choice of airway is important. A size too small is too short to bypass the relaxed tongue; a size too long does not fit comfortably into the mouth and contacts the back of the pharynx, thereby causing the patient to retch and possibly vomit unless he is deeply unconscious (Figures 25.1 to 25.9).

DANGERS OF THE AIRWAY

The presence of an airway can lull the resuscitator into a feeling of false security. Several misfortunes can befall the patient if suitable adjustments are neglected. For example, movement of the head or the airway may upset the relative position of the airway with the tongue and pharyngeal wall causing partial or total respiratory obstruction. Furthermore, movement may rub the distal end of the airway against the posterior pharyngeal wall, causing the patient to retch or try to 'spit

out', that is to extrude the airway whereupon the natural response of
the attendant is to pull it out of the mouth. This action is justified and
correct, provided the muscle tone of the tongue is adequate to maintain the natural clear airway of the conscious patient. If, however, the
patient is still semiconscious, he may become hypoxic and reinsertion
of the airway rapidly becomes a necessity. In such circumstances full
reinsertion of the airway may again cause the same result and the
sequence of retching–removal of airway–retching is repeated. Two
alternatives are possible. An airway one size smaller may suffice but
the easiest and quickest manoeuvre is to replace the original airway
but to leave 1–1.5 cm of the proximal end of the airway protruding
from the mouth. In fact, the anaesthetist, seeing the patient retching
or gagging on the airway, usually withdraws the airway a little, to
break its contact with the pharyngeal wall, and waits a few seconds to
see if the patient accepts it in its new position.

The advantages of these manoeuvres are that the airway still
bypasses possible obstruction by lips and tongue, and oral catheter
suction is possible. Also, should vomiting of solid material occur, a
mouth gag can be inserted in the gap between the teeth alongside the
airway, to grant access to, and allow removal of the vomit.
Withdrawal of the airway to the extent of 1 – 1.5 cm is stipulated because
if pulled out too far, beyond the limits of the metal framework in its
proximal part, its lumen can be obliterated by the clenched teeth, thus
rendering its presence almost useless so that obstruction once more
occurs.

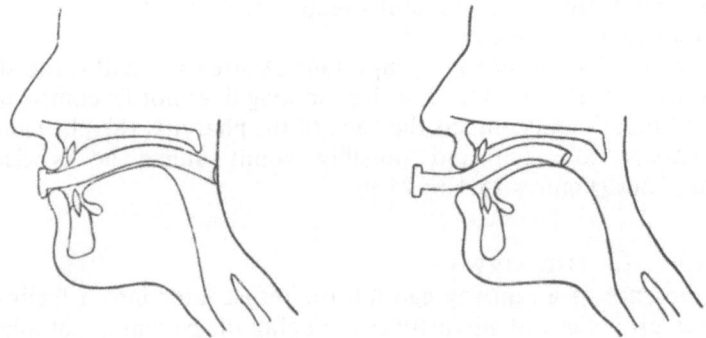

Figure 25.1 Airway in contact with
the pharynx can produce vomiting on
recovery from anaesthesia

Figure 25.2 Airway pulled away from
the pharyngeal wall which is
therefore not stimulated

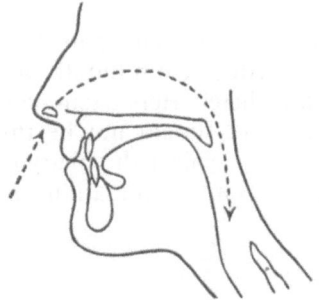

Figure 25.3 Lips together. Air can enter through nose

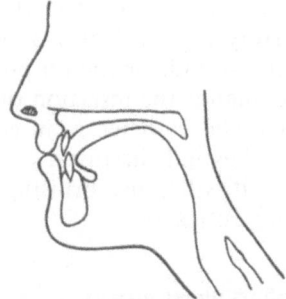

Figure 25.4 Lips together, nose obstructed. Air cannot enter through lips or nose. Remedy – separate lips and insert airway

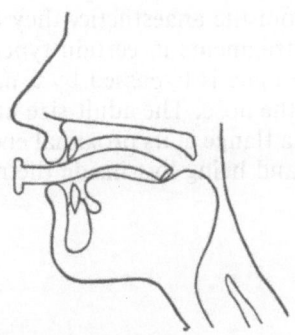

Figure 25.5 Too small an airway pushes tongue against the pharyngeal wall

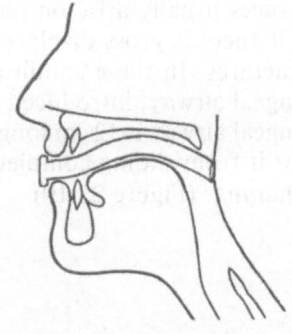

Figure 25.6 Too large an airway. Blockage due to pressing against the pharyngeal wall

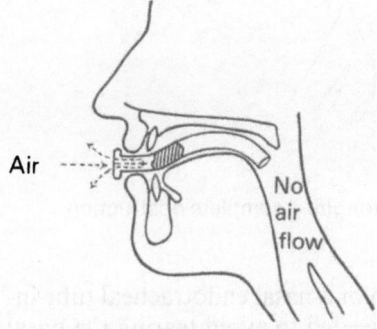

Air

No air flow

Figure 25.7 Blocked airway

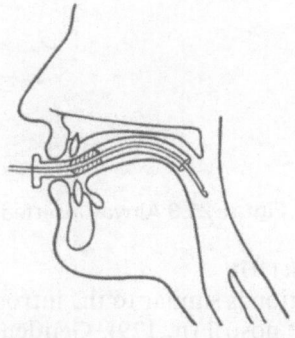

Figure 25.8 Catheter inserted allows air to pass. Obstruction relieved

SUCTION THROUGH THE AIRWAY

An airway is useful only as long as its lumen remains patent. Any bubbling sound, or the outpouring of secretions from mouth or airway, demands the insertion of a suction catheter. Here again, care is needed. The catheter is inserted gently, and should not be thrust roughly beyond the distal end of the airway against the pharyngeal wall, or it will cause bruising of the mucosa and stimulation of the vomiting reflex.

Nasopharyngeal airway

INDICATIONS

Occasions arise when the patient is too light (that is too awake) to tolerate an oral airway, yet has insufficient tone in his tongue to guarantee an unobstructed respiratory exchange. Although such circumstances usually arise on recovery from the anaesthetic, they also occur if there is gross displacement of fragments in certain types of jaw fractures. In these conditions the tongue is bypassed by a nasopharyngeal airway, introduced through the nose. The adult-size nasopharyngeal airway is 12 cm long and has a flange at its proximal end to prevent it from sliding completely into and being lost inside the nose and pharynx. (Figure 25.10).

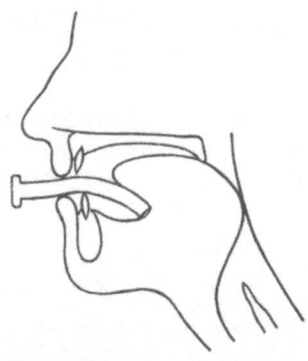

Figure 25.9 Airway inserted under tongue – complete obstruction

INSERTION

Insertion is similar to the introduction of a nasal endotracheal tube into the nostril (p. 179). Gentleness is needed to avoid tearing the nasal mucous membrane, because pooling of blood in the nasopharynx can lead to aspiration, laryngeal spasm and asphyxia.

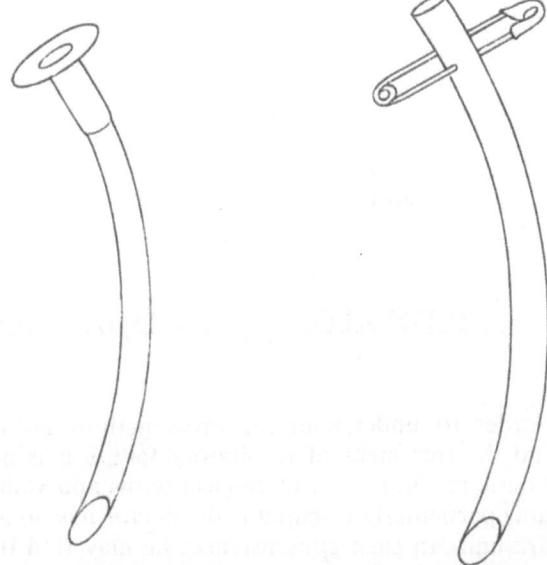

Figure 25.10 Naso-pharyngeal airway   **Figure 25.11** Cut down endotracheal tube with safety pin

Introduction of a nasopharyngeal airway in a conscious patient is unpleasant and may lead to struggling, with further displacement of jaw fragments and hypoxia. Attempts should be made to provide analgesia by squirting 2–3 ml 4% lignocaine up the chosen nostril and also by lubricating the nasopharyngeal airway with a similar cream or gel. Once inserted it is well tolerated.

If an actual nasopharyngeal airway is unobtainable, a shortened endotracheal tube is perfectly satisfactory. Insertion of a large safety-pin through its proximal end is an effective, if less elegant, way of preventing the tube being aspirated. (Figure 25.11).

26

Respiratory pathophysiology

In order to understand the investigations needed for the diagnosis and the treatment of respiratory failure it is necessary to understand basic respiratory physiological terms and values. A clear appreciation is particularly essential if the doctor has no access to an intensive care unit. In such circumstances he may find that nursing staff change frequently and he has to explain the meaning of definitions and symbols concerned with both the pulmonary interchange of gases and the handling of ventilation.

Use of symbols in respiratory pathophysiology
As explained later (p. 303), PO_2 and PCO_2 refer to the partial pressures of oxygen and carbon dioxide respectively but sometimes it is obviously necessary to denote the particular locality in the body to which the partial pressure refers.

In order to clarify the situation, symbols are classified as *primary* and *secondary*. Primary symbols are written in *large capital letters* and secondary symbols in *small capital letters*. The symbols are followed by the formula of the respective gas. For example,

P = gas pressure, and A = alveolar gas

$\therefore PA$ = partial pressure in alveolar gas

and PAO_2 = partial pressure of oxygen in alveolar gas

Other examples are found on p. 211.

Symbols frequently encountered in resuscitation are:

Gases   Primary symbols (large capitals)

→P = gas pressure

→V = gas volume

→F = fractional concentration

Secondary symbols (small capitals)

↳I   = inspired gas

↳E   = expired gas

↳A   = alveolar gas

T   = tidal gas

D   = dead space gas

Examples of their combination, illustrated by the arrows above are:

P_ACO_2 = partial pressure of carbon dioxide in the alveoli

V_E = volume of expired gas

F_IO_2 = fractional concentration of inspired oxygen. This is another way of expressing the percentage concentration by volume. For example $F_IO_2 = 0.209$ means that the inspired gas contains 20.9% oxygen.

Blood   Primary symbols (large capitals)

Q = volume of blood

S = percentage saturation of Hb with O_2

For example

SO_2 = percentage saturation of Hb with O_2 or CO

Secondary symbols (small letters)

a   = arterial blood

v   = venous blood

c   = pulmonary capillary blood

For example

$P\text{a}O_2$ = partial pressure of O_2 in arterial blood

$P\acute{c}O_2$ = partial pressure of O_2 in end (pulmonary) capillary
            blood

$P\text{c}O_2$ = partial pressure of O_2 in mixed (pulmonary)
            capillary blood

$P\bar{v}O_2$ = partial pressure of O_2 in mixed venous (pulmonary)
            artery) blood

            (The superscript $^-$ indicates 'mean', average or mixed
            but is omitted when referring to mixed pulmonary
            capillary blood.)

$P(\text{A}-\text{a})O_2$ = alveolar − arterial O_2 pressure difference

It must be stressed that *P* stands for partial pressure. It is *not* an
abbreviation for 'pulmonary'.

PARTIAL PRESSURE (TENSION)
Provided that the concept of partial pressure is clear (p. 303) and the
concentrations of the various components in a mixture of gases are
known it is easy to calculate the individual partial pressures. For example:

total atmospheric pressure at sea level = 760 mmHg (101 kPa)

dry atmospheric air (inspired air) contains
    oxygen   20.95%
    carbon dioxide   0.04%
    nitrogen   79.01%

Therefore, in dry inspired air:

partial pressure of oxygen,

P_IO_2, is $\dfrac{20.9}{100} \times 760 = 159\,mmHg$, or $\dfrac{20.9}{100} \times 101 = 21\,kPa$

partial pressure of carbon dioxide,

P_ICO_2, is $\dfrac{0.04}{100} \times 760 = 0.3\,mmHg$ or $\dfrac{0.04}{100} \times 101 = 0.04\,kPa$

partial pressure of nitrogen,

P_IN_2, is $\dfrac{79}{100} \times 760 = 601\,mmHg$, or $\dfrac{79}{100} \times 101 = 79.8\,kPa$

sum of partial pressures = 760 mmHg (101 kPa)

In measurements involving the volumes and concentrations of respiratory gases containing water vapour it must be remembered that the volumes are expressed dry, that is without their water vapour, at standard temperature and pressure. Therefore, the individual gases are expressed as percentages of the dry volume. So, in converting the concentration of a gas to its partial pressure, the partial pressure of any water vapour present must be deducted from the atmospheric pressure before the partial pressure of the gas is calculated. For example, in the alveoli:

normal atmospheric pressure   = 760 mmHg   (101 kPa)

partial pressure of water vapour P_AH_2O = 47 mmHg   (6.3 kPa)

Therefore, pressure of dry air   = 713 mmHg   (94.7 kPa)

and if a sample of alveolar air contains 5.6% CO_2

partial pressure, P_ACO_2, = 5.6 (760 − 47) mmHg ($\dfrac{5.6}{100}(101-6.3)$ kPa)

$$= \dfrac{5.6}{100} \times 713\,mmHg \text{ or } \dfrac{5.6}{100} \times 94.7\,kPa$$

$$= 40\,mmHg\ (5.3\,kPa)$$

Table 26.1 shows a comparison of partial pressures.

Table 26.1 Comparison of partial pressures in alveolar air, mixed systemic arterial blood, and mixed venous blood

	mmHg	kPa
Alveolar air		
Oxygen, P_AO_2	= 104	13.8
Carbon dioxide, P_ACO_2	= 40	5.3
Nitrogen, P_AN_2	= 569	75.7
Water vapour, P_AH_2O	= 47	6.3
Sum of partial pressures including water vapour	= 760	101.1
Mixed systemic arterial blood		
Oxygen, P_aO_2	= 100	13.3
Carbon dioxide, P_aCO_2	= 40	5.3
Nitrogen, P_aN_2	= 573	76.2
Water vapour P_aH_2O	= 47	6.3
Sum of partial pressures including water vapour	= 760	101.1
Mixed venous blood		
Oxygen, $P_{\bar{v}}O_2$	= 40	5.3
Carbon dioxide, $P_{\bar{v}}CO_2$	= 46	6.1
Nitrogen, $P_{\bar{v}}N_2$	= 573	76.2
Water vapour, $P_{\bar{v}}H_2O$	= 47	6.3
Sum of partial pressures including water vapour	= 706	93.9

Blood leaving the pulmonary capillaries, that is at the start of the pulmonary veins, is in equilibrium with the alveolar gases, and therefore they have similar tensions. But this region is usually inaccessible, and mixed arterial blood is chosen because its gaseous contents show the closest, easily available, approximation to those in the blood leaving the pulmonary capillaries. The oxygen content of mixed systemic arterial blood is slightly lower because of the addition to it of venous blood which has bypassed the pulmonary capillaries (see Table 26.1).

The discrepancy of 54 mmHg (7.2 kPa) between the sum of the partial pressure of 706 mmHg (93.9 kPa) in mixed venous blood and their sum of 760 mmHg (101 kPa) in atmospheric air and systemic arterial blood is due to the fact that the removal of 5 ml oxygen from 100 ml mixed arterial blood by the tissues causes a fall in oxygen tension of 60 mmHg (100 mmHg − 40 mmHg) or 8 kPa (13.3 − 5.3 kPa), whereas addition of 4 ml of carbon dioxide per 100 ml of blood leaving the

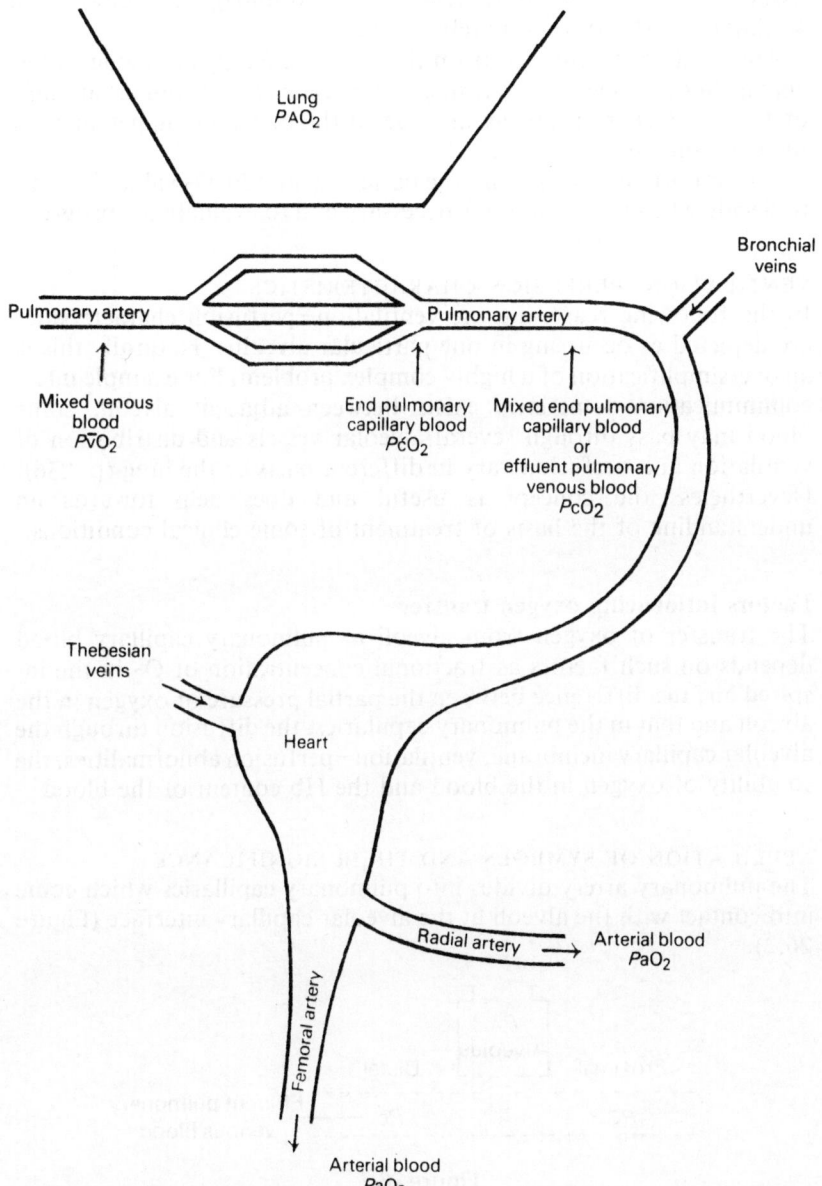

Figure 26.1 Symbols used in respiratory physiology applicable to oxygen tension

tissues causes the PCO_2 to rise by only 6 mmHg (0.08 kPa) from 40 mmHg (5.3 kPa) to 46 mmHg (6.1 kPa).

The vastly different effects on the PO_2 and PCO_2 of gaseous interchange in the tissues due to losing and gaining almost similar amounts of O_2 and CO_2 respectively are due to the different shapes of their dissociation curves (p. 312).

It is important to memorize the basic PO_2 and PCO_2 values in order to decide when resuscitation is necessary and to evaluate the progress.

VENTILATION–PERFUSION CHARACTERISTICS
In the following reasoning the ventilation–perfusion characteristics are depicted as occurring in one particular alveolus. Naturally this is an oversimplification of a highly complex problem. For example intercommunication sometimes exists between adjacent alveoli, some blood may pass through several alveolar vessels and distribution of ventilation and perfusion vary in different parts of the lung (p. 236). Nevertheless the concept is useful and does help towards an understanding of the basis of treatment of some clinical conditions.

Factors influencing oxygen transfer
The transfer of oxygen from alveoli to pulmonary capillary blood depends on such factors as fractional concentration of O_2 in the inspired air, the difference between the partial pressure of oxygen in the alveoli and that in the pulmonary capillaries, the diffusion through the alveolar capillary membrane, ventilation–perfusion abnormalities, the solubility of oxygen in the blood and the Hb content of the blood.

APPLICATION OF SYMBOLS AND THEIR SIGNIFICANCE
The pulmonary artery divides into pulmonary capillaries which come into contact with the alveoli at the alveolar capillary interface (Figure 26.2).

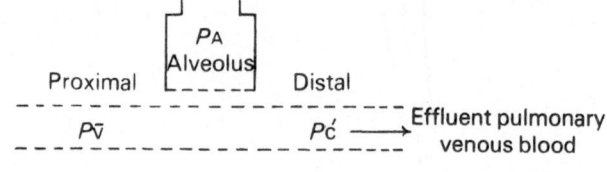

Figure 26.2

The proximal end of the pulmonary capillary is the terminal part of the pulmonary artery and the partial pressure therein is symbolized as

$P\bar{v}$; $\bar{v}$ denotes mixed venous blood. The partial pressure of O_2 at the entrance of every capillary is the same because of the thorough mixing of the deoxygenated blood in the right side of the heart. The distal end of the pulmonary capillary is the beginning of the pulmonary vein and the partial pressure therein is symbolized $P\acute{c}$. The blood emerging from the pulmonary capillary is also termed effluent pulmonary venous blood.

In the normal lung there is a difference between the relatively high partial pressure of oxygen in the alveolus, PAO_2, and that in the mixed venous blood, $P\bar{v}O_2$, entering the pulmonary capillary. In the 0.75 s taken for a corpuscle to pass through the pulmonary capillary it becomes almost fully oxygenated so that, to all intents and purposes, in the healthy young adult the oxygen tension in the corpuscle and plasma leaving the pulmonary capillary, $P\acute{c}O_2$, is equal to that in the alveolus. In fact there is usually a difference of only 1 mmHg (0.13 kPa) or less in pressure between the PAO_2 and $P\acute{c}O_2$. This slight difference (ignored in Figures 26.3 to 26.10) existing between PAO_2 and $P\acute{c}O_2$ is known as the alveolar-end pulmonary capillary difference $P(A - \acute{c})O_2$ which progressively increases as the patient ages. However, the addition of venous blood from the bronchial veins into the pulmonary veins and the drainage of small myocardial veins into the left ventricle causes a fall of 5 mmHg (0.66 kPa) in the oxygen tension of the blood leaving the left ventricle as systemic arterial blood. This shunt component (p. 220) accounts for the difference between the PAO_2 and PaO_2 and is referred to as the alveolar–arterial oxygen pressure gradient or the $P(A - a)O_2$ difference (p. 221).

Breathing air
The $P(A - a)O_2$ difference may reach

In young healthy adults	10 mmHg (1.3 kPa)
Middle-aged people	20 mmHg (2.7 kPa)
Old people	25 mmHg (3.3 kPa)
In disease	50 mmHg (6.6 kPa) or more

NORMAL VALUES

PAO_2	=	104 mmHg (13.8 kPa)
$P\bar{v}O_2$	=	40 mmHg (5.3 kPa)
$P\acute{c}O_2$	=	104–103 mmHg (13.8–13.7 kPa)

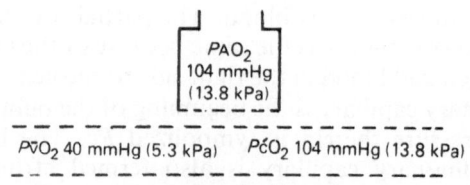

Figure 26.3

These values remain fairly constant provided that ventilation of the alveolus is normal and the flow of blood (the perfusion) is normal within the adjacent pulmonary capillary.

The ventilation–perfusion ratio

If ventilation is represented by $\dot{V}$ (p. 127), which is the amount of air per minute entering the alveoli, and if perfusion is represented by $\dot{Q}$, which is the volume of blood per minute perfusing the alveoli, than a relationship can be established between $\dot{V}$ and $\dot{Q}$, and this is known as the ventilation–perfusion ($\dot{V}/\dot{Q}$) ratio.

Normally the $\dot{V}/\dot{Q}$ ratio is equal to

$$\frac{4 \; l/min}{5 \; l/min} = \frac{4 \; l}{5 \; l} = 0.8$$

If ventilation is lowered relative to perfusion the patient has a lowered ventilation–perfusion ratio. This occurs in hypoventilation due to a variety of conditions such as in an overdosage of narcotics (p. 123). If perfusion is lowered relative to ventilation the patient has a raised ventilation–perfusion ratio. This occurs in shock following pulmonary embolus (p. 21).

Although the $\dot{V}/\dot{Q}$ ratio is a useful concept, it can be misleading unless it is remembered that the lungs are composed of a myriad of units, each with an alveolus and a capillary, and its own. $\dot{V}/\dot{Q}$ ratio. The $\dot{V}/\dot{Q}$ ratio for the whole patient is a mean of all these ratios which vary in different parts of the lung.

ABNORMAL VALUES
It is easy to comprehend what happens if circumstances arise that alter the normal values (p. 215) in an alveolus and its capillary.
For example,

Diminished ventilation

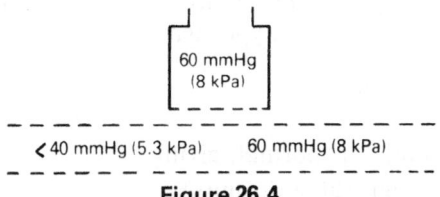

Figure 26.4

if the $P\text{A}O_2$ falls to 60 mmHg (8 kPa) then the $P\text{c}O_2$ falls to 60 mmHg (8 kPa) and the PaO_2 will be even lower at about 55 mmHg (7.3 kPa).

Adequate oxygenation of the tissues may still be obtained, but the $P\bar{v}O_2$ value will be <40 mmHg (5.3 kPa), (Figure 26.4) perhaps 25 mmHg (3.3 kPa). Further tissue oxygen requirement, however, such as occurs in exercise or the increased muscular effort of hyperpnoea following near drowning (p. 64) cannot be met and tissue hypoxia will develop.

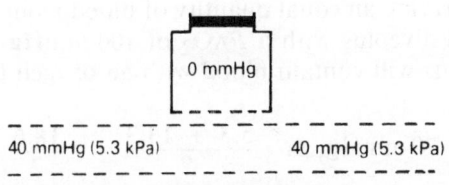

Figure 26.5

Complete blockage of the alveolus reduces the alveolar oxygen tension to zero so that the blood passes through the pulmonary capillary without change in its oxygen tension. The blood is said to be shunted past that alveolus and an absolute shunt is said to exist. Because ventilation of the alveolus is zero, although perfusion is full, the ventilation–perfusion ratio of that aveolus is also zero.

$$\dot{V}/\dot{Q} \; = \; 0/\dot{Q} \; = \; 0$$

Diminished perfusion

Complete obstruction to the flow of blood through the pulmonary capillary prevents any oxygenation from taking place so that perfusion $\dot{Q}$ is zero even if ventilation of the alveolus is normal (Figure 26.6). However, pulmonary arterial blood meeting such an obstruction is usually redirected through patent capillaries, and provided that the transit time through the perfused capillaries is adequate there may be no change in PaO_2 and $PaCO_2$. But compensation may be incomplete and in some patients with pulmonary embolism the diffusion impairment in areas of lung with high blood flow and a consequent short transit time frequently causes hypoxaemia.

Therefore, in Figure 26.6

$\dot{Q}$ = 0 and $\dot{V}$ is normal, giving
$\dot{V}/\dot{Q}$ a high value (infinity)

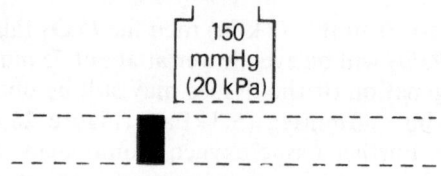

Figure 26.6

If the shunted blood is then joined by another pulmonary capillary (Figure 26.7) carrying an equal quantity of blood from an almost normally ventilated alveolus with a PAO_2 of 100 mmHg (13.3 kPa) the combined streams will contain blood with an oxygen tension of

$$\frac{40 + 100}{2} = 70\,\text{mmHg, or} \quad \frac{5.3 + 13.3}{2} = \frac{18.6}{2} = 9.3 \text{ kPa}$$

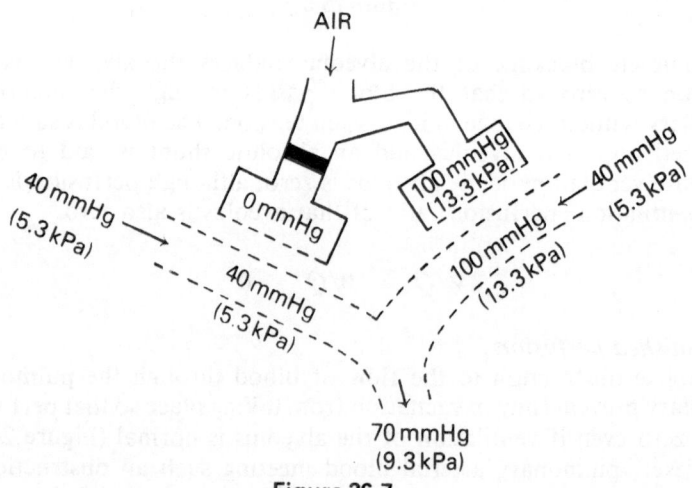

Figure 26.7

If the patient then breathes an oxygen-enriched mixture (Figure 26.8), so that the PAO_2 of the aerated alveolus is raised to 160 mmHg

(21.2 kPa), the combined streams with equal flow rates will have an average oxygen tension of approximately

$$\frac{40 + 160}{2} = 100 \text{ mmHg, or } \frac{5.3 \times 21.2}{2} = \frac{26.5}{2} = 13.3 \text{ kPa}$$

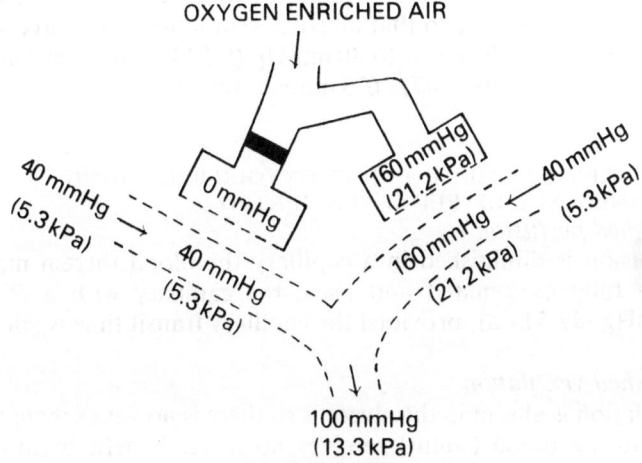

Figure 26.8

The effects of breathing 100% oxygen

NORMAL PATIENT BREATHING SPONTANEOUSLY

Administration of 100% oxygen displaces the nitrogen of atmospheric air, so the partial pressure exerted by the pure oxygen in the alveolus is equal to 760 mmHg (101.3 kPa) minus the sum of the $PACO_2$ and the PAH_2O (Figure 26.9). Therefore, the PAO_2 achieved when breathing 100% oxygen is $760 - (40 + 47) = 673$ mmHg, that is $101.3 - (5.3 + 6.3) = 89.5$ kPa. As a result the PaO_2 reaches around 660 mmHg (87.8 kPa), the $P(A-a)O_2$ difference increasing with the elevated FIO_2.

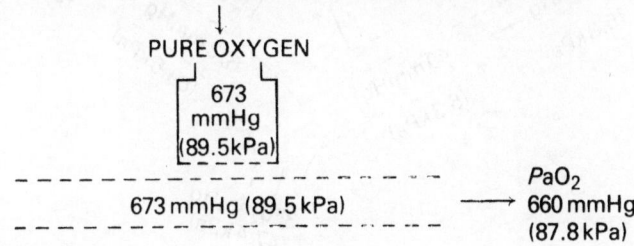

Figure 26.9

PATIENT HYPOVENTILATING, BREATHING
SPONTANEOUSLY 100% OXYGEN
Normal perfusion
Hypoventilation leads to a rise in PACO$_2$ to say 60 mmHg (8 kPa).
Provided that perfusion is normal the administration of 100% oxygen
raises the PAO$_2$ to $760 - (60 + 47) = 653$ mmHg, that is, $101.3 - (8 +
6.3) = 87$ kPa and the PaO$_2$ to around 640 mmHg (85 kPa). If the pa-
tient is then ventilated, so that alveolar ventilation is restored to normal, the PACO$_2$ will return to 40 mmHg (5.3 kPa) and the PaO$_2$ will
rise towards $760 - (40 + 47) = 673$ mmHg, that is, $101.3 - (5.3 + 6.3) =
89.5$ kPa.

NORMOCAPNIC PATIENT ON 100% OXYGEN BREATHING
SPONTANEOUSLY OR BEING VENTILATED
Diminished perfusion
If perfusion is diminished in a capillary the blood therein may still
become fully oxygenated and leave the capillary with a PċO$_2$ of
673 mmHg (89.5 kPa), provided the capillary transit time is adequate.

Diminished ventilation
If ventilation is absent in the alveolus so there is no gas exchange, then
the perfusing blood (shunt) receives no direct benefit because it is
denied contact with a normal aerated alveolus. Therefore, addition of
blood from this shunted blood to that from the well-ventilated
alveolus will give an average or mean oxygen tension whose value is
always less than the PcO$_2$ in the capillary of the well-oxygenated
alveolus.

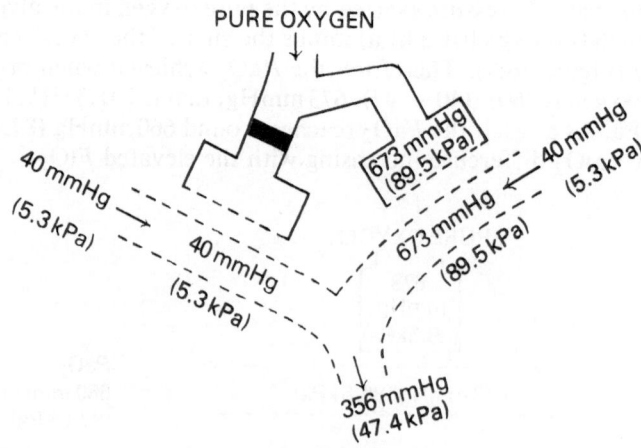

Figure 26.10

Figure 26.10 shows that in these circumstances administration of 100% oxygen gives, for these two capillaries, an average $P\acute{c}O_2$ of $(40 + 673)/2$ = approximately 356 mmHg, that is $5.3 + (89.5/2)$ = 47.4 kPa.

Therefore, when an absolute shunt is present the administration of oxygen does raise the PaO_2, but it is impossible to raise the PaO_2 to the level of the PAO_2. Even when breathing pure oxygen there is a large $P(A-a)O_2$ difference. The presence of an absolute shunt is the only condition where the PaO_2 value is more than a few mmHg below that of the PAO_2.

USE OF OXYGEN IN DIAGNOSIS

From the previous reasoning it can be seen that the administration of 100% oxygen can help to differentiate between a low PaO_2 due to a shunt and a low PaO_2 due to other causes.

In all measurement and assessments of PaO_2 values it is essential to known the FIO_2, on which it depends, in the inspired gases. The FIO_2 is measured by means of an oxygen analyser, or in the case of disposable oxygen masks, it is obtainable from charts (p. 68). The FIO_2 is important in the determination of PIO_2 (p. 211) which is necessary for assessing the alveolar – arterial oxygen difference ($P(A-a)O_2$) which is derived below.

DERIVATION OF THE ALVEOLAR–ARTERIAL OXYGEN DIFFERENCE ($P(A-a)O_2$)

Changes in the alveolar–arterial oxygen difference $P(A-a)O_2$ help to assess the effectiveness of treatment in conditions where a shunt exists. To obtain its value the PaO_2 is obtained from the acid–base laboratory, and the PAO_2 is derived from a simplification of Comroe's alveolar air equation:

$$\text{Alveolar oxygen tension} = \text{inspired oxygen tension} - \frac{\text{alveolar carbon dioxide tension}}{\text{respiratory quotient}}$$

$$\text{or } PAO_2 = PIO_2 - \frac{PaCO_2}{R}$$

$$R = \text{the respiratory quotient} = \frac{\text{oxygen intake/min}}{\text{carbon dioxide output/min}} = 0.8$$

$$\therefore PAO_2 = PIO_2 - \frac{PACO_2}{0.8}$$

The PIO_2 is calculated from the FIO_2, measured by means of an oximeter; the $PACO_2$ is equal to $PaCO_2$ and is measured by arterial puncture.

The equation $PAO_2 = PICO_2 - \dfrac{PACO_2}{0.8}$ is now reversed

in other words,

$$PIO_2 - \frac{PACO_2}{0.8} = PAO_2, \text{ or } PIO_2 - \frac{PaCO_2}{0.8} = PAO_2$$

Substituting in the equation for a normal patient breathing air

PIO_2 is 150 mmHg (20 kPa) and the $PACO_2$ (or $PaCO_2$) is 40 mmHg (5.3 kPa)

then $150 - \dfrac{40}{0.8} = 100$ mmHg, that is a PAO_2 of 100 mmHg

or $\quad 20 - \dfrac{5.3}{0.8} = 13.3$ kPa, that is a PAO_2 of 13.3 kPa.

A rise in $PACO_2$ *influences* PAO_2 because raising the $PACO_2$ to 60 mmHg (8 kPa) reduces the PAO_2 to 75 mmHg (10 kPa), that is

$$150 - \frac{60}{0.8} = 75 \text{ mmHg or } 20 - \frac{8}{0.8} = 10 \text{ kPa}$$

A rise in inspired oxygen concentration influences PAO_2 because administration of 30% oxygen increases the PIO_2 to 30/100 × 760=228 mmHg or 30/100 × 95 = 30 kPa, and thereby raises the PAO_2 to 178 mmHg (23.4 kPa), that is

$$228 - \frac{40}{0.8} = 178 \text{ mmHg, or } 30 - \frac{5.3}{0.8} = 23.4 \text{ kPa}$$

or, if the $PACO_2$ is 60 mmHg the PAO_2 is 153 mmHg or 13.4 kPa.

27

Respiratory failure

Respiratory failure exists if the patient is unable to carry out an adequate respiratory exchange. It is present if there is a fall in PaO_2 to less than 60 mmHg (8 kPa), a rise in $PaCO_2$ to more than 50 mmHg (6.6 kPa), or a combination of the two, when breathing air. Respiratory failure can occur as a result of hypoventilation, mismatching of ventilation and perfusion, or a combination of both.

Hypoventilation

Hypoventilation occurs principally:

(1) When the airways are normal but there is injury or depression of the respiratory centre, spinal cord, peripheral nerves, neuromuscular junction, respiratory muscles or chest wall (p. 73). Examples are head injury, overdosage of narcotics, poliomyelitis or the Guillain–Barré syndrome.
(2) Where there is airway obstruction due to bronchial narrowing caused by secretions, oedema of the mucous membrane or hypertrophy of the bronchial musculature. Bronchial obstruction can arise in most pulmonary diseases as a result of infection, the commonest conditions being acute bronchitis, chronic bronchitis with emphysema, and asthma.

Ventilation–perfusion mismatching

This is explained on p. 216.

Resuscitation in respiratory failure

Much of the treatment, particularly emergency treatment, of respiratory failure is the same irrespective of the pulmonary condition responsible for the inadequate respiratory exchange. Whether there is hypoxaemia and hypercapnia due to hypoventilation or to ventila-

223

tion–perfusion inequalities the immediate aim is to ensure adequate delivery of oxygen to, and the removal of carbon dioxide from, the lungs. Therefore, in the emergency situation it is best to start resuscitative measures as soon as possible, leaving the establishment of the finer points of diagnosis for a little later on.

One problem, however, remains unsolved, and this is how far to proceed with resuscitative measures. An acute pneumonia or bout of acute bronchitis on a previously active chronic bronchitic usually responds well even if controlled ventilation has to be instituted for a few hours or days. On the other hand one must question the wisdom of starting prolonged IPPV on a respiratory cripple. This type of patient may spend days or weeks on a ventilator, necessitating a tracheostomy, only to find then that he cannot maintain his own ventilation unaided for more than a few hours. He is then condemned to relying on the ventilator for most of the day with the added burden of being unable to speak, with the obvious distressing effects on both the patient and the relatives.

Resuscitation starts by attention to the mouth, nose and pharynx. In the unconscious patient removal of secretions and other foreign material is best done with the help of a laryngoscope. This allows the operator to remove secretions quickly and effectively without damaging the pharyngeal mucous membrane. It also avoids getting the uvula stuck in the suction catheter, thus preventing bruising and swelling which can change its size and colour within a few seconds to resemble that of a damson in both size and appearance.

During suction, care must be taken to avoid stimulating the posterior pharyngeal wall otherwise retching and vomiting may occur. Provided care is exercised it is often possible to get a quick look at the larynx, and this may show the presence of a foreign body, a laryngeal growth or laryngeal oedema; purulent secretions may be seen oozing upwards between the vocal cords, indicating that bronchial suction, endotracheal intubation and possibly tracheostomy should be considered.

USE OF AIRWAY

Edentulous patients in particular need an oral or nasopharyngeal airway. Babies, in addition, have small nares and because they cannot blow their noses they soon obstruct; this, combined with the fact that they are natural nose breathers, often results in them becoming cyanosed before they condescend to open their mouths.

Clearance of the upper airways as described above may suffice to restore adequate ventilation but further treatment may be required.

BLOOD GAS ESTIMATION
Measurement of blood gases is essential because it gives the clinician valuable help in establishing a diagnosis and also helps him to assess the effect of treatment.

Whenever blood gases are estimated it is essential to record whether the patient is breathing air and/or oxygen and in what percentage. The first blood sample, if the patient's condition allows, is taken with him breathing air.

TEMPORARY ENDOTRACHEAL INTUBATION
Endotracheal intubation is easy in the moribund patient with respiratory failure. If, however, the patient is conscious he needs a prior injection of thiopentone (thiopental) and a relaxant (p. 194). Indications for intubation are the moist chest with râles and rhonchi, the typical 'bubbling chest', or the localized absence of breath sounds, particularly when the patient is unable to clear his secretions spontaneously. Often an endobronchial catheter instantly delivers $10 - 30$ ml of purulent sputum with an immediate improved air entry and general condition.

Provided that continued intubation is not considered necessary after the initial suction it is sometimes advisable, when the effect of the relaxant is wearing off, to move the endotracheal tube gently up and down. This action makes the patient cough and often delivers more secretions into the reach of a suction catheter. Finally, when no more secretions can be aspirated the tube is again agitated and withdrawn as the patient is coughing. Usually this results in him producing an explosive cough which helps to dislodge further secretions. Occasionally the patient may then develop extubation laryngeal spasm, and it is always wise to give him a few breaths of 100% oxygen before extubation. This concentration in the lungs will then provide him with enough oxygen for the next minute or two whilst his laryngeal spasm disappears, thus avoiding the possibility of hypoxia.

The first few minutes following extubation are very important. The mouth and pharynx are again examined and cleared of secretions, and the patency of the airway is ensured by the patient's own efforts, by insertion of an oral or nasopharyngeal airway, or by separation of the lips by the fingers of the resuscitator.

Reinsertion of the endotracheal tube
If ventilatory movements appear inadequate, or are inadequate as measured by the respirometer (p. 122 and Figure 18.1), or if the condition deteriorates, it is essential to ventilate the patient with bag and

mask and usually reinsert the endotracheal tube. Reinsertion is preceded by spraying the larynx with 4% lignocaine or by smearing the
tube with lignocaine cream or gel. This enables the patient to tolerate
the tube without coughing. Bypassing the obstructing lips or tongue,
reducing the dead space, and endobronchial suction, may result, within
a few minutes or hours, in an increase in the tidal volume and an
improvement in the general condition when extubation may again be
attempted.

Repeated blood gas measurements
It is essential to repeat blood gas measurements, especially if
oxygen is administered, otherwise carbon dioxide retention may
become more profound than before treatment was started because of
the abolition of the hypoxic drive.

HYPOXIC DRIVE WHEN BREATHING AIR
Retention of carbon dioxide stimulates the respiratory centre so that
hyperpnoea is obvious. If the CO_2 accumulation is long-lasting or the
body is unable to excrete it in adequate amounts so that it gradually
rises, there comes a stage where the respiratory centre is no longer sensitive to its presence. Furthermore the increased $PaCO_2$ causes a
lowered PaO_2 (p. 67) which in turn causes hypoxaemia, which takes
over the role of stimulating the respiratory centre.

Effect of oxygen therapy on hypoxic drive
Administration of 100% oxygen results in the oxygen replacing the
nitrogen in the alveoli but the CO_2 is still being produced in the same
amount as before the start of the oxygen therapy. The increased PaO_2
removes the hypoxic drive. The respirations begin to fail but the
patient appears uncyanosed because oxygen diffusion is more than
adequate to provide a high PaO_2. On the other hand the hypoventilation fails increasingly to eliminate the carbon dioxide so that the
$PaCO_2$ progressively rises. Eventually carbon dioxide narcosis supervenes and the patient dies unless IPPV is started.

Administration of 24 – 28% oxygen often relieves hypoxaemia
without removing the hypoxic drive, but vigilance must be maintained
to see that such a concentration does not result in a rising PCO_2 level
and eventual apnoea. Cessation of breathing is less likely to occur
than if higher oxygen concentrations are given but if warranted they
should be given; however, the resuscitator must be capable of ventilating the patient by bag and mask.

Choice of oxygen concentration

This depends on the response of the PaO_2 and $PaCO_2$ and must be adjusted to changing circumstances. Although hard and fast rules cannot be stated it is helpful to proceed as follows:

(1) Patient conscious and breathing spontaneously – give 24–28% oxygen by mask.
(2) Patient unconscious, breathing spontaneously with well-established respiratory movement – give 24–28% oxygen through endotracheal tube; give 100% oxygen if improvement is not quickly established.
(3) Patient unconscious with poor respiratory excursions – give 100% oxygen and IPPV.

When the hypoxaemia is corrected as confirmed by the PaO_2 the oxygen percentage can be reduced accordingly.

SECTION III
THE HEART AND
CIRCULATION IN HEALTH
AND DISEASE

28

Physiology of the heart and circulation

The human vascular system is really two separate circulations, the high pressure systemic circulation, and the low pressure pulmonary circulation, driven by the left and right ventricles respectively. The adequacy of the circulation is dependent on the pumping action of the heart and the maintenance of normal circulating volume and vascular reflexes.

The heart as a pump

Since the systemic and pulmonary circulations are in series, in health the output from the left and right ventricles must be the same. Were this not the case, blood would build up on the venous side of the ventricle that was pumping less than the other, thereby producing 'backward failure', because the ventricle would be unable to pump away all the venous return. Acute left ventricular failure (LVF), therefore, leads to pulmonary venous congestion and often frank pulmonary oedema, whereas right ventricular failure (RVF) leads to systemic venous congestion and oedema.

The mechanisms that maintain the output of the two ventricles at the same level are not completely understood, but their derangement is thought to be responsible for the pulmonary oedema which can occur without apparent reason following head injury. The efficiency of the myocardium as a pump depends on venous return, myocardial contractility and peripheral resistance or afterload.

VENOUS RETURN

An adequate venous return is needed to give a suitable ventricular end diastolic pressure or 'preload'. As this pressure increases, according to Starling's Law, the more stretched the myocardial fibres become, and to a certain limit, the greater is the contraction developed. The venous return depends on:

(1) blood volume,
(2) sympathetic tone of arteries and veins,
(3) position of patient (compensated in health by (2)),
(4) intrathoracic pressure (including mechanical factors such as pericardial tamponade),
(5) muscle pump,
(6) absence of obstruction to venous return; obstruction can occur in the supine hypotensive syndrome or following a pulmonary embolus.

MYOCARDIAL CONTRACTILITY
This depends on the following factors:

The amount of healthy myocardium available
Loss of 40% of left ventricular function usually results in cardiogenic shock and death.

Action of drugs
These may be positively inotropic, augmenting contraction (for example, dopamine and isoprenaline), or negatively inotropic, depressing contraction (for example barbiturates or disopyramide).

Acidosis
Acidosis whether metabolic or respiratory in origin is cardio-depressant. Raised CO_2 levels can precipitate dysrhythmias.

Sympathetic outflow
In shock this is often maximal, and use of sympathomimetic drugs is often limited by the development of tachydysrhythmias.

Oxygenation and nutrition of the cell
Adequate oxygenation and supply of high energy compounds such as ATP (adenosine triphosphate), are as essential for the myocardial cell as for any other. The maintenance of the sodium pump and normal electrolyte levels (especially K^+, Ca^{2+}, Mg^{2+}) within and outside the cell are vital for normal contractility.

PERIPHERAL RESISTANCE OR AFTERLOAD
If the resistance against which the heart must pump rises excessively, cardiac output falls.

Systemic circulation and changes in disease

The systemic circulation is a high pressure system (typical pressure 125/75 mmHg), driven by the left ventricle, and subdivided into several secondary circulations, arranged in parallel (Figure 28.1).

This arrangement means first, that the perfusion pressure, whose value is equal to the difference between mean arterial and venous pressure, is the same for all organs and tissues and provides the maximal head of pressure possible across the organs at any given blood pressure. Second, with the system arranged in parallel the blood flow through individual organs can be increased or decreased in response to tissue requirements without necessarily influencing the blood flow to other organs.

A simple electrical analogy may be used to illustrate the circulatory changes in shock (Figure 28.1).

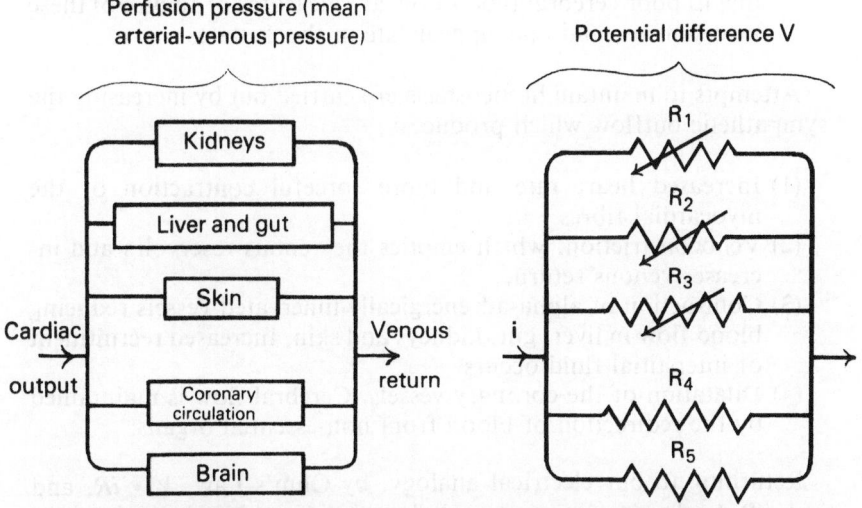

Figure 28.1 Electrical analogy to the systemic circulation

V, the potential difference across the resistances, is analogous to the perfusion pressure.

i, the current flowing through the system, is analogous to the cardiac output.

R_1, R_2, etc. the values of the resistances in the circuit are analogous to the resistance of each organ.

Those organs that are well supplied by sympathetic vasoconstrictor innervation of their vessels, such as the kidney, liver and gut, and skin, are represented by variable resistances. The brain and heart, on the other hand, have very few vasoconstrictor fibres passing to their vessels; the coronary vessels, in fact, have sympathetic vasodilator fibres. Consequently their resistance and blood flow change very little in the presence of generalized vasoconstriction, and so may be represented by fixed resistances.

The two major functions of cardiovascular homeostasis mechanisms are:

(1) To maintain blood pressure, pulse pressure, and circulating fluid volume.
(2) To maintain the cerebral and cardiac circulations. If necessary these are sustained at the expense of adequate performance of other organs, such as the liver, gut, and kidneys. Therefore a severe fall in blood pressure or clouding of the consciousness due to poor cerebral blood flow are measures of failure of these mechanisms, and may appear late in shock states.

Attempts to maintain homeostasis are carried out by increasing the sympathetic outflow which produces:

(1) Increased heart rate and more forceful contraction of the myocardial fibres.
(2) Venoconstriction, which empties the venous reservoirs and increases venous return.
(3) Contraction of alpha-adrenergically innervated vessels reducing blood flow in liver, gut, kidneys and skin. Increased recruitment of interstitial fluid occurs.
(4) Dilatation of the coronary vessels. Cerebral flow is maintained by the redirection of blood from non-essential organs.

Returning to our electrical analogy, by Ohm's Law, $V = iR$, and $i = V/R$. In the circulation as a whole, then, V tends to be maintained even if the value of i declines because the value of R, the total peripheral resistance, compensates by increasing its own value. Since V is unchanged or only slightly decreased, the current flow V/R_4 and V/R_5 through R_4 and R_5 (the blood flow through the heart and brain) is normal or only slightly decreased, although the current flow through R_1, R_2 and R_3, the blood flow through the kidneys, liver and gut, and skin, is considerably reduced. The net result is that the circulation to the heart and brain is sustained as long as the compensating mechanisms function effectively but at the expense of increasing the work done by the heart and of reducing the perfusion of some organs to a dangerous level.

THE VENOUS SYSTEM IN SHOCK

The importance of the venous side of the circulation has been emphasized in recent years. Although formerly the veins were thought to be the passive conduits from the tissues back to the heart, their function as a venous reservoir and their ability to transfer blood to the rest of the circulation in times of stress are now recognized. More than half the circulating blood at any time is in the systemic veins, while only 8% is in the systemic arteries.

Pulmonary circulation, functions, and changes in disease

The total blood flow through the lungs per minute is of course the same as the systemic output, that is about 5.5 l/min in a fit man at rest. Of the total blood volume 8% is in the pulmonary circulation, mostly in the pulmonary veins which act as a reservoir. In the adult, with the action of sitting up from the supine position, 400 ml of blood are discharged from the pulmonary veins into the systemic circulation. The pulmonary circulation is a low pressure system, and pulmonary artery pressure usually has a value of about 25/10 mmHg with a mean pressure of 15 mmHg. Pressure in the left atrium is about 7 mmHg, so the pressure head across the pulmonary circulation between the right ventricle and the left atrium averages only 8 mmHg, compared with about 90 mmHg in the systemic circulation.

Factors causing a rise in pressure in the systemic circulation have little effect on the pressure in the pulmonary circulation. This is because the resistance of the pulmonary circulation is only a tenth that of the systemic, and as flow through the pulmonary circulation increases, following an increase in systemic flow due to exercise, the resistance drops further by increasing the number of capillaries utilized (capillary recruitment), and distension of the capillaries already in use.

FUNCTIONS OF THE PULMONARY CIRCULATION

(1) To circulate blood to the alveoli to provide gas exchange of O_2 and CO_2.
(2) To act as a blood reservoir.
(3) To perform as a filter for particulate matter; it prevents emboli of fat, air or thrombus from the systemic veins reaching the brain or coronary arteries.

CHANGES IN DISEASE

Shock

When the cardiac output falls or the perfusion pressure across the lung drops, as in hypovolaemia or cardiogenic shock, the flow through the lung tends to diminish most in the uppermost parts of the lung due to a gravitational effect. This means that some ventilated areas will be underperfused thus increasing the dead space, and causing decreased efficiency in gas exchange. The PaO_2 therefore declines.

Pulmonary oedema
The causative factors are (see also p. 25):

(1) increased capillary permeability, as occurs in bacteraemic shock,
(2) increased net capillary hydrostatic pressure, as in left ventricular failure,
(3) decreased capillary osmotic pressure, as in hypoproteinaemia,
(4) decreased lymphatic drainage, as in carcinomatous infiltration.

As previously mentioned, the precise cause of pulmonary oedema following head injury has not been clearly identified.

Pulmonary embolism

Massive embolism — If an embolus blocks off a large enough part of the pulmonary circulation, the pressure rises in the pulmonary artery, and the right ventricle may show signs of strain or failure; arrhythmias may develop. The alveolar dead space increases and $\dot{V}/\dot{Q}$ mismatching decreases the efficiency of the parts of the lung still perfused. The main objective of treatment is to remove the block, or failing that, to move it more distally in the vascular tree.

Microemboli — Impaction of microemboli can produce an insidious deterioration of lung and circulatory function by gradual reduction of the numbers of functioning capillaries.

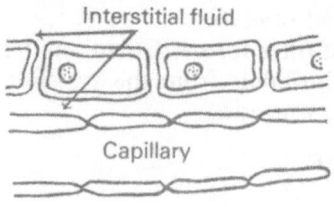

Figure 28.2 The cellular circulation

The microcirculation in health and disease
PHYSIOLOGY
The cell is the fundamental unit of all organisms. The integrity of the cell is dependent on the maintenance of its metabolic processes which enable the sodium pump to maintain the ionic gradients and electrical potential across the cell membrane. To sustain cellular function there must be:

(1) Adequate transport of nutrients and oxygen across the interstitial fluid from the capillaries to the cells (Figure 28.2), and of metabolic products and CO_2 to the capillaries for excretion.
(2) Normal ionic composition of the interstitial fluid bathing the cells. (The interstitial fluid has essentially the same ionic composition as other extracellular fluid, but differs from plasma in containing little protein.)

Satisfying both of these requirements is the essential function of the capillaries. Although only 5% of the circulating blood volume is in the capillaries at any one time, they are perhaps the most important part of the circulation, because they are directly responsible for the supply of nutrients to, and removal of waste products from, the cells via the interstitial fluid. It is thought that a volume of fluid equal to the plasma volume leaves the capillaries every minute to enter the interstitial fluid and an equal volume returns. The interstitial fluid, therefore, is not a static, sluggish volume of fluid, but a dynamic body of fluid constantly undergoing change in composition and often also in volume. The two major forces acting along every capillary to produce this massive exchange of fluid and materials are the net hydrostatic pressure, and the net osmotic pressure of the plasma proteins.

Net hydrostatic pressure
The hydrostatic pressure in the capillary at its arteriolar end is about 36 mmHg, while the interstitial fluid pressure is only about 1 mmHg; in other words the net hydrostatic pressure forcing fluid out of the capillary at its arteriolar end is 35 mmHg. This pressure diminishes along the capillary to a net 15 mmHg at the venular end, which is not enough to counteract the net osmotic pressure of the plasma proteins (Figure 28.3).

Net osmotic pressure of the plasma proteins
This pressure, of about 25 mmHg, acts along the whole length of the capillary to pull fluid back into the capillary. The balance of the

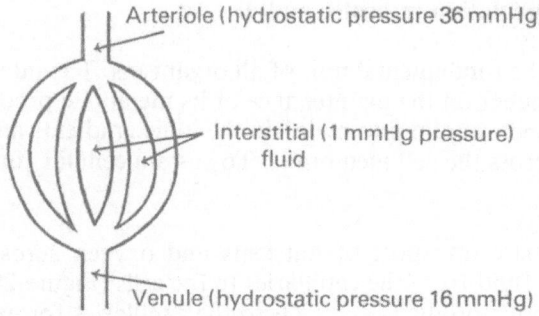

Figure 28.3 Pressures acting across the capillaries

opposing forces determines whether a net amount is lost to or gained by the circulation; a fall in the plasma osmotic pressure should cause a net loss of fluid from the circulation into the tissues, while a fall in the net hydrostatic pressure in the capillaries should cause a net gain to the circulation. Nowadays this is considered to be an oversimplification, and a great deal of active pumping of solutes is believed to occur across the capillary walls in addition to the purely passive effects described.

At any given time the majority of capillaries in a tissue are unused, but in response to local or systemic stimuli the flow through them can be increased or decreased to match tissue demands (capillary recruitment). Control is achieved by increasing or decreasing the resistance to either inflow to or outflow from the capillary bed.

There are three areas of variable resistance in the microcirculation:

(1) arterioles,
(2) precapillary sphincters,
(3) postcapillary sphincters.

All are controlled both by local reflex and metabolic activity and also by the systemic sympathetic outflow.

EFFECTS OF RESISTANCE CHANGES IN THE MICROCIRCULATION
If the tone of the precapillary sphincters or the arterioles is increased, the net hydrostatic pressure is decreased along the capillaries, and there is a net flow of tissue fluid into the capillaries. If, instead, the postcapillary sphincter tone is increased, then the net hydrostatic pressure along the capillary increases, and fluid is lost from the circulation (Figure 28.4).

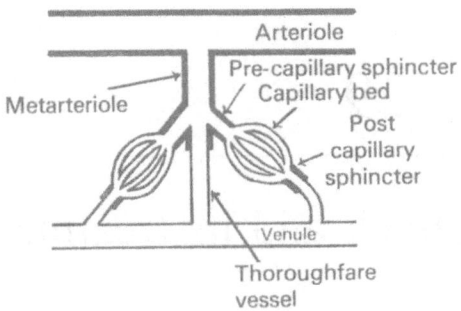

Figure 28.4 Diagrammatic representation of the microcirculation

It is said that in hypovolaemic shock the precapillary sphincters constrict in response to sympathetic stimuli more effectively than the postcapillary sphincters, so the circulation tends to gain fluid, an obvious benefit in hypovolaemia. However, if the constriction of the precapillary sphincters is prolonged, local tissue hypoxia occurs and acidotic products of metabolism collect in sufficient amounts to cause relaxation of the more sensitive precapillary sphincters while the postcapillary sphincters remain constricted. As a result, there is a net loss of fluid from the circulation; a vicious circle may develop in which increasing interstitial fluid pressure causes capillary closure, which in turn produces capillary cell hypoxia with swelling and increased permeability. Plasma-rich fluid is lost into the interstitial fluid, and the situation becomes more and more difficult to reverse.

The microcirculation can also be damaged insidiously by disseminated intravascular coagulation (DIC), particularly in prolonged hypovolaemia and in septic shock. Microemboli impact in the capillaries, causing signs and symptoms due to increasing circulatory embarrassment and to generalized cellular hypoxia and dysfunction.

29

Shock and its treatment

Definition and diagnosis of shock

Shock may be defined as inadequate perfusion of the tissues which is severe enough to lead to cellular damage.

It is important to emphasize the cellular level of the shock syndrome because the pathology is primarily in the microcirculation, and an adequate understanding of the pathophysiology is necessary before logical treatment can be applied to the individual case. There are classically four categories:

(1) hypovolaemic (haemorrhagic),
(2) septicaemic, bacteraemic or endotoxic,
(3) cardiogenic,
(4) anaphylactic.

Other conditions producing a shock-like state can occasionally give rise to confusion, for example:

(1) restricted venous return, as occurs in tension pneumothorax, cardiac tamponade, and supine hypotension of pregnancy;
(2) loss of vasomotor tone, as in spinal cord transection;
(3) adrenal insufficiency, following steroid withdrawal;
(4) psychological reactions, due to pain, grief or fear.

Hypovolaemic shock

AETIOLOGY AND PATHOPHYSIOLOGY

This kind of shock is caused by loss of circulating fluid volume usually through blood loss which may be internal or external; it may also be due to plasma loss as occurs in burns or in sequestration of plasma-rich fluid in the gut, or even extracellular fluid loss as in cholera.

The initial and most important symptoms and signs in hypovolaemic shock are not due directly to the loss itself, but to the attempts of the homeostatic mechanisms of the body to minimize the

240

effects of the loss, and to maintain adequate function of priority organs such as the brain and heart. Increased sympathetic outflow causes:

(1) raised heart rate and increased myocardial contractility.
(2) peripheral vasoconstriction in organs not immediately essential for survival, such as the kidneys, liver and gut, and skin. Shunting of blood occurs through arteriovenous shunts bypassing the capillary beds, and tone is increased in the arteriolar and precapillary sphincters which increases fluid recruitment from the interstitial fluid.
(3) venoconstriction, which augments the circulation by shifting blood to the arterial side of the circulation;
(4) the coronary and cerebral flow to be maintained by shunting blood from other circulations and shortening the circulation time.

There is also a massive increase in the output of other hormones, particularly glucocorticoids and mineralocorticoids causing:

(1) increased glucose production from glycogen and protein breakdown.
(2) water and sodium retention,
(3) increased potassium and nitrogen loss.

The above changes due to increased sympathetic outflow lead to increasing tissue hypoxia. Cellular metabolism is disrupted, and cellular oedema and increased permeability appear. Fluid is lost from the circulation, and the capillaries become blocked by oedema and slow-moving viscous blood. This perpetuates a vicious circle of hypoxia→poor metabolism→further hypoxia (Figure 29.1).

SIGNS OF A FAILING CIRCULATION
These are due to, in order of their appearance:

(1) The responses of the compensatory mechanisms such as tachycardia and peripheral vasoconstriction which maintain circulating volume and pressure;
(2) poor cellular and tissue function in non-priority organs, such as kidneys, liver and guts, and skin;
(3) the deterioration of myocardial and brain function—in cardiogenic shock the myocardial function is obviously grossly impaired from the outset.

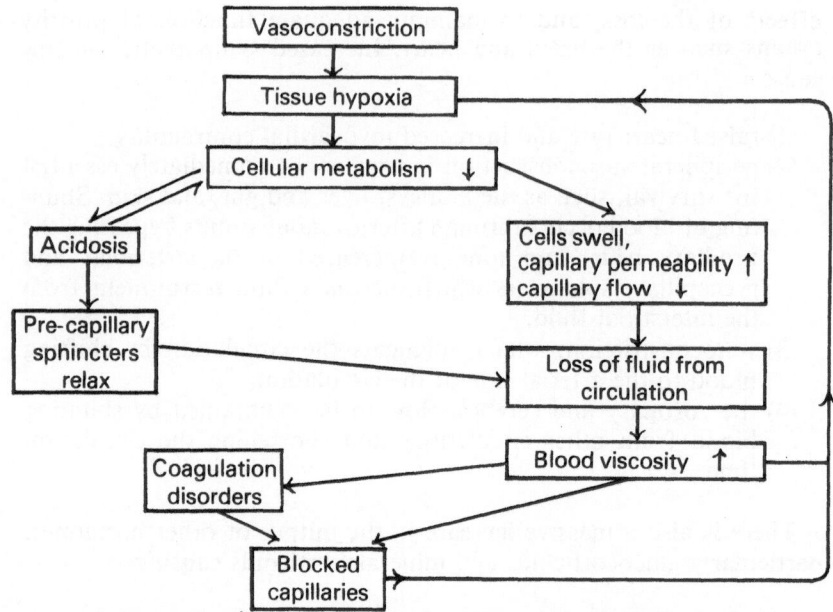

Figure 29.1 Flow diagram – microcirculation in shock

Signs of circulatory compensation
Increased sympathetic activity is the first sign of compensation.
Pulse – A rising pulse rate, becoming 'thready', is usually the first
sign of the loss of 10% or more of the circulating volume. However,
the pulse can be altered by many other factors, such as emotion, head
injury, or drugs.
Blood pressure – Since the homeostatic mechanisms tend to maintain the blood pressure, it can be temporarily normal or even elevated.
However, when more than 20% of the blood volume has been lost, the
blood pressure usually begins to fall. Old or sick people with less flexible vascular systems decompensate more rapidly. In cardiogenic and
septicaemic shock the blood pressure can be low from the outset.

It is common practice to equate the blood pressure with the cardiac
output. But this is very misleading, because the two are very different,
blood pressure being proportional to cardiac output multiplied by
peripheral resistance. Therefore, in the presence of a falling cardiac
output, the blood pressure can be maintained at least initially by increasing the peripheral resistance.

The blood pressure must never be considered in isolation – for instance, a patient whose blood pressure is normally 210/110 mmHg

may be in severe shock if it falls to an *apparently* normal 120/70 mmHg.

Peripheral resistance – The extent of the peripheral resistance can often be estimated in a warm environment by feeling the temperature of the arms and legs. In low output states, the skin is usually cold and often clammy. Increasing skin warmth is frequently used as a fairly sensitive guide to progress in treatment. A temperature sensor is applied to the foot, and another is inserted in the rectum or oesophagus to record the core temperature. As the condition improves the temperature difference narrows, and vice versa.

The three signs above should be considered together in the assessment of the circulation, because cardiac output is dependent on them all, and no two patients are alike. For example, in endotoxic shock, one patient may at the outset have profound hypotension with warm extremities (appropriately named 'warm hypotension') while another may have a normal blood pressure with cold extremities and oliguria. Yet, in both patients, the actual measured cardiac output may be identical.

The central venous pressure (CVP)

This may be another useful guide to the assessment of the circulation. The CVP is the pressure of the blood measured in the great veins leading to the right side of the heart or in the right atrium itself. The pressure in the right atrium is normally 0 to 5 cmH$_2$O, but may be greatly increased in mitral valve disease or cardiac failure. In clinical practice the CVP is measured in relation to a fixed point. This is either the sternal angle (considered to be 5 cm anterior to the right atrium) giving normal values of -5 to 0 cm, or the midaxillary line (taken to be at the level of the right atrium) giving values of 0 to $+5$ cm in the normal person.

The central venous pressure depends on three factors:

(1) The amount of blood returning to the heart, which in turn depends on:
   (a) the blood volume,
   (b) venoconstriction,
   (c) the intrathoracic pressure,
   (d) the muscle pump, driving the blood towards the heart.
(2) The ability of the heart to pump away the venous return.
(3) The position of the patient; the CVP should always be measured with the patient in the same position, and the value must always be referred to the same fixed point, either the sternal angle or the midaxillary line, as above.

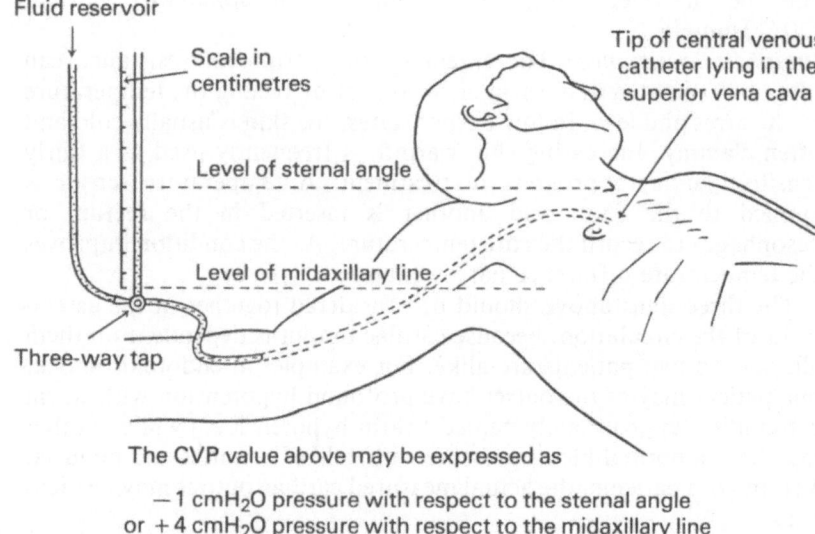

The CVP value above may be expressed as

−1 cmH₂O pressure with respect to the sternal angle
or +4 cmH₂O pressure with respect to the midaxillary line

Figure 29.2 The CVP line and reference levels

It is therefore an oversimplification to say that the CVP will fall
with blood loss, and the extent of its fall will always be proportional to
the blood loss. Although loss of blood decreases the venous return and
tends to reduce the CVP, the compensatory venoconstriction improves the venous return, and the CVP may well return to normal
despite the continuing hypovolaemia. Consequently, the value must
never be examined uncritically or in isolation from other signs of circulatory adequacy.

On the other hand, in the late stages of peripheral circulatory
failure, there is often progressive myocardial dysfunction which
causes a rise in the CVP due to the 'backward failure' of the right ventricle, despite persisting hypovolaemia.

A low CVP in the presence of warm, well-perfused extremities is
likely to be of less significance than a normal or even a high value in
the presence of oliguria and cold extremities. In recent years it has
been increasingly recognized that in CVP measurement the values obtained are of the venous side of the right ventricle when the concern is
primarily with the venous return to the left ventricle, and consequently
the pressure on the venous side of the failing systemic circulation.
Although in health the pressures on the venous side of the left and
right ventricles should be similar, this is not necessarily the same in
disease, where one ventricle may fail with respect to the other. This is

particularly likely in cardiogenic shock, where a better estimate of left atrial pressure can be made by floating a flow-directed balloon-tipped catheter (Swan–Ganz catheter) via the superior vena cava, right atrium and ventricle and pulmonary artery until it impacts in a distal branch of the pulmonary artery. As the catheter blocks the minor artery in which it lies, the pressure measured at its tip reflects the pressures distal to it in the arteriole, capillaries, venule, and vein, which in turn reflect the pressure in the left atrium.

A useful function of a CVP line is to note the response of the circulation to a fast infusion of 200–300 ml colloid. If the CVP falls back to its previous level quickly the circulation is normal or hypovolaemic, the myocardium can cope, and more may be infused. However, if the CVP rises and stays high the circulation is overloaded, the myocardium cannot cope with the increased load and no more should be infused. Finding the value of the CVP or the pulmonary capillary wedge pressure which produces the optimum output enables the clinician to find the optimum preload for the individual patient. This may be as high as $15\,cmH_2O$ measured at the midaxillary line, following cardiac surgery or in the patient with mitral valve disease.

Signs of poor tissue flow
These are as follows:

(1) Cold, clammy skin; delayed filling of skin capillaries after blanching with pressure.

(2) Oliguria or anuria; it is often said that pink, warm feet means pink, warm kidneys. Certainly in the absence of intrinsic renal disease, a fall in urine output in peripheral circulatory failure is a good indicator of inadequate renal perfusion, and a rise in the output following treatment of the underlying circulatory cause is an early sign of improvement. Hourly urine output should be charted. Urinary urea concentration is usually increased, and sodium concentration is low. The treatment is that of the extrinsic cause, that is, the poor circulation. Diuretics in this situation are of little value, and serve to confuse the clinician who may attribute an increased urinary flow to an improving circulation, when it is due entirely to the diuretic.

The use of loop diuretics such as frusemide may shorten the period of oliguria if it persists after correction of the circulation. Frusemide, however, can be nephrotoxic and ototoxic and large doses should not be given routinely, particularly if cephalosporin or aminoglycoside antibiotics are being used.

(3) Deteriorating acid–base balance with increasing metabolic acidosis and a rising lactate level.

Deterioration of myocardial and cerebral function
Myocardial function – Deterioration of myocardial function may
be either primary, as in cardiogenic shock, or secondary, as in
hypovolaemic and endotoxic shock, where accumulation of
metabolites, endotoxins and acidosis can depress the myocardium and
make effective treatment difficult. The development of arrhythmias,
the continuing deterioration of organ and circulatory function despite
appropriate treatment associated with a rising CVP, and the inability
of the heart to cope with small increments of colloid intravenously,
are bad prognostic signs.

The ECG – The usefulness of the ECG in assessing the failing circulation is limited but it is useful in:

(1) diagnosing treatable arrhythmias which produce inefficient
    myocardial activation;
(2) diagnosing characteristic appearances of specific or generalized
    myocardial damage or of pulmonary embolus;
(3) assessing electrolyte disorders and their treatment, particularly
    disorders of potassium.

TREATMENT OF HYPOVOLAEMIC SHOCK
The cornerstone of treatment of hypovolaemic shock is the adequate
replacement of the type of fluid which has been lost. This may be
blood, plasma, other extracellular fluid (ECF) or mixed losses from all
the compartments, including intracellular fluid (ICF). Where trauma
is the cause of blood loss, other problems such as a crushed chest or a
head injury may require urgent attention. As in other emergencies, the
airway and the circulation are the two priorities.

FLUID REPLACEMENT AND BODY COMPARTMENTS
In fluid replacement, the first consideration is restoration of the
plasma volume, followed by the rest of the ECF, and then if necessary
by the ICF. The main guide to adequate replacement is the improvement in the general condition of the patient as restoration of the body
compartments proceed (Figure 29.3).

Plasma
The plasma is separated from the rest of the ECF by the capillary wall,
which allows free passage of water and ions, but only a minimal

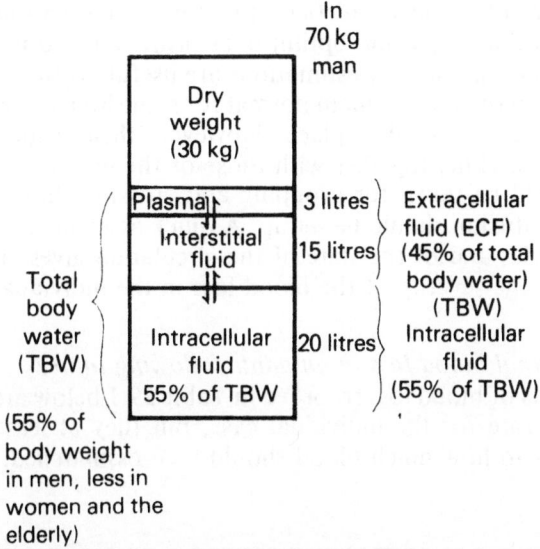

Figure 29.3 Body compartments

amount of protein. Essentially it has the same ionic composition as the rest of the ECF.

Interstitial fluid
This undergoes rapid and constant turnover in the tissues, except for the small part sequestrated in bones and ligaments. The main cation is sodium and the main anion is chloride. In health its ionic composition is maintained remarkably constant.

Intracellular fluid
This has a high potassium and phosphate content and is separated from the ECF by cell membranes. The ionic differences and electrical charge across the cell membrane are maintained by the sodium pump.

ESTIMATION OF BLOOD AND PLASMA LOSS
Of the circulating blood volume 10% can usually be lost without noticeable effects, although old people tolerate blood loss poorly. Loss of more than 20% causes a decline in cardiac output and blood pressure (p. 242).

Blood loss can be internal, external or both. Even when it is wholly external the volume lost is difficult to estimate. Patients usually exaggerate, and doctors, being optimists at heart, tend to underestimate the losses. Few laboratory estimations are useful, as the haemoglobin and haematocrit values remain normal for some hours after blood loss until haemodilution takes place. However, their values should be taken as a baseline, together with those of the urea and electrolytes. Blood should be taken for grouping and crossmatching, and an intravenous infusion should be set up. A quick assessment of the extent of the injuries and of the state of the circulation gives an initial impression of the severity of the blood loss in the individual patient.

Likely internal blood loss in an adult following injury
The amounts of blood loss recorded in Table 29.1 below are inevitably very inaccurate for the individual case, but they at least give some guidance as to how much blood should be crossmatched.

Table 29.1

Injured area	Moderate injury	Severe injury
Arm	500 ml	1000 ml
Lower leg	500 ml	2000 ml
Thigh	1000 ml	3500 ml
Pelvis	1000 ml	4000 ml
Abdomen	1000 ml	5000 ml
Chest	1000 ml	4000 ml

REPLACEMENT OF BLOOD LOSS
The normal blood volume at birth is 85 ml/kg, falling to about 70 ml/kg in adults. Therefore, an adult man of 70 kg should have a circulating blood volume of 5.0 l (composed of about 2.2 l red blood cells, and 2.8 l plasma).

Blood, plasma, or plasma substitutes are usually given when 10–20% of circulating blood volume has been lost. Circulating volume is of greater importance than the total red cell mass; indeed, many authorities recommend the initial administration of plasma or plasma substitutes to maintain the blood volume, and suggest that the reduced viscosity of the blood due to the haemodilution leads to improved tissue perfusion. Frequent assessment of the circulation is necessary particularly when the blood loss is heavy, or the extent of the loss is unknown. Central venous or pulmonary wedge pressure measurements are useful to control replacement under these circumstances, or when myocardial function is impaired.

Plasma losses
Major losses of plasma occur after burns. Lesser amounts are often sequestrated in loops of strangulated gut in patients with obstruction.

Plasma loss after burns
The plasma loss in burns is proportional to the area of skin involved, and may be estimated in adults by the 'rule of nine' (Figure 29.4). Many

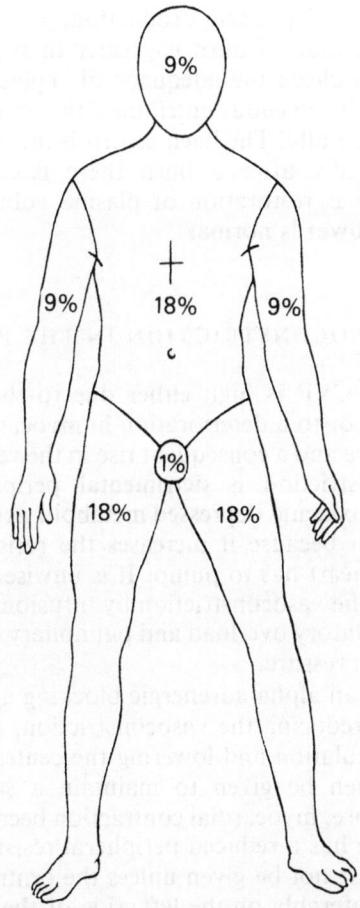

Figure 29.4 Skin areas as percentage of total surface area

regimes are available to indicate the amount of plasma or plasma substitute required. The following is one such scheme: The volume to be given over the first 48 hours following a burn is 120 ml for each per cent of the body burned, to an initial maximum of 6.0 l. Half of this volume should be given in the first 8 hours. Thus a person sustaining a 25% burn requires 3.0 l plasma or substitute, 1.5 l being given in the first 8 hours. In addition, the patient is given his normal fluid requirements.

Red cell loss

Whole blood is frequently indicated in deep burns to compensate for red cell destruction, depressed production, and increased red cell fragility. When the area of burn is greater than 30% a CVP line is useful, not only to check the adequacy of replacement, but also to provide a route for intravenous nutrition if the patient is unable or unwilling to be fed enterally. The haematocrit is the most useful guide to improvement; initially after a burn there is considerable haemoconcentration, but as restoration of plasma volume progresses, the haematocrit falls towards normal.

Problems in shock

PERSISTENT VASOCONSTRICTION IN THE PRESENCE OF AN ELEVATED CVP

In these cases the CVP is high either due to therapy with plasma volume expanders, or to a deterioration in myocardial function causing backward failure and a consequent rise in the venous pressure. The persistent vasoconstriction is detrimental peripherally because it causes cellular hypoxia and depressed metabolic activity, and centrally to the myocardium because it increases the resistance or afterload against which the heart has to pump. It is unwise in this situation to attempt to reduce the vasoconstriction by infusion of plasma because it may lead to circulatory overload and pulmonary oedema, by further raising the venous pressure.

Judicious use of an alpha-adrenergic blocking agent can 'open-up' the circulation by reducing the vasoconstriction, thus increasing the capacity of the circulation and lowering the central venous pressure. More fluid can then be given to maintain a suitable myocardial preload. Furthermore, myocardial contraction becomes more efficient as the left ventricle has a reduced peripheral resistance to overcome. Alpha-blockers must not be given unless the central venous pressure on the right, or preferably on the left, side of the heart is known by means of a central line or a Swan–Ganz catheter. The systolic blood pressure must be at least 90 mmHg since the major hazard of the technique is the production of severe hypotension with reduced coronary artery perfusion. The following drugs are suitable for reducing vasoconstriction.

Phentolamine
This is an alpha-adrenergic blocker with a length of action of 10–15 minutes. It is given intravenously in doses of 1 mg/min and is usually the drug of choice due to its effectiveness and short action; it also improves myocardial contractility to a minor degree.

Chlorpromazine
This drug has a milder alpha-blocking effect than phentolamine, but a longer action. It is given intravenously in doses of 5 mg/h until a suitable effect is obtained.

ACIDOSIS AND BICARBONATE THERAPY
Acidosis in shock is due to inadequate cellular metabolism in the presence of tissue hypoxia, usually caused by a sluggish or obstructed microcirculation. The effectiveness of the buffer systems of the body is also decreased in shock, and if kidney function is depressed, the excretion of acid products is limited. It is often customary to treat the acidosis, repeatedly if necessary, with bicarbonate solution, using the formula below to estimate the appropriate amount:

$$\frac{\text{Body weight (kg)} \times \text{base deficit (mmol/l)}}{4} = \text{mmol of bicarbonate required}$$

The reasoning behind the above formula is that the deficit of base is distributed throughout the extracellular fluid, whose volume is approximately one-fourth of the body weight.

Advantages and disadvantages of bicarbonate therapy
The advantage is that the myocardial and brain cells which are still being adequately perfused in the shock situation function more satisfactorily in a less acid environment.

The disadvantages are:

(1) Although the acid–base state of the patient (as measured in arterial blood) may return to normal after bicarbonate therapy it is essential to remember that the acidosis has merely been *buf-*

fered, not *cured.* Bicarbonate penetrates cells poorly, so they are no less acidic. The cause of the acidosis must be treated by improving cell perfusion and metabolism (p. 252).

(2) A decreasing acidosis indicates both an improving microcirculation and oxygenation, a sign which may be obscured by bicarbonate therapy.

(3) A *slight* acidosis improves tissue oxygen uptake by causing a shift to the right in the haemoglobin dissociation curve.

(4) The sodium load when bicarbonate is given may be considerable, and this is contraindicated in some patients; 100 ml of 8.4% sodium bicarbonate solution contains 100 mmol of sodium ions as well as 100 mmol of bicarbonate ions, while the normal adult daily requirement of sodium is only 50–100 mmol.

The advantages and disadvantages of bicarbonate therapy must be considered in every patient with acidosis. If the acidosis is severe, with a base deficit of 8 mmol/l or more, a single infusion of bicarbonate following the formula

$$\frac{\text{Body weight (kg)} \times \text{base deficit (mmol/l)}}{4} = \text{mmol bicarbonate required}$$

may be given to improve the acid–base status of the ECF while strenuous efforts are being made to improve the tissue circulation and metabolism.

GLUCOSE–POTASSIUM–INSULIN REGIMEN (GKI)

Cellular metabolism in shock can often be improved in the presence of an adequate microcirculation by the use of a mixture of 50% glucose, potassium salts, and insulin (GKI regimen). The logic behind the use of this solution is that the insulin moves the glucose intracellularly to stimulate the metabolic processes within the cells. Since potassium enters the cells with the glucose, hypokalaemia can occur unless a potassium salt is added to the solution. A phosphate salt of potassium is included since phosphate is a component of the high energy compounds such as ATP (adenosine triphosphate) which are required for the maintenance of cellular function.

A suitable solution in a patient with normal potassium and blood sugar levels is

80 mmol potassium, half as potassium chloride and
    half as potassium dihydrogen phosphate   ⎫
                                           ⎬   in 450 ml
                                           ⎪   50%
80 units soluble insulin   ⎭   dextrose

Initially 100 ml of this solution can be given over 1 hour, under ECG monitoring, to provide an early warning of hyperkalaemia or hypokalaemia. Due to its high osmolality the solution is extremely irritant if given into a peripheral vein.

POOR MYOCARDIAL FUNCTION

Myocardial contractility is invariably depressed after myocardial infarction, usually diminished in septic shock, and often reduced in the late stages of hypovolaemic shock. If the blood pressure is low and the cardiac output appears to be deteriorating as indicated by the appearance of oliguria, metabolic acidosis and cold extremities, myocardial function may require support with positive inotropic drugs. Therapy to restore and maintain myocardial function is directed to the improvement of cell environment, abolition of arrhythmias, and the use of positive inotropic drugs.

Improvement of cell environment

All necessary measures are taken to improve oxygenation and restore the PO_2 of the arterial blood to at least 60 mmHg (8 kPa), to reduce acidosis, correct electrolyte disorders, and improve cell metabolism.

Control of arrhythmias

Arrhythmias (p. 14) may require urgent treatment, particularly fast arrhythmias which prevent adequate ventricular filling in diastole, and slow arrhythmias which limit the cardiac output.

Beta-adrenergic agonists

All have short biological halflives, and are given by continuous intravenous infusion.

Isoprenaline (Isoproterenol) – This drug (dose $0.02 - 0.2$ (μg/kg)/min) has both beta-1 and beta-2 actions, causing an increase in myocardial contractility and heart rate, and a decrease in peripheral resistance, due largely to the shunting of blood through dilated muscle arterioles. Renal blood flow may be reduced.

Dopamine – The effects of dopamine on the circulation and the heart depend on the dosage. Infusions of $0.5 - 2$ (μg/kg)/min improve renal blood flow and glomerular filtration rate (dopaminergic receptors).

At infusion rates of $2 - 10$ (μg/kg)/min heart rate and myocardial contractility are increased, and the peripheral resistance is lowered or unchanged (beta-1-receptors). At dose rates above 20 (μg/kg)/min the peripheral resistance is raised and the renal blood flow is reduced (alpha-receptors).

Dopamine is less likely to cause arrhythmias and sinus tachycardia than isoprenaline, and is also less likely to extend any area of infarction. *Dobutamine* – This recently introduced drug (dose 4 – 40 (μg/kg)/min has not yet been fully assessed for use in shock. It is said to selectively increase contractility without altering the heart rate.

At present, dopamine is the agent of choice in shock, except where there is bradycardia, when isoprenaline should be used because of its greater chronotropic effect. In states of hypotension high dosage rates of dopamine may be required initially for its alpha-agonist effect to produce a systolic blood pressure of at least 90 mmHg and so maintain adequate coronary perfusion. This dose rate should, however, be reduced as soon as possible to reduce the left ventricular afterload.

Other agents
Glucagon – Glucagon (dose 5 – 10 mg/h by continuous infusion) has an inotropic effect, and may be used if the sympathomimetic agents prove inadequate.

Digoxin – This drug should probably not be used in shock because of its long halflife, and its uncertain metabolism and excretion.

BLEEDING PROBLEMS
In shock, bleeding may be due to activation of the fibrinolytic system or to dilution or consumption of the clotting factors. Early advice from a haematologist should be sought whenever there is an unexplained bleeding problem. Disseminated intravascular coagulation (DIC) which often occurs in shock, is discussed more fully in Chapter 30; in brief, the clinician should be alerted to the possibility of DIC whenever bleeding is associated with:

(1) A predisposing cause
    (a) hypoxia, such as in prolonged hypotension,
    (b) infection, particularly with septicaemia,
    (c) trauma,
    (d) massive transfusion.
(2) Unexplained and generalized deterioration of organ function, including deterioration of conscious level, urinary output, cardiac output, and arterial oxygenation.
(3) A low platelet count.

OLIGURIA OR ANURIA
Precipitating factors must be treated, for example:

(1) inadequate renal perfusion which may be due to hypovolaemia, DIC or cardiogenic shock,
(2) septicaemia or toxaemia,
(3) electrolyte or acid−base disturbances.

If prolonged, deterioration in renal function due to circulation problems (prerenal causes) can lead to renal damage through ischaemia. Differentiation between prerenal and renal causes of depressed renal function is difficult, as a degree of both is often present. Table 29.2 is a useful guide.

Table 29.2

	Prerenal uraemia	*Ischaemic renal failure*
Urinary sodium (mmol/l)	< 20	> 50
Urine/plasma urea ratio	> 10	< 10
Urine/plasma osmolal ratio	> 1.2	< 1.1
Urine osmolality (mosmol/kg)	> 500 usually	similar to plasma

Use of diuretics
There is no evidence that diuretics such as frusemide have any effect on renal function once failure is established, and the use of diuretics in these circumstances remains controversial. In high doses frusemide can itself cause renal damage, especially in the presence of other potentially nephrotoxic agents such as cephaloridine or the aminoglycoside antibiotics. It is suggested that no more than one dose of frusemide should be given (a maximum of 250 mg intravenously) and the patient should be treated as for acute renal failure as outlined below.

Management of acute renal failure
Conservative management − The initial steps are:
    (1) control fluid and electrolyte balance;
    (2) control any hyperkalaemia;
    (3) reduce catabolism and therefore urea production by high calorie intake.
Haemodialysis or peritoneal dialysis − This is contemplated when:
    (1) the patient has a gross fluid overload;
    (2) when the blood urea is rising rapidly, and approaching 30 mmol/l.

HYPERKALAEMIA

Hyperkalaemia can occur in shock, especially in the presence of massive tissue damage or in association with renal failure. In the ECG the first signs are tall, peaked T waves, followed, as the potassium level continues to rise, by absent P waves and prolonged QRS complexes. These are followed by ventricular tachycardia and fibrillation.

Treatment
  (1) To transfer some of the potassium intracellularly 100 ml 50% glucose with 20 units soluble insulin is given.
  (2) To protect the heart against the dysrhythmic properties of potassium 10 ml 10% calcium chloride is given intravenously; this should be given slowly because too rapid infusion may itself cause arrhythmias.
  (3) To increase the excretion of the potassium ion 60 g calcium resonium should be given either rectally or orally.

Bicarbonate solution to combat the acidosis present is contra-indicated as it may induce hypocalcaemic convulsions or tetany, and constitutes a considerable sodium load.

Septicaemic shock

AETIOLOGY, INCIDENCE AND MORTALITY

Septicaemic, bacteraemic and endotoxic shock are terms often used synonymously. More precisely:

Septicaemia exists when pathogenic bacteria are actively multiplying in the circulation and produce symptoms of disease.

Bacteraemia exists when bacteria are present in the bloodstream; this is common, and no problems usually ensue.

Endotoxaemia exists when toxins, circulating in the bloodstream, produce symptoms and signs of disease. These are released by the disruption of the cell walls of gram-negative bacteria, sometimes as a result of antibiotic treatment. Toxins are also produced by gram-positive bacteria, giving a clinical picture usually indistinguishable from that of gram-negative toxaemia. Although they usually coexist, toxaemia can be present without overt sepsis, and sepsis can exist without toxaemia.

Incidence. Septicaemic shock is said to affect at least 1% of all hospital admissions.

Mortality depends on the state of the patient when therapy is commenced. It is greater than 60% when hypotension is associated with poor peripheral perfusion and oliguria.

CLINICAL FEATURES

These are only mentioned because the symptomatology can be protean, and vary from an insidious onset with hypotension and warm extremities ('warm hypotension', p. 243) to acute collapse with tachypnoea which may mimic myocardial infarction or pulmonary embolism.

(1) The patient may by pyrexial and have rigors, or be hypothermic.
(2) The patient may have peripheral vasoconstriction and hypotension ('cold hypotension') with other signs of reduced cardiac output, or 'warm hypotension', associated with a normal or even elevated output.
(3) The patient may present with signs and symptoms of multiorgan failure, bleeding, polyuria or oliguria, jaundice, vomiting and diarrhoea, confusion or coma, or deteriorating lung function with hypoxia and tachypnoea.

PREDISPOSING CONDITIONS

(1) Infection of any body system.
(2) Instrumentation, including urinary catheterization and insertion or presence of venous cannulae.
(3) Recent operation or anaesthetic.
(4) Blockage or suppression of the reticuloendothelial system, such as in immunosuppressive therapy, agranulocytosis and neoplasia.
(5) Portosystemic bypass. In cirrhosis or following portocaval bypass procedures, blood and toxins can pass from the portal system to the systemic circulation without being filtered by the reticuloendothelial system.

PATHOPHYSIOLOGY

The end result of the septicaemia and toxaemia is similar to that in other causes of shock, namely deterioration of function in many tissues due to damage to the microcirculation, followed by cellular hypoxia and deranged metabolism. The initial damage to the circulation by the toxaemia becomes self-sustaining in a vicious circle of vasoconstriction, hypoxia and acidosis, which eventually prove fatal.

EFFECTS OF ENDOTOXINS

(1) Release of histamine and kinins produces vasodilatation and increased capillary permeability, which may be severe enough to lead to extravasation of protein-rich fluid from the capillaries, and eventually hypovolaemia. The release often occurs early in the illness, causing 'warm hypotension', which if allowed to progress becomes 'cold hypotension' with circulatory failure.

(2) Vasoconstriction, both as a direct effect on the vessel walls and by stimulation of the sympathetic nervous system, and also by activation of the renin−angiotensin system.

(3) Pyrogenic effect.

(4) Antagonism to the actions of glucocorticoids.

(5) Depression of cellular respiration in general; leukocytes and platelets are also damaged.

(6) Activation of the coagulation system and inhibition of protective fibrinolysis.

(7) Damage to the capillary endothelium; the latter three effects tend to induce disseminated intravascular coagulation (DIC).

(8) Decrease of protective phagocytosis.

(9) Production of disturbances of carbohydrate and fat metabolism, leading eventually to hypoglycaemia.

To summarize: there is widespread tissue damage, due not only to the direct effects of the toxaemia, but also to the indirect effects on the circulation and the myocardium. There is obstruction to the microcirculation by emboli and thrombus formation due to DIC and swelling of the endothelial cells due to hypoxia and acidosis. A bleeding diathesis may appear.

AIMS OF TREATMENT
Removal of infection
This may be difficult if the organism is unknown. If the identity of the causal organism is known or suspected from the history, the appropriate narrow spectrum antibiotic can be given, once appropriate specimens including blood have been taken for bacteriological culture. Gram-negative bacteraemia is now more common in hospitals than Gram-positive infections. Anaerobic organisms are increasing in frequency.

Endotoxaemia can come from the patient's own gut flora, especially when the reticuloendothelial cells of the liver are functioning poorly, or are bypassed. When the bowel mucosa is hypoxic, endotoxins may pass from the mucosa into the peritoneal cavity and thence into the bloodstream. If the source of the infection is uncertain, any focus for infection should be removed, including urinary catheters and central venous catheters, and replaced, if essential, under strict asepsis. Surgery may be required to drain an abscess or repair a ruptured anastomosis. This should be carried out sooner rather than later if surgery is necessary, as operation can sometimes result in dramatic improvement, while delay can mean death.

If a broad-spectrum antibiotic has to be used initially a combination such as clindamycin and gentamycin or chloramphenicol and gentamycin may be used. Metronidazole is very useful if anaerobes are suspected. A further problem is that the antibiotics may increase the endotoxaemia temporarily by disrupting the cell walls of the causative organisms.

Maintenance of the circulation

The aim must be to provide the optimum conditions of preload, myocardial function and afterload in the heart and circulation (see p. 250). Central venous pressure monitoring, or pulmonary wedge pressure monitoring if myocardial function is compromised, is essential.

Maintenance of organ function

Respiratory function – Septic shock is a well recognized cause of 'shock lung', or the adult repiratory distress syndrome. Microembolization of pulmonary capillaries, interstitial and often intra-alveolar pulmonary oedema, and damage to the surfactant-producing cells occur. As a result the lungs become less efficient at effecting gaseous exchange, while the work of respiration is increased by the reduction in pulmonary compliance. Initially the impaired efficiency of the lungs is masked as far as blood gases are concerned if the patient is on added oxygen (by MC mask (p. 69), for example), and the best guides to deterioration – which may be rapid – are the clinical signs of respiratory distress and increased respiratory work, such as a rising respiratory rate, mouth breathing, the use of accessory respiratory muscles, anxiety and restlessness. The $PaCO_2$ is often normal or even below normal until the respiratory homeostatic mechanisms of the body are overwhelmed, and the decision to institute mechanical ventilation is best taken on the clinical picture rather than on laboratory data.

General cellular function – This may be improved by the infusion of a glucose and insulin regimen as discussed previously (p. 252). The amount of potassium added depends on the serum potassium levels, which can be high or low in septic shock; ECG monitoring is essential. Hypoglycaemia and hypophosphataemia are both common in septic shock, while hypocalcaemia may also require correction. The regimen is particularly useful to support myocardial and hepatic function, and should be used as a preliminary for full parenteral nutrition, with glucose as the main nutrient. Fat emulsions, which may block the reticuloendothelial system, are contraindicated.

Renal function – This may deteriorate due to prerenal or renal causes, and require treatment. Urine output, plasma electrolyte and urea levels should be closely monitored.

Steroids
Steroids in pharmacological doses:

(1) encourage peripheral vasodilatation;
(2) have a membrane-stabilizing effect;
(3) encourage endotoxin detoxification;
(4) may preserve surfactant production in the lungs.

Methylprednisolone, in two doses of 1 g each 6 hours apart, is often given in septic shock. However, the value of this therapy remains controversial.

Two doses only should be given due to the undesirable side-effects of steroids, particularly immunosuppression.

Other aspects of treatment
Disseminated intravascular coagulation (DIC) may require treatment with heparin or blood components (p. 271).

Other aspects of septicaemic shock may require treatment, for example acidosis, arrhythmias, or liver failure (10% of cases of septic shock are jaundiced, and a much higher percentage have abnormal liver function tests). Cimetidine infusion in non-trauma patients reduces the risk of gastrointestinal bleeding.

Cardiogenic shock
DEFINITION
Cardiogenic shock is defined as myocardial infarction complicated by:

(1) Hypotension of 90 mmHg systolic or less; if the patient has previously been hypertensive, shock may be present at a higher pressure.

(2) Signs of inadequate tissue perfusion (p. 245).
(3) Peripheral vasoconstriction.

The presence of cardiogenic shock implies that at least 40% of the left ventricular myocardium is no longer functioning. The mortality, once cardiogenic shock has developed, is greater than 90%.

PRIMARY TREATMENT
Once cold hypotension has developed, treatment becomes extremely difficult. Therefore, to be effective, therapy should be started as soon as possible. Again, as the main basis of therapy is to give the myocardium the optimal conditions for proper function, the following must be ensured:

(1) Adequate oxygenation. Mechanical ventilation may be required if the patient remains hypoxic on high O_2 concentration by mask.
(2) Arrhythmias, acidosis, and electrolyte disorders must be treated. Glucose−potassium−insulin infusions (p. 252) may improve myocardial cell metabolism.
(3) Any hypovolaemia present must be treated to obtain the optimal preload (p. 245). A Swan−Ganz catheter (p. 245) is required, or failing that a central venous pressure (CVP) line (p. 243).

OTHER FORMS OF TREATMENT
Drug therapy to stimulate the myocardium is disappointing. However, if the systolic blood pressure is less than 80 mmHg a dopamine drip should be used $(10 - 20 \,(\mu g/kg)/min)$ in an attempt to raise it to at least 80 mmHg and improve coronary perfusion (p. 253). Alpha-adrenergic stimulants such as noradrenaline (norepinephrine) have little place in cardiogenic shock, except very occasionally to raise the systolic blood pressure to 80 mmHg if dopamine proves inadequate by itself, and should be discontinued as soon as possible. In the presence of a Swan−Ganz catheter which measures the left ventricular filling pressure, alpha-blocking agents such as phentolamine may be used to reduce the afterload on the heart and promote a more efficient circulation. The left ventricular filling pressure should be maintained at least at 15 cmH$_2$O by infusion of colloid. To be effective, the afterload must be reduced before the clinical picture of 'cold hypotension' appears.

Mechanical assistance or cardiac surgery
Although the appropriate use of these facilities, for example intra-aortic balloon pumping, can limit extension of the area of infarct and support the circulation, they are not generally available except in specialized units.

Anaphylactic shock
AETIOLOGY
This is a severe systemic condition due to an antigen–antibody reaction following administration of an antigen to which the individual is sensitized.

The reaction, known as type I or the immediate hypersensitivity reaction, is mediated by IgE (reaginic) antibodies, which bind strongly to mast cells. When the antigen to which the patient is sensitized is injected, an antigen–antibody reaction takes place on the surface of the mast cell, causing the release of vasoactive substances, which include:

(1) Histamine, producing:
   (a) vasodilatation,
   (b) increased capillary permeability,
   (c) smooth muscle contraction.
(2) Slow-Reacting-Substance A (SRS-A), producing smooth muscle contraction.
(3) Serotonin, producing:
   (a) vasoconstriction,
   (b) increased capillary permeability.
(4) Various kinins, producing:
   (a) vasodilatation,
   (b) increased capillary permeability.

The signs and symptoms which appear depend on the relative amount of each substance released, and the individual reaction of the patient. Similar clinical appearances can occur that have a pharmacological rather than an immunological basis, in which case these reactions are usually termed anaphylactoid. Many drugs are known to release histamine or kinins. The term anaphylactic should be reserved for cases which are proven to be immunological.

DIAGNOSIS AND CLINICAL FEATURES
The clinical picture varies considerably in patients; some exhibit a severe hypotension, while others present with rapidly progressing air-

way obstruction due to laryngeal oedema, or with severe bronchospasm, and still others have all three. Skin rashes are usually present and there is frequently diarrhoea and vomiting. Because of the differing emphasis on the body systems from patient to patient, and the lack of useful specific antagonists to most of the factors released, both the diagnosis and the treatment have to be symptomatic in the acute situation. The condition is usually self-limiting provided the vital functions can be maintained.

AIMS OF TREATMENT AND INITIAL MANAGEMENT
The essentials are:

(1) Stop further infusion or injection of the presumed antigen (if relevant).
(2) Maintain airway, ventilation and circulation.
(3) Give 0.5 ml 1 in 1000 solution of adrenaline subcutaneously, 500 mg hydrocortisone hemisuccinate intravenously, and an antihistamine such as chlorpheniramine 10 mg slowly intravenously after dilution with 10 ml of blood.

SPECIAL POINTS TO REMEMBER
Airway
If the airway is threatened by the onset of laryngeal oedema intubation should be considered early rather than late, since acute airway obstruction can supervene very suddenly, especially in the comatose patient. Tracheostomy may be necessary, and facilities for this should be available during intubation lest failure occurs. Tracheal or cricothyroid puncture may occasionally be lifesaving (p. 97).

Adequate pulmonary function
Bronchospasm is one of the commonest problems in anaphylactoid reactions, and if severe, with impending exhaustion or hypoxia, may require intubation and ventilation. Drug treatment of the bronchospasm consists of agents such as aminophylline (intravenous loading dose 250 mg given over 15 minutes, then 250 mg every 4 – 6 hours by infusion), salbutamol (intravenous dose 2 – 4 µg/kg by slow injection, and steriods (see also asthma, p. 60). Milder attacks may well settle down on the above drugs without recourse to artificial ventilation, but adequate oxygenation should be maintained with 40 – 50% oxygen by means of a mask (p. 69).

Circulation
Severe hypotension in this condition is mainly due to a sudden expansion of the capacity of the circulation following the vasodilatation, but circulating fluid is also lost due to increased capillary permeability. It is therefore logical to treat the hypotension both by infusion of fluid, including plasma expanders such as dextran 70, and by decreasing the vasodilatation through the use of an adrenergic stimulant such as ephedrine (alpha and beta effects), 5 mg intravenously every 5 minutes up to 30 mg. An alternative is metaraminol (alpha and beta effects) 1.5 to 5 mg intravenously. ECG monitoring is advisable. Arrhythmias may require appropriate therapy (p. 14).

30

Blood transfusion, bleeding, and plasma substitutes

Blood transfusion and associated problems

Blood for transfusion is maintained between 2 °C and 6 °C, and is available anticoagulated with either ACD (acid–citrate–dextrose) solution or with the more commonly used CPD (citrate–phosphate–dextrose) solution. A unit of whole CPD blood contains approximately 430 ml blood and 60 ml CPD solution. Plasma-reduced blood, from which 100–180 ml plasma has been removed, is being increasingly used. No drug should be added to blood prior to use, and blood which has been out of the blood refrigerator (or an insulated box) more than 60 minutes should be discarded unless it is to be used within the next few hours. One unit of blood should raise the haemoglobin level by about 1 g/100 ml. The urgency of a situation in which blood is required may preclude enough time for a full crossmatch which takes a minimum of 1 hour. Where this is the case, but with decreasing safety levels, other alternatives are:

(1) Patient's ABO and Rh groups determined, and an accelerated crossmatch technique performed, which takes 30 minutes.
(2) Patient's ABO and Rh groups determined, which takes 10 minutes. Blood of the appropriate group is then given.
(3) Group O Rh negative blood is given without grouping or crossmatching.

In (2) and (3) no compatibility studies of the donor blood are carried out with the patient's serum. This is obviously a dangerous practice, and should only be considered if exsanguination seems to be imminent. In obstetric emergencies, the patient's blood group has usually been ascertained in pregnancy as part of her antenatal care. It is safer in this type of patient to give blood of the same group rather than the traditional O Rh negative blood, provided that the patient's ABO and Rh types are clearly documented. If group O blood is given in quantities over two units (or four units of plasma-reduced blood) to a patient with a different blood group the anti-A and anti-B agglutinins present in the transfused blood may give rise to difficulties when crossmatched blood of the patient's own group subsequently becomes available and is transfused. Every effort should therefore be made to establish the patient's own ABO group and to use blood of this group. Group O and blood of other groups must never be allowed to mix in the giving set.

PROBLEMS WITH BLOOD TRANSFUSIONS
Effect of storage (CPD blood unless specified)
  (1) Red cells die at the rate of about 1% per day. At least 70% should be still viable after 21 days (ACD blood) or 28 days (CPD blood).
  (2) Neutrophils lose all phagocytic activity after 48 hours, but lymphocytes can survive 2 to 3 weeks. Platelets in whole blood are non-viable after 24 hours.
  (3) Factors V, VIII (antihaemophilic globulin) and XI decline rapidly in concentration and low levels are found after only 1 to 2 days storage. Factors IX and X decline in concentration after a week.
  (4) Metabolic and electrolyte changes in stored blood are considerable. The pH of the stored blood falls due to the continuing metabolism of the corpuscles, with utilization of the dextrose and production of lactate and ammonia. The cells gradually become depleted of ATP, necessary for continued function of the cellular processes, and 2,3-DPG (2,3-diphosphoglycerate), required for the proper functioning of haemoglobin as an oxygen carrier. Eventually they die, releasing potassium and free haemoglobin into the plasma. In those which survive, ATP and 2,3-DPG levels in the red cells are back to normal within 16 to 24 hours after transfusion.

Changes on storage	*On collection*	*Day 21*
Potassium level (mmol/l)	4	20 (30 in ACD blood)
Lactate (mg/dl)	20	100
Free haemoglobin (mg/dl)	0–10	20 (60 in ACD blood)

Haemolytic reactions
These are either specific incompatibilities between the blood of the donor and the recipient, often due to clerical error in the labelling of

blood samples or in form-filling, or non-specific, for example following the use of expired blood or blood which has been frozen or overheated.

Symptoms and signs – These include: pain and heat along the vein used for transfusion, chest tightness and pain, lumbar pain, flushing of the face, cardiovascular collapse with hypotension, haemoglobinuria, oliguria, an abnormal bleeding tendency, and symptoms due to microembolic phenomena.

Treatment – Stop transfusion, support circulation and/or respiration as required, give 500 mg methylprednisolone if the symptoms are severe, and treat symptomatically. A mannitol-induced diuresis reduces the likelihood of renal failure, which may, together with DIC, require specific treatment. Take blood samples in a plain tube and a sequestrene anticoagulated sample, and save the remainder of the blood being transfused for later investigation. A sample of urine should also be obtained and tested for free haemoglobin.

Transmission of disease
Syphilis, brucellosis, malaria, toxoplasmosis and various viruses causing post-transfusion hepatitis can be transmitted by banked blood. Since the advent of screening donor blood for serum hepatitis antigen (HBsAg) the incidence of serum hepatitis in the United Kingdom has fallen dramatically.

Bacterial contamination
Up to 2% of blood bags are contaminated with bacteria, which usually happens at the time of collection of the donor blood. Most bacteria cannot survive the acidic and cold (2 °C–6 °C) conditions of storage, but some of those which do can produce endotoxins. An immediate pyrexia with profound cardiovascular collapse can occur after only a few millilitres of blood have been given, leading to a misdiagnosis of severe haemolytic reaction due to incompatible blood. Treatment is as for endotoxic shock (p. 258). Acute disseminated intravascular coagulation (DIC) may occur following the endotoxaemia. Contaminated blood may have an area of haemolysis in the plasma above the red cells if they are allowed to settle, but may appear quite normal.

Mild allergic and pyrogenic reactions
These are rarely of importance clinically, and the symptoms are usually controllable with an antihistamine and/or a steroid such as hydrocortisone.

Particular problems with rapid or massive transfusions
Danger of overloading the circulation – A central venous pressure
(CVP) line is essential when the blood loss is massive or concealed, as
in a leaking aortic aneurysm, to prevent possible fluid overload during
replacement. Auscultation of the lung bases may also be useful, since
appearance of moist sounds indicates overtransfusion.
Use of cold blood – Hypothermia and cardiac arrhythmias can occur.
If more than two units of blood are needed per hour, the blood should
be warmed by a thermostatically controlled proprietary blood warmer
to prevent the blood temperature exceeding 39 °C or 40 °C.
Acidity – The pH of stored blood can fall as low as 6.6, so a massive
transfusion can lead to a considerable metabolic acidosis. In the
presence of an adequate circulation with good tissue and particularly
good liver function, this is not a problem, and the acidosis resolves
over several hours. If the patient is shocked or has poor hepatic function bicarbonate may be given to combat a severe acidosis (p. 251). A
mild acidosis, however, encourages the release of oxygen from
haemoglobin in the tissues; 24 hours after transfusion, there is often a
mild alkalosis due to metabolism of citrate to bicarbonate.
Potassium intoxication – Although the potassium concentration in
stored blood close to the expiry date may be 30 mmol/l, the cells act as
a potassium sponge during transfusion and there is little danger of
hyperkalaemia unless a large amount is given via a central venous cannula; this produces a bolus effect which can be dangerous.
Hypokalaemia is often found the day after a massive transfusion.
Citrate toxicity – Transfused blood contains an excess of citrate,
which reduces the patient's ionized calcium. Normally this is not a
problem since the patient can mobilize calcium from the skeleton, and
metabolize citrate in the liver to bicarbonate. These mechanisms can,
however, be overwhelmed due either to impaired liver perfusion and
function or a massive citrate load. Signs of hypocalcaemia then appear such as cardiovascular depression, muscle tremors, and
characteristic ECG changes. If the clinician is in doubt about the adequacy of hepatic function, or blood is to be given more rapidly than a
litre every 15 minutes, 10 ml 10% calcium gluconate should be given
for every litre transfused.
Filtration – Stored blood, particularly CPD blood, contains a large
amount of aggregated matter which is filtered out by the pulmonary
capillaries as the blood passes through the lungs. This embolization
may cause serious disturbances in lung function leading to respiratory
failure, and can be prevented by the use of a micropore filter (pore size
20 – 40 μm). The value of filtration is questionable if less than four
units of blood are being given.

Loss of clotting factors – Banked blood which has been stored for several days has no viable platelets and low concentrations of factors V, VIII and XI. Because the patient's levels of these factors is diluted by the transfusion of such blood (if the amount of blood transfused is comparable to the patient's own blood volume), bleeding can readily occur. Platelet concentrate and fresh frozen plasma may have to be given to replace these clotting factors. Following large transfusions thromboplastic substances in banked blood can sometimes initiate the coagulation cascade and cause DIC.

Other problems such as air embolism, thrombophlebitis, over-heating of blood and extravenous haematomata can be caused by poor technique or inadequate care.

Abnormal bleeding

The investigation of clotting disorders is difficult and full of pitfalls for the unwary. This brief summary attempts to give some idea of the main causes of inadequate blood clotting likely to be encountered in emergency situations.

Blood is maintained in a fluid state within the circulation by a number of inhibitors and through the removal of any inappropriate fibrin formation by the enzymes of the fibrinolytic system. In health there is a dynamic equilibrium such that neither excessive clotting nor clot lysis occurs.

Abnormal bleeding can be due to reduced or inadequate clotting due to absence or inhibition of one or more of the factors necessary for normal coagulation. Massive blood transfusion can cause this by dilution of the patient's own factors. Bleeding can also occur in anticoagulant therapy due to inhibition of coagulation factors, and in diseases such as classical haemophilia due to deficiency of a specific factor. However, a state of pathologically increased coagulation, or consumptive coagulopathy, can occur, where excessive clotting in the circulation consumes platelets and other factors necessary for normal coagulation, and so gives rise to abnormal bleeding.

Excessive fibrinolysis also causes abnormal bleeding. This can be primary fibrinolysis, when it happens in the presence of a normal coagulation cascade, or secondary fibrinolysis, which is induced by an accelerated clotting process, such as is mentioned in the previous paragraph.

The three common causes of pathological bleeding likely to require urgent treatment are:

(1) disseminated intravascular coagulation (DIC).

(2) anticoagulant therapy with heparin or oral anticoagulants,
(3) massive transfusion leading to dilution of factors (DIC is also often present to some degree).

DISSEMINATED INTRAVASCULAR COAGULATION (DIC)

This is acute transient coagulation occurring in the circulation, causing embolization and obstruction of the microcirculation. There are two principal results: firstly, abnormal bleeding, and secondly, deterioration of organ function produced by the obstruction and damage to the microcirculation throughout the body.

The abnormal bleeding has several causes:

(1) Consumption of clotting factors and platelets by the coagulopathy produces low fibrinogen and platelet levels.
(2) Secondary activation of the fibrinolytic system by the coagulopathy.
(3) The presence of fibrin degradation products (FDPs) in the circulation due to breakdown of fibrin by the fibrinolytic system; these FDPs have anticoagulant activity.

The patient may show only a tendency to ooze from wounds, but in severe cases may have generalized purpura and bruising, with oozing from intravenous cannula and injection sites, wounds and incisions.

The impaction of microemboli in the small vessels of the lung, brain, liver, kidneys and other organs produces widespread disruption of organ function, with falling PaO_2 levels, oliguria, altered consciousness, metabolic acidosis, and a deteriorating cardiovascular status. status.

Predisposing conditions

(1) Haemolytic syndromes, such as following mismatched transfusion or massive transfusion.
(2) The following obstetric conditions:
    (a) intrauterine death,
    (b) concealed antepartum haemorrhage,
    (c) amniotic fluid embolism,
    (d) abortion.
(3) Septicaemia.
(4) Miscellaneous causes – pancreatitis, prolonged shock, etc.

Diagnosis

Generalized bleeding or bruising occurring in any of the above predisposing conditions, particularly in association with unexplained general deterioration of consciousness, renal function or PaO_2 levels, should alert the clinician to the possibility of DIC. Usually there are also low fibrinogen and high FDP levels, a low platelet count, a prolonged prothrombin time, thrombin time and partial thromboplastin time. An exception is in pregnancy where high fibrinogen levels are normal, so an apparently normal level does not exclude hypofibrinogenaemia. A haematologist should be involved at an early stage.

Treatment
The aim is to sustain the patient through the period of defibrination and where possible to treat the precipitating cause. In concealed antepartum haemorrhage or intrauterine death the delivery of the fetus usually ends the defibrination. Fresh blood, fresh frozen plasma, or fibrinogen may sustain the patient long enough for this to be done. In severe cases of DIC a low dose heparin infusion can interrupt the vicious circle of accelerating coagulation and fibrinolysis by inhibiting the coagulation cascade and thus preventing further fibrin deposition and lysis and FDP formation. However, there is still much disagreement among experts as to when heparin is indicated in DIC. The general opinion is that it may be lifesaving particularly in the following conditions:

(1) In amniotic fluid embolism (p. 24). This condition may have such an acute and severe onset that heparin may have to be given on clinical suspicion, before the results of tests are available, if the best response is to be obtained.
(2) In severe incompatibility reactions during transfusion, heparin may prevent renal shutdown in such cases.
(3) In neoplastic causes of DIC, for example acute leukaemia or carcinoma with multiple metastases.
(4) In septicaemia.

The dose of heparin should usually be low, 500 to 1000 units/h by intravenous infusion except in severe cases of very acute onset, where an initial dose of 5000 units should be given to counteract the anti-heparin factor released by platelet breakdown.

BLEEDING DUE TO ANTICOAGULANT THERAPY WITH HEPARIN OR ORAL ANTICOAGULANTS
Bleeding due to heparin therapy is reversed by the slow intravenous administration of protamine sulphate in a dose of 1 mg for every 1 mg

heparin (1 mg = approximately 100 units heparin). The halflife of heparin is 1 – 2 hours depending on the dose given. Oral anticoagulants, usually coumarin or indanedione derivatives, act by decreasing the synthesis of the clotting factors which are dependent on vitamin K_1, prothrombin (factor II) and factors VII, IX, X.

The effects of oral anticoagulants are reversed by vitamin K_1, but this takes at least 12 hours. If bleeding is severe, fresh frozen plasma should be given in the intervening period to provide the missing factors. The dose of vitamin K_1 is 20 mg if anticoagulation is to be stopped completely, or 5 mg if anticoagulation is to be continued once the immediate bleeding tendency is over. The effect is monitored by means of the prothrombin time, or the thrombotest, or the British Comparative Ratio (BCR).

MASSIVE TRANSFUSION LEADING TO DILUTION OF FACTORS
Clotting factors reduced by massive transfusion of banked blood can be replaced, if a bleeding tendency exists, by the use of fresh frozen plasma and platelet concentrate. Massive transfusion, however, can induce DIC, so the picture may be more complicated than at first appears.

Plasma and plasma substitutes
The advantages and disadvantages of plasma and plasma substitutes are shown in Table 30.1 below.

Table 30.1

	Advantages	*Disadvantages*
Dried pooled plasma (less often available nowadays)	Good and physiological blood volume expander; shelf-life of 8 years (unless reconstituted); good fibrinogen content	Has to be reconstituted with sterile water; increased risk of serum hepatitis (due to preparation from ten-donor pool)
Plasma protein fraction (PPF)	Ready for infusion; physiological blood volume expander; no risk of serum hepatitis; shelf-life of 2 years	Has to be kept in blood refrigerator; no fibrinogen or gammaglobulin present; expensive; limited amounts available from blood donations (four units of blood are required for 400 ml PPF)

	Advantages	Disadvantages
Dextran		
Available as dextran 40, 70, and 110 in dextrose or saline; polysaccharide; dextran 40 remains 4–6 hours in circulation, dextran 70 remains 8–12 hours and dextran 110 remains > 12 hours.	Good plasma expander; useful for reducing plasma viscosity; said to reduce incidence of thromboembolism; long shelf-life; cheap substitute for plasma	Dextran 110 may interfere with crossmatching – blood for crossmatching should be taken before dextran is given; dextran 40 has been associated with renal failure, especially with hypovolaemia or pre-existing renal disease, and may seriously interfere with platelet function; hypersensitivity occurs but is uncommon; no clotting factors are present
Haemaccel		
Gelatin preparation	Ready-madeup solution; no interference with crossmatching techniques; long shelf-life; cheap	Short plasma life of 4–6 hours; hypersensitivity reactions have been reported, and are probably more common than with dextran solutions

31

Practical techniques

Peripheral vein infusion

The following are the steps used in setting up an intravenous infusion.

(1) First find a suitable vein. The most satisfactory veins for infusion are usually in the upper limb. If possible avoid those overlying the wrist joint and elbow joint. Usually a suitable vein becomes visible or can be palpated after a venous tourniquet or a sphygmomanometer cuff is applied to the arm at a pressure midway between the arterial systolic and diastolic pressures. A vein well supported by sub-cutaneous tissue is ideal, and this is often found on the radial side of the forearm just proximal to the wrist.

(2) Shave the skin if necessary distal to the proposed entry site, and clean the area thoroughly with spirit. Stretch the distal skin to fix vein (Figure 31.2), estimate skin entry site about 5 mm distal to site of proposed entry into vein and inject enough 0.5% or 1% lignocaine (lidocaine) intradermally to raise a small bleb. Relax skin and wait for the local analgesic to take effect, meanwhile checking that the cannula and needle to be used separate from one another easily.

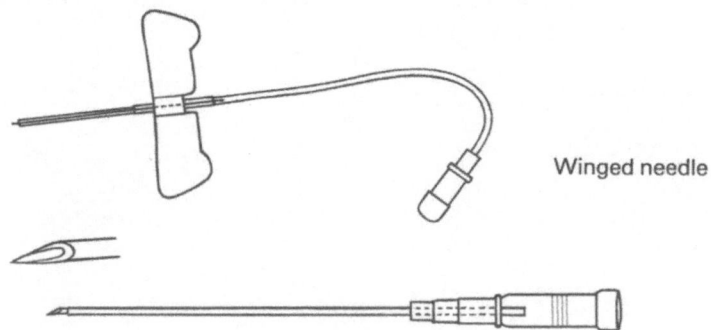

Winged needle

Figure 31.1 Typical needle-through-cannula device for venous and arterial cannulation

(3) If a small cannula (20 SWG or smaller) is to be used as perhaps for a child, or when the skin is thick and difficult to penetrate, it is often a good idea to incise the skin entry site with the tip of a scalpel blade. This minimizes any crumpling of the cannula over the needle, which can easily occur when needle and cannula are thrust through intact skin, and allows a more controlled entry into the vein.

(4) Insert the needle (and cannula) through the anaesthetized skin at an angle of about 20° to the skin surface, with the needle bevel upwards, maintaining skin tension with the thumb of the other hand to help fix the vein (Figure 31.2). Pass the needle-in-cannula into the vein – it usually enters with a definite 'give' – and then along the vein for a further 5 mm. Blood should then 'flashback' or be easily aspirated through the needle, depending on the type of cannula used.

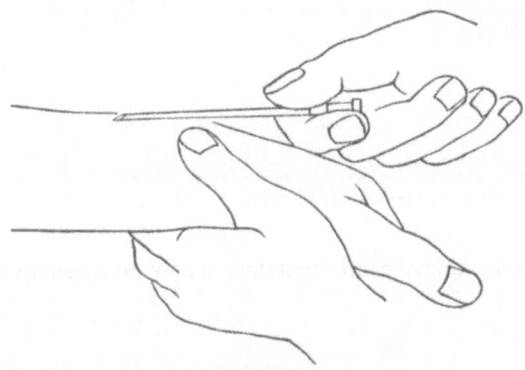

Figure 31.2 Insertion of the needle-through-cannula device after stretching skin with left hand to fix vein

(5) Hold the needle steady in relation to the skin with one hand, and with the other slide the cannula down the needle further into the vein. Most beginners find this manoeuvre the most difficult (Figure 31.3).

(6) Connect to drip set and fix well (Figure 31.4).

POINTS TO REMEMBER
(1) Winged needles (Figure 31.1) are often preferred for insertion into scalp veins in small children although they tend to block, or penetrate the vein wall.

(2) Veins in the lower limbs are very prone to spasm, are more likely to become thrombosed, and should only be used if there is no alternative.

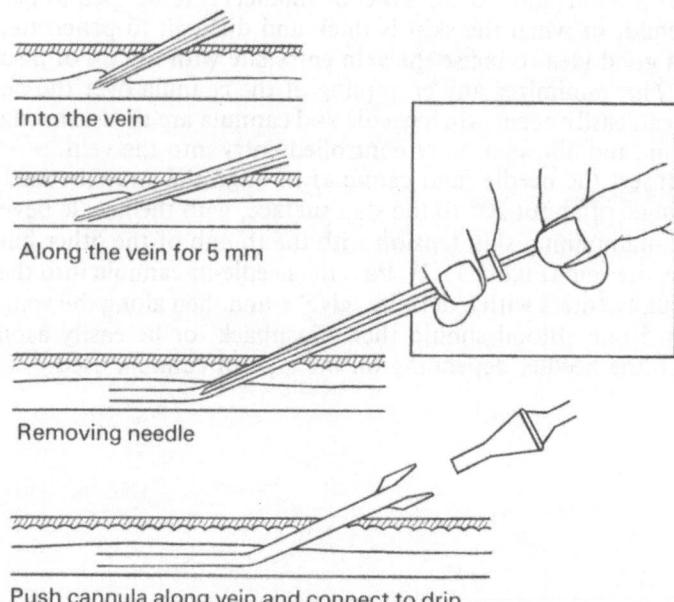

Into the vein

Along the vein for 5 mm

Removing needle

Push cannula along vein and connect to drip

Figure 31.3 Diagrammatic representation of peripheral venous cannulation

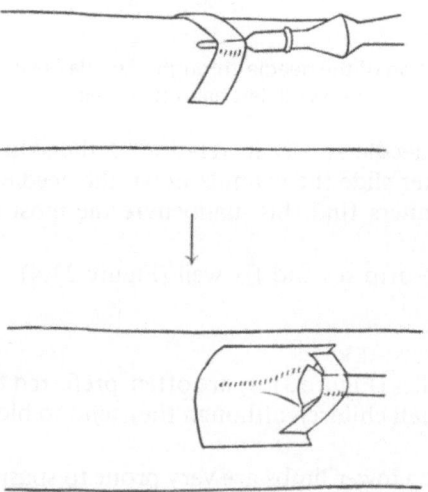

Figure 31.4 Securing the cannula in position

(3) In old patients, and patients on treatment with steroids, the skin is often papery, with the veins fragile and poorly supported by the surrounding tissues. It is often easiest to puncture the vein wall where two veins come together in a 'Y' formation. An alternative is first to penetrate the skin beside a vein rather than directly over it, and then to enter the vein from the side.

(4) In cardiac arrest following myocardial infarction the external jugular veins are frequently grossly distended, and are much easier to cannulate than more peripheral veins, which in fact are usually intensely constricted.

Central venous catheterization

Central venous pressure, to be accurate, should be measured central to the first venous valve on the venous side of the right atrium (p. 243). In practice, this means that the tip of the central cannula should lie in the superior vena cava, a subclavian vein, or an innominate vein.

The insertion sites for central venous catheterization are:

(1) the internal jugular veins,
(2) the subclavian veins,
(3) the antecubital veins.

Catheterization of the inferior vena cava via leg veins have an unacceptably high incidence of infection, thrombosis and embolism.

The external jugular vein is sometimes used for central venous cannulation, but it penetrates deep fascia before it enters the subclavian vein, often at an angle which makes passing a catheter difficult. However, it is an excellent site for inserting a simple needle-through-cannula for an emergency infusion in cardiac arrest (p. 11).

INTERNAL JUGULAR VEIN
Anatomy and landmarks
The internal jugular vein on each side passes down the neck in the carotid sheath to join the subclavian vein and form the innominate vein. With the head turned to the opposite side, the surface markings can be represented by a broad line drawn from the lobe of the ear to the medial end of the clavicle. There are two main landmarks:
The carotid artery – The vein is behind the external carotid artery in the upper third of the neck, lateral to the common carotid in the middle third, and anterolateral to it in the lower third.
The sternomastoid muscle – The sternomastoid muscle (Figure 31.5)

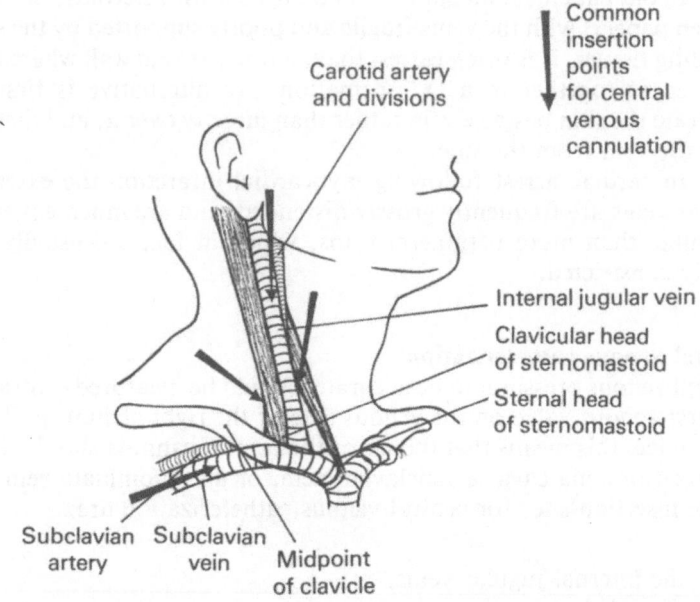

Figure 31.5 Anatomy and landmarks for cannulation of the internal jugular and subclavian veins. The part of the sternomastoid muscle overlying the internal jugular vein and the carotid artery has been omitted for clarity

overlaps the vein in its upper course. In its lower course the vein lies deep and just lateral to the medial edge of the clavicular head of the sternomastoid muscle.

When the patient is relaxed and in a steep head-down position, the vein may often be palpated deep to the sternomastoid muscle. In its lower course the vein is often 25 mm wide.

Procedure
The patient is tilted head down at least 20° to distend the veins and prevent air embolism. The head is turned to the side opposite to that of the proposed cannulation. The right internal jugular vein is usually used because:

(1) the internal jugular vein, the innominate vein and the SVC are almost in a line on the right side;
(2) right-handed operators tend to find it easier;

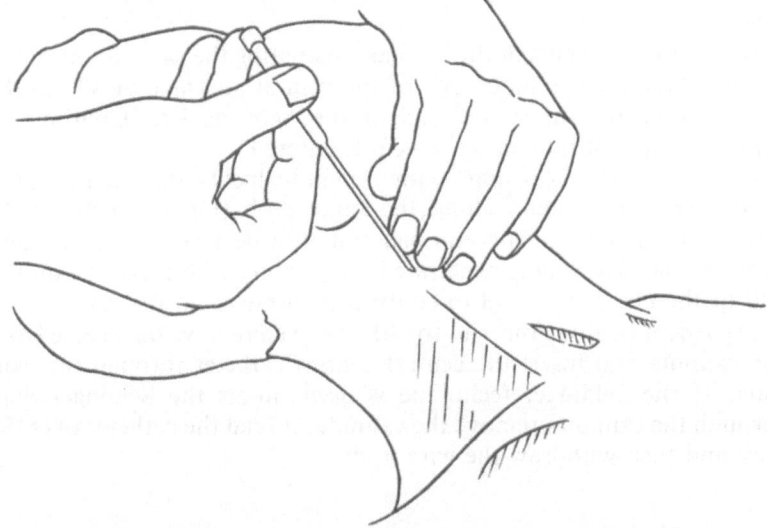

Figure 31.6 Internal jugular cannulation (high approach)

(3) the thoracic duct is on the left side, and can be punctured if insertion on the left side is attempted.

The left vein can of course be used if necessary, or if found more satisfactory by the individual operator. A local analgesic such as 1% lignocaine plain (lidocaine) should always be used to infiltrate the tissues in a conscious patient; many find it helpful to attempt to find the vein while infiltrating, by aspiration with the syringe and needle along the line of the intended insertion – this gives a guide to the direction of the subsequent insertion of the cannula. Care must, however, be taken to avoid intravenous injection of the lignocaine. At least three approaches have been described, with different advantages and disadvantages.

All methods demand an absolutely sterile technique – there is no place for a 'quick swab-down and jab'. It is advisable to try to visualize the line of the vein before inserting the needle, remembering also that the most important decision to be made is where to enter the skin.

Upper technique
(1) Palpate the carotid artery about halfway down the neck with the patient in the position described above, and infiltrate the skin just

lateral to that point with a 23 SWG needle and lignocaine in a 5 ml syringe.

(2) With the fingers of the left hand palpating the carotid, insert the needle along the presumed line of the vein at an angle of 30° to the skin, aiming for the sternal end of the right clavicle. Continue to aspirate and infiltrate until the vein is entered.

(3) Enlarge the entry point with a small scalpel blade, and insert the needle-through-cannula along the same path (Figure 31.6). Slight resistance is felt as the operator penetrates the deep cervical fascia and again as the vein wall is penetrated. Aspirating with a syringe on the end of the needle is useful to confirm its presence in the vein.

(4) Advance along the vein for 10 mm, then remove the needle from the cannula and insert the central venous catheter through the cannula. If the Seldinger technique is used, insert the Seldinger wire through the cannula, remove the cannula, thread the catheter over the wire and then withdraw the wire itself.

Lower techniques
Two methods are commonly used.
Method 1
   (1) Raise wheal of lignocaine (lidocaine) at the apex of the triangle formed by the clavicular and sternal heads of the sternomastoid muscle.
   (2) Continue to aspirate and infiltrate with local analgesic inserting the 23 SWG needle at an angle of 30° to the skin surface, deep to the medial edge of the clavicular head of sternomastoid until the vein is penetrated (about 20–30 mm beyond the point of entry in the skin).
   (3) Enlarge the entry point, and insert the needle-through-cannula along the same line until the vein is penetrated (Figure 31.7). Then proceed as above.

Method 2 – A further lower technique has been described, with an entry point along the posterior border of the sternomastoid muscle, 30 mm above the clavicle, with insertion deep to the sternomastoid muscle aiming for the suprasternal notch.

SUBCLAVIAN VEIN
Anatomy
The subclavian vein is a continuation of the axillary vein, and passes behind the medial third of the clavicle, where it joins the internal jugular vein to become the innominate vein. The vein is bound down

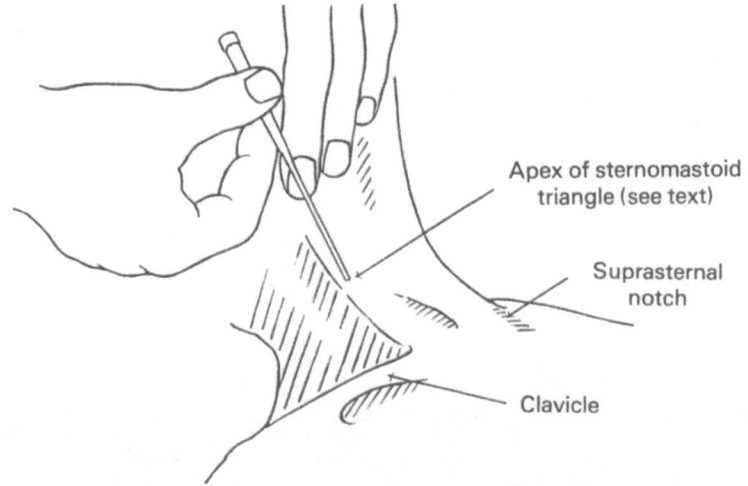

Figure 31.7 Internal jugular cannulation (low approach)

by fascia where it passes between the clavicle and the first rib, and is at its widest at this point. The surface marking is a broad line drawn convexly upward along the clavicle from just medial to its midpoint to the medial edge of the clavicular head of the sternomastoid muscle at its insertion. The subclavian artery, which runs deep, lateral, and cephalad to the vein, can in thin individuals sometimes be palpated in the supraclavicular fossa. The vein passes over the apical pleura after it has crossed the first rib. The left side is said to be easier to cannulate.

Procedure: infraclavicular technique
A variety of techniques has been described, which suggests that many people have difficulty with the procedure. A popular technique is:

(1) Infiltrate the skin with a local analgesic at a point just lateral to the midpoint of the clavicle and 2 cm caudal to it.
(2) Infiltrate further, with aspiration, from that point in the direction of a point midway between the upper border of the thyroid cartilage and the suprasternal notch, as far as the underside of the clavicle.
(3) Enlarge the entry point with a scalpel blade, and insert the needle-with-cannula along the line of infiltration, first to the underside of the clavicle, then continue in the same direction

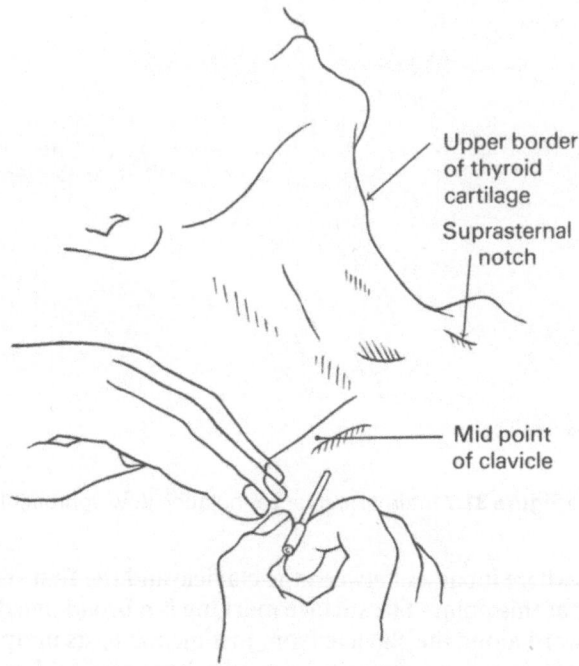

Figure 31.8 Subclavian vein cannulation (see text)

keeping close to the underside of the clavicle until there is entry into the vein (Figure 31.8).

(4) Advance the needle-with-cannula a further 5 mm or so, remove needle, and insert the catheter through the cannula.

ANTECUBITAL VEINS
It is said that it is easier to pass a catheter into the superior vena cava via the cephalic vein rather than the basilic, in other words using a large vein on the lateral side of the antecubital fossa rather than on the medial side. However, the personal experience of one of the authors (WGP) is that the basilic route is more likely to be successful.

The vein is penetrated in a manner similar to setting up a peripheral infusion, but a long catheter is passed through the cannula; there is often difficulty where the vein passes through fascial layers. Further advance can sometimes be effected by abducting the arm while insertion proceeds, or by injecting saline through the catheter to distend the vein.

ADVANTAGES AND DISADVANTAGES OF DIFFERENT TECHNIQUES
These are shown in Table 31.1 below.

Table 31.1

Site	Ease of insertion (some individual variation)	Predictability of placement	Possible damage	Ease of management
Basilic	Usually easy; patient does not need to lie down	Poor; often passes up internal jugular vein	Rare	Tends to kink and block; short term only
High jugular	Less easy	Good	To carotid artery, nerves, thoracic duct	Tends to kink; short term only
Low jugular	Moderately easy	Good	To pleura	Fairly useful for medium term
Subclavian	Less easy	Good	To pleura, subclavian artery	Easy, good for long term

Before accepting a CVP line as giving a valid reading of central venous pressure:

(1) when aspirated, blood must flow freely back along the catheter;
(2) the readings must fluctuate with respiration, rising with expiration or a Valsalva manoeuvre, and falling with inspiration;
(3) the position of the tip of the central line should be checked by a chest X-ray. The tip should lie in the superior vena cava or the subclavian vein. If it lies within a heart cavity arrhythmias may occur, and cardiac tamponade has been described following perforation of the atrial wall by the catheter tip. A central venous line provides an excellent route to the circulation for bacteria, particularly if intravenous nutrition is being undertaken. Therefore, strict aseptic conditions must be observed not only during insertion of the catheter, but also when drip sets and infusion solutions are changed. Ideally no drug should be injected into a central line, but any that is must be given extremely slowly to prevent a bolus effect on the heart. This particularly applies to electrolyte solutions containing potassium and calcium salts, and drugs acting on the myocardium.

Arterial punctures for blood gas and acid – base analysis
The arteries most frequently used for arterial sampling are the radial, the brachial and the femoral. The dorsalis pedis artery is useful if it is readily palpable. Arteries:

(1) tend to be sited deeper than veins;
(2) have more muscular walls than veins, and are more sensitive to pain;
(3) often constrict after injury, making attempts progressively more difficult after initial failure;
(4) are sometimes effectively end arteries, so that if they thrombose, necrosis of the distal part of the limb may occur. Such arteries should never be used for arterial sampling.

Probably the most frequent artery used is the radial. Because of the danger of arterial occlusion, the patency of the ulnar artery which provides a collateral supply to the hand should be tested before puncture. This can be done in the conscious patient by asking him to clench his hand tightly. The radial and ulnar arteries are then occluded by digital pressure, and the patient told to open his hand. The relative contribution of the ulnar artery to the blood supply of the hand is clearly seen by the time taken for the palm to flush following removal of the pressure on the ulnar artery.

TECHNIQUE OF RADIAL ARTERY PUNCTURE
The radial artery is palpated and a suitable point chosen for insertion, usually at the level of, or just proximal to, the wrist joint. The palm is dorsiflexed by an assistant to bring the tissues and artery at the front of the wrist under tension, so that the artery is less likely to move laterally during attempted puncture. After cleansing the skin, local analgesic solution without adrenaline (epinephrine) is injected into the skin and down to the level of the artery with a fine needle (SWG 25); the angle of insertion of the needle for the sample is usually steeper (30 – 40°) than for venepuncture (Figure 31.9). If arterial puncture has occurred the blood flows freely back into the syringe without active aspiration, particularly if a glass syringe is used. Similar techniques are used for other arteries.

If an artery is to be cannulated for frequent sampling with a needle-through-cannula device as used for veins, essentially the same procedure as the above is used. If a small gauge cannula is to be inserted it is useful to incise the anaesthetized skin with a scalpel blade before the introduction of the cannula and needle. Many people find they are more successful if they first transfix the artery with the needle-through cannula (in other words, pass through the lumen and out the other side of the artery), then remove the needle, slowly pull back the cannula until blood rushes back – as it certainly will if it is in

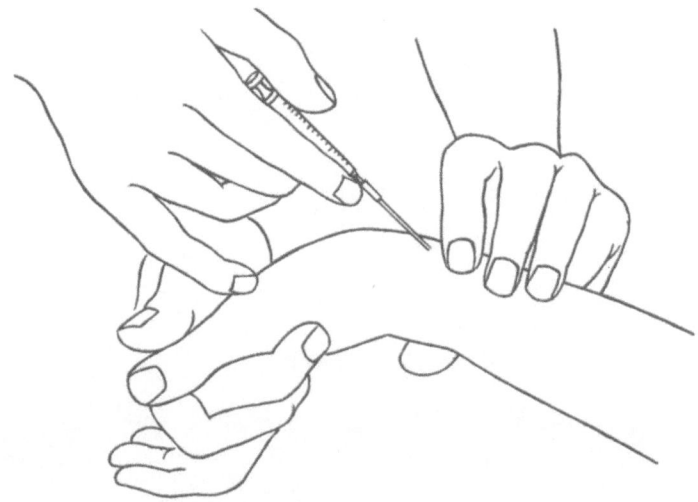

Figure 31.9 Radial artery puncture

the lumen of an artery – and then push it up the lumen. This is slightly easier than it reads!

SAMPLES FOR ANALYSIS

Bubbles of air should always be excluded from syringes before and after taking samples for blood gas analysis. A minimum of heparin is used as anticoagulant; heparin is acidic, and an excess will give rise to misleading acid–base results. If the dead space of the nozzle and barrel of the syringe is filled with heparin, this is adequate. Samples are traditionally taken in glass syringes, sealed to prevent entry of air, and taken to the laboratory surrounded by ice. These precautions to minimize both the loss of dissolved gas and the continuing metabolism of the samples are only required if analysis is delayed. Nowadays, blood gas analyses are often carried out by automatic machines operated by the person taking the sample and are therefore done almost immediately. In this situation samples can be taken by plastic syringes and no ice is required, but the requirement for an air-free sample is still absolute.

SECTION IV
pH AND SI UNITS

32

Acid−base laboratory (analyser) readouts − terminology

Table 32.1 shows the readings obtained in the acid−base laboratory (analyser) from a sample of normal arterial blood.

The purpose of this chapter is to clarify the meaning of the above reading, because without such knowledge it is impossible to appreciate how and why their values vary in health and disease. A basic knowledge of such measurements is essential to those who need to correct acid−base disturbances.

Acid−base balance is a complex subject which is difficult to understand even by those who encounter it daily. It poses a much greater problem to those who meet it less frequently, and just as revision of a language needs a return to basic grammar the understanding of pH etc. needs the revision of basic chemistry and mathematics. Every heading in this chapter could provide enough material to fill a separate book and were it the intention to provide absolute scientific accuracy in all statements an enormous number of footnotes would be necessary. However, the authors hope that the general information provided is enough for an understanding of acid−base balance.

This chapter and Chapter 33 form two parts of the same theme. This chapter explains, step by step, the derivation of the Henderson−Hasselbalch equation from the atom, the ion, the Law of Mass Action and the logarithmic values of ionic concentrations. An understanding of the Henderson−Hasselbalch equation is vital when interpreting acid−base balance disorders, and although some authorities substitute the molar concentration of hydrogen ions to denote the degree of acidity of the blood, the recording of hydrogen ion concentration in pH form is well established and is likely to remain so for many years to come.

Chapter 33 discusses briefly the common disturbances in acid−base balance and their interpretation, under the headings of the various conditions in which they occur.

Table 32.1 Readings obtained in the acid−base laboratory (analyser) from a sample of normal arterial blood

	Normal values breathing air
Hb	15 g
pH	7.4
PCO_2	40 mmHg (5.3 kPa)
PO_2	97 mmHg (13.0 kPa)
HCO_3	24 mmol/l
TCO_2	25.2 mmol/l
BE	−2.5 to +2.5 mmol/l
SAT	97%
SBC	24 mmol/l

Readings actually measured by the acid−base laboratory apparatus

Hb	the concentration of haemoglobin in g/100 ml
pH	actual pH
PCO_2	actual PCO_2 in mmHg (or kPa)
PO_2	actual PO_2 in mmHg (or kPa)

Readings calculated by the acid−base laboratory apparatus

HCO_3	plasma bicarbonate in mmol/l plasma
TCO_2	total CO_2 in mmol/l blood
BE	base excess in mmol/l blood
SAT	oxygen saturation as a percentage
SBC	standard bicarbonate in mmol/l plasma

Definition of terms used

THE ATOM

An atom consists of a nucleus and an electron or electrons. Except in hydrogen, which has only one proton, the nucleus consists of neutrons and protons.

Neutrons, as the name suggests, have no electrical charge. They do not influence the chemical properties of the atom and are therefore not discussed further in this chapter.

Protons, however, have a positive electrical charge, and *electrons* have a negative electrical charge.

There is always present in an atom an equal number of protons and electrons (that is, an equal number of positive and negative electrical charges) which electrically cancel out or neutralize one another, so an atom is electrically neutral.

THE ION
When an atom forfeits its neutrality it becomes an *ion*. An atom which loses an electron, with its negative charge, becomes positively charged and is called a *cation*. On the other hand, if an atom gains an electron it becomes negatively charged and is called an *anion*. An ion is therefore an electrically charged atom or group of atoms.

Dissociation of molecules into ions
Dissociation means a reversible breakdown of a molecule into ions, which in biological systems occurs in aqueous solutions. Dissociation is important in maintaining acid–base balance, especially in the reaction $H_2CO_3 \rightleftharpoons H^+ HCO_3^-$ which is explained on p. 292.

The hydrogen ion H^+
This is a hydrogen atom H which has lost its electron 'e'.

Hydrogen atom − electron　　=　hydrogen ion

that is　　　　　　　　H − e　=　H^+

Because the hydrogen atom H consists of one electron and one proton, removal of the electron e leaves the proton

∴　　　H − e　=　the proton H^+

Therefore proton is another name for the H^+ ion.

Hydrogen ions in solution make the solution acid and, provided that other factors do not alter, the higher the concentration of hydrogen ions the more acid the solution becomes. This fact leads to the definition of an acid as something which dissociates in solution and which can supply hydrogen ions H^+ (protons). More concisely, an acid is a hydrogen ion generator.

Carbonic acid is an acid because it breaks up or dissociates into hydrogen ions and bicarbonate ions.

$$H_2CO_3 \rightleftharpoons H^+ + HCO_3^-$$

Similarly hydrochloric acid dissociates into hydrogen ions and chloride ions

$$HCl \rightleftharpoons H^+ + Cl^-$$

There is, however, an important difference between the two acids because of the extent to which they break up or dissociate. In the case of HCl in solution almost complete dissociation takes place which produces a greater number of H^+ ions; its acidity, therefore, is strong – it is a *strong acid*. On the other hand, a relatively smaller proportion of the H_2CO_3 dissociates to produce a relatively smaller number of H^+ ions; so its acidity is weak – it is a *weak acid*.

BASES
Conjugate base
In the reaction

$$H_2CO_3 \rightleftharpoons H^+ + HCO_3^-$$

the H_2CO_3 dissociates into H^+ and HCO_3^-. H_2CO_3 is an acid because it donates an H^+ ion.

In the reverse direction

$$H^+ + HCO_3^- \rightleftharpoons H_2CO_3$$

the HCO_3^- receives a H^+ ion, so it is known as a base because a base is defined as a substance that will combine with or accept H^+ ions. A base can also be regarded as that part of the acid which remains after the hydrogen ion or ions have been removed. Because the base HCO_3^- is intimately related to H_2CO_3 it is known as the conjugate base of H_2CO_3.

Although ions such as H^+ and HCO_3^- are shown in formulae to be unattached, such a state exists only momentarily. Ions are very 'promiscuous' and become attached to any other ion bearing a different charge; for example HCO_3^- readily combines with Na^+ to become $NaHCO_3$.

Buffer base – buffers
The body is intolerant towards changes in hydrogen ion concentration. So, because the production of H^+ in the body is variable, and since excretion from the body is not immediate, the excess of H^+ ions has to be buffered until it can be excreted to avoid any ill-effects.

For example, in diabetes the ketone bodies acetoacetic acid and β-hydroxybutyric acid are strongly acidic. If these strong acids can be converted into weaker acids then less H^+ ions are available to disturb the normal acidity of the body. This is precisely what happens. For example, the strong acid acetoacetic acid CH_3COCH_2COOH readily dissociates with H^+ ions and $CH_3COCH_2COO^-$ ions.

$$CH_3COCH_2COOH_2 \rightarrow H^+ + CH_3COCH_2COO^-$$

and is converted by sodium bicarbonate $NaHCO_3$ into sodium acetoacetate CH_3COCH_2COONa and carbonic acid.

$$CH_3COCH_2COOH + NaHCO_3 \rightarrow CH_3COCH_2COONa + H_2CO_3$$

The latter being a weak acid dissociates into a smaller number of H^+ ions and so produces a smaller rise in H^+ ion concentration than would the acetoacetic acid which it has replaced.

The extra H_2CO_3 formed is broken down mainly in the red blood cells into CO_2 and H_2O.

that is $$H_2CO_3 \rightarrow CO_2 + H_2O$$

This reaction is reversible and is usually written

$$H_2CO_3 \rightleftharpoons CO_2 + H_2O$$

The CO_2 is eliminated, usually by increasing the ventilation, the hydrogen ion and acetoacetic radical are excreted later and the bicarbonate is reabsorbed by the kidney to restore the acid—base equilibrium of the body.

To summarize
(1) A strong acid is converted into a weak acid.
(2) In this case the weak acid H_2CO_3 is broken down into CO_2 and H_2O. The CO_2 is disposed of by the lungs, and the kidney eliminates some of the H^+ ions.
(3) The rise in H^+ ion concentration is minimized.

The HCO_3^- in association with a cation such as Na^+ has reduced or *buffered* the effect of the added strong acetoacetic acid. So the HCO_3^- radical is known as the *buffer base*. Other examples of physiological buffer bases are HPO_4^{2-} and groups associated with haemoglobin and proteins.

Buffer base — buffer pairs
In the reaction

$$H_2CO_3 \;\rightleftharpoons\; H^+ + HCO_3^-$$

the acid H_2CO_3 and its conjugate base HCO_3^- are together referred to as a buffer pair and are written

$$HCO_3^-/H_2CO_3$$
bicarbonate

Other examples are

$$HPO_4^{2-}/H_2PO_4^- \qquad Pr^-/HPr \qquad Hb^-/HHb$$
phosphate   protein   haemoglobin

When the actual base and acid is not specified the buffer pairs are usually collectively depicted base/acid, which therefore implies that several buffer pairs are involved, and although most attention is paid to the plasma bicarbonate buffer pair HCO_3^-/H_2CO_3 it is obviously not solely responsible for the buffering of changes in the concentration of H^+ ions caused by addition to or loss of acids from the body. All the other buffer systems play their part and are in equilibrium with the bicarbonate system so that the effect of the respiratory control (p. 295) on the bicarbonate system is transmitted to all the others.

A buffer pair is sometimes depicted as consisting of a weak acid, such as H_2CO_3, poorly dissociated, and a salt of that acid. This means that a salt is formed when the H^+ ion of an acid is replaced by an ion such as the cation Na^+ or K^+. The cations are always lurking around the body fluids or cells where they combine with negatively charged ions such as HCO_3^-; for example

$$Na^+ + HCO_3^- \;\rightleftharpoons\; NaHCO_3$$

The $NaHCO_3$ can then react with a strong acid such as CH_3COCH_2COOH to form the weak acid H_2CO_3 (p. 293).

Together the buffer pairs constitute the buffer system.

From the above it can be seen that 'base' is a term which is often modified, taken for granted or omitted, and as a result can cause considerable confusion. For example, in the reaction

$$H^+ + HCO_3^- \;\rightleftharpoons\; H_2CO_3$$

the HCO_3^- ion is referred to as:

(1) simply the 'base' because it accepts H^+ ion;

(2) the 'conjugate base' which is the non-hydrogen part of the acid;
(3) the 'buffer base' because, besides accepting H^+ ion, it helps to buffer the effects of stronger acids;
(4) a component of the 'buffer pair' HCO_3^-/H_2CO_3;
(5) a component of the 'buffer system' $BHCO_3/H_2CO_3$ or salt/acid where B is an abbreviation for cations such as Na^+ and K^+.

The efficiency of buffer pairs — It should be apparent that if a strong acid or strong base is added to a buffer pair such as HCO_3^- /H_2CO_3 such a pair will be most efficient in buffering pH changes if it consists of equal concentrations of HCO_3^- and H_2CO_3. If, for example, 50% of the HCO_3^- /H_2CO_3 pair consists of HCO_3^- and 50% of H_2CO_3 there is equal opportunity for both numerator and denominator of dealing with added solutions which tend to upset the H^+ ion concentration. If, however, there is 20 times as much HCO_3^- as H_2CO_3 the buffer pair can deal with much more added acid than it can added base, so it is far less efficient. The ratio of HCO_3^- /H_2CO_3 in blood at a pH 7.4 is 20:1, so this buffer pair is inefficient in states of alkalaemia but relatively efficient in states of acidaemia (the more common situation in health and disease) when hydrogen ions need to be buffered. A further reason why the HCO_3^- /H_2CO_3 pair is most important is because it exists in greater quantities than do the others and any derangement can quickly be corrected, especially by alterations in respiration. The HCO_3^- /H_2CO_3 system is the pillar of acid—base balance but it must be remembered that any addition or removal of H^+ ions affects all buffers, and because the latter participate in acid—base balance the final pH following the addition of a strong acid depends on their efficiency and their concentrations. The buffer systems become markedly depleted only when compensatory replenishment mechanisms fail and significant changes then occur in the blood pH.

CONCENTRATION
When H_2CO_3 exists in a state of equilibrium with H^+ ions and HCO_3^- ions

$$H_2CO_3 \;\rightleftharpoons\; H^+ + HCO_3^-$$

in a given volume at constant temperature, the amount of H_2CO_3 is proportional to the amounts of H^+ ions and HCO_3^- ions and vice versa. To denote the amount of reagent in a given volume, that is the *concentration,* it is enclosed in square brackets. Therefore, [H^+] and

$[HCO_3^-]$ denote the concentrations of hydrogen and bicarbonate ions respectively whereas $[H_2CO_3]$ denotes the concentration of carbonic acid.

The Law of Mass Action

This leads to one version of the Law of Mass Action which states that when a reaction such as $H_2CO_3 \rightleftharpoons H^+ + HCO_3^-$ has reached equilibrium, the product of the concentrations on one side of the equation is proportional to the product of the concentrations of reagents on the other side of the equation. The reaction can be written

$$[H_2CO_3] \propto [H^+] \, [HCO_3^-]$$

It will be noticed that when the reaction $H_2CO_3 \rightleftharpoons H^+ + HCO_3^-$ is replaced by a reaction involving concentrations, the concentrations of the reagents in the square brackets on the right side of the equation are multiplied and not added; in other words:

$$[H_2CO_3] \rightleftharpoons [H^+] \times [HCO_3^-]$$

and the reader should remember that in such chemical situations concentrations are always multiplied and never added.

Proportionality constant

In reactions such as

$$[H_2CO_3] \propto [H^+] \, [HCO_3^-]$$

the proportion sign $\propto$ can be replaced by the equality symbol $=$ if a suitable constant K (known as the proportionality constant) can be inserted – hence

$$K \, [H_2CO_3] = [H^+] \, [HCO_3^-]$$

which can then be rewritten

$$K = \frac{[H^+] \, [HCO_3^-]}{[H_2CO_3]}$$

and then by rearranging the equation

$$\text{H}^+ = K \, \frac{[\text{H}_2\text{CO}_3]}{[\text{HCO}_3^-]} \qquad \text{or} = K \, \frac{[\text{acid}]}{[\text{base}]}$$

Any reagent on the left side of the original equation

$$K[\text{H}_2\text{CO}_3] = [\text{H}^+] \, [\text{HCO}_3^-]$$

is called a reactant. Those reagents on the right side of the equation are called products. By convention, in a rearrangement of the equation, the products are always placed as the numerator and the reactants as the denominator.

K – the dissociation constant – When a proportionality constant is associated with dissociation it is known as a dissociation constant. K is sometimes written K_a or K_b where a or b implies that either an acid or a base is dissociating.

Since different acids dissociate to different extents the value of K varies according to the acid concerned. For H_2CO_3, K has the rather forbidding value 7.2×10^{-7}

or
$$\frac{7.2}{10\,000\,000}$$

To render such values more acceptable and manageable their logarithmic values are used. When two numbers are multiplied together their logarithmic values are added. For example,

$1000 \times 100 \qquad = 10^3 \times 10^2 = 10^5 = 100\,000$ (in these circumstances the 3, 2, and 5 are also referred to as the power or exponent of 10, that is the base on which they rest or act)

$3 =$ the log of 10^3

$2 =$ the log of 10^2

$5 =$ the log of $10^5 =$ the log of $100\,000$

if $K = 7.2 \times 10^{-7}$ and log $7.2 = 0.8573 =$ approximately 0.9

and log $10^{-7} = -7$

then the log of $K = \log 7.2 + \log 10^{-7}$

$$= 0.9 + (-7)$$

$$= 0.9 \quad -7$$

$$= -6.1$$

Therefore log $K = -6.1$.

pK − negative logarithms − If negative logarithms are taken the signs preceding the logarithmic values are altered from plus to minus or from minus to plus as the case may be

If log $K = -6.1$

then negative log K = positive 6.1

that is $-\log K = 6.1$

The prefix '−log' before a letter is signified by the letter 'p' which is chosen to represent the negative power of something; for example:

$$-\log K \text{ is written } pK$$

that is $pK = -\log K$

and pH $= -\log$ H$^+$ ion concentration

$$= -\log [\text{H}^+]$$

As indicated above the entire purpose of taking logarithmic values followed by negative logarithmic values is to make the numbers easier to handle; 'p' is merely an abbreviation of '−log'; nothing else is gained or intended. It is necessary, however, to appreciate how and why negative logarithmic values are taken to understand the Henderson−Hasselbalch equation

$$\text{pH} = pK + \log\frac{[\text{HCO}_3^-]}{[\text{H}_2\text{CO}_3]}$$

which features so prominently in acid−base balance.

The Henderson—Hasselbalch equation in acid—base balance
DERIVATION
The equation

$$[H^+] = K\frac{[H_2CO_3]}{[HCO_3^-]}$$

was derived on p. 297. If logarithmic values are taken, log is written before every value in the equation; in other words:

$$\log [H^+] = \log K + \frac{\log [H_2CO_3]}{\log [HCO_3^-]}$$

which is usually abbreviated to

$$\log [H^+] = \log K + \log\frac{[H_2CO_3]}{[HCO_3^-]}$$

If negative logarithms are now taken, all the values being positive have their signs changed to negative.

$$-\log [H^+] = -\log K - \log\frac{[H_2CO_3]}{[HCO_3^-]}$$

but $-\log$ before a letter such as K or $[H^+]$ can be abbreviated to p;

therefore

$$pH = pK - \log\frac{[H_2CO_3]}{[HCO_3^-]}$$

To convert

$$pH = pK - \log\frac{[H_2CO_3]}{[HCO_3^-]} \quad to\; pH = pK + \log\frac{[HCO_3^-]}{[H_2CO_3]}$$

– when a number is divided by another number the logarithmic value of the denominator is subtracted from the logarithmic value of the numerator; for example:

$$\frac{10^5}{10^3} = 10^2 = 100$$

$$5 = \text{the log of } 10^5$$

$$\underline{3} = \text{the log of } 10^3$$

$$2 = \text{the log of } 10^2 = \text{the log of } 100$$

Then let the value of $[H_2CO_3]$ be 1.2 units (mmol), and the value of $[HCO_3^-]$ be 24 units (mmol);

then the ratio $[H_2CO_3]/[HCO_3^-]$ $= \frac{1.2}{24} = \frac{1}{20}$

Now log 20 = 1.3

and log 1 = 0

Thus $\log \dfrac{[H_2CO_3]}{[HCO_3^-]} = \dfrac{\log 1}{\log 20} = 0 - 1.3 = -1.3$

Similarly if we turn the ratio $\frac{1}{20}$ upside down to $\frac{20}{1}$ and take logs as before

log 1 = 0

log 20 = 1.3

and log 20 − log 1 = 1.3 −0 = 1.3

therefore $\log \dfrac{[HCO_3^-]}{[H_2CO_3]} = \log \dfrac{20}{1} = 1.3 - 0 = 1.3$

whereas $\log \dfrac{[H_2CO_3]}{[HCO_3^-]} = \log \dfrac{1}{20} = 0 - 1.3 = -1.3$

Thus, transposing numerator and denominator causes a change in the sign before the logarithmic value. The importance of this is that in the derivation of the Henderson–Hasselbalch equation from the expression

$$-\log [H^+] = -\log K -\log \frac{[H_2CO_3]}{[HCO_3^-]} \text{ (p. 299).}$$

the value $- \log \dfrac{[H_2CO_3]}{[HCO_3^-]}$ is the same value as

$$\log \frac{[HCO_3^-]}{[H_2CO_3]}$$

so the relationship can be written

$$-\log [H^+] = -\log K + \log \frac{[HCO_3^-]}{[H_2CO_3]}$$

The negative sign originally here has been eliminated.

To summarize

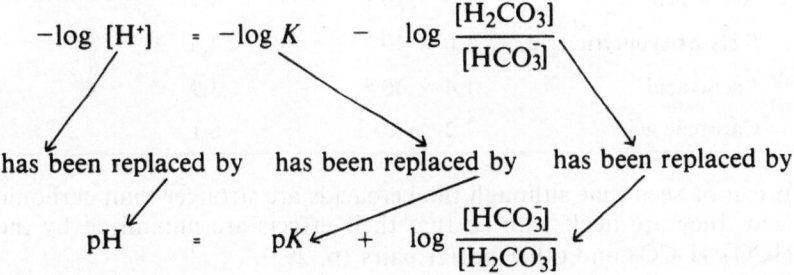

$$-\log [H^+] = -\log K - \log \frac{[H_2CO_3]}{[HCO_3^-]}$$

has been replaced by   has been replaced by   has been replaced by

$$pH = pK + \log \frac{[HCO_3^-]}{[H_2CO_3]}$$

the value of $pK = 6.1$ (p. 298),

and the value of $\log \dfrac{[HCO_3^-]}{[H_2CO_3]} = 1.3$ (p. 300),

therefore pH = 6.1 + 1.3 = 7.4

so pH of plasma in arterial blood = 7.4

THE SIGNIFICANCE OF THE VALUE OF pK (OR pK_a)
pK is often mentioned in acid–base balance, particularly with regard
to the derivation of the Henderson–Hasselbalch equation and to the

efficacy of buffer pairs. It is also important in the mechanisms of drug
absorption.

The value of the dissociation constant K gives the strength of the
acid. The stronger the acid, the higher is its K but because pK is the
negative logarithm to the base 10, the lower is its pK. The converse is
also true, the weaker the acid the lower is the value of K but the higher
the value of pK.

STRONG OR WEAK ACIDS

To know which acids are strong or weak the reader must look up the
values of K and pK for the acids of biological importance in a
physiology book and compare them with the value for carbonic acid
(Table 31.2).

Table 32.2

	K	pK
Acetoacetic acid	2.6×10^{-4}	3.6
Acetic acid	1.8×10^{-5}	4.7
β-Hydroxybutyric acid	1.6×10^{-5}	4.8
Lactic acid	1.4×10^{-4}	3.9
Carbonic acid	7.2×10^{-7}	6.1

It can be seen that although the ketoacids are stronger than carbonic
acid, they are dealt with so that their effects are minimized by the
HCO_3^-/H_2CO_3 and other buffer pairs (p. 293).

FACTORS DETERMINING THE VALUE OF [H_2CO_3]

To understand the significance of pH changes it is necessary to
understand how the value of [H_2CO_3] is derived, so it is necessary
once more to revert to

$$H_2O + CO_2 \rightleftharpoons H_2CO_3$$

from which it is plain to see that the value of [H_2CO_3] depends on
whether the blood is brought into contact with much or little carbon
dioxide. More scientifically, it depends on whether the blood is
exposed to a low or a high pressure of carbon dioxide (that is, the
partial pressure of carbon dioxide).

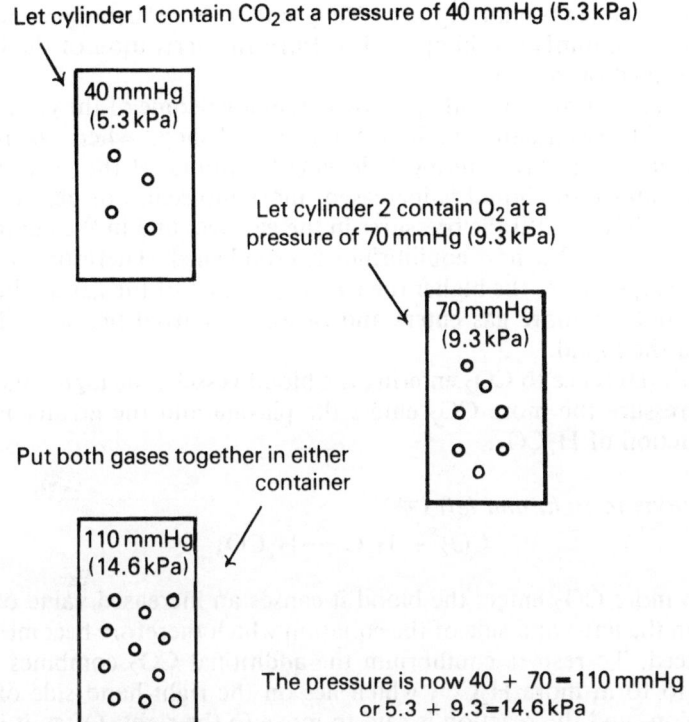

Let cylinder 1 contain CO_2 at a pressure of 40 mmHg (5.3 kPa)

40 mmHg
(5.3 kPa)

Let cylinder 2 contain O_2 at a
pressure of 70 mmHg (9.3 kPa)

70 mmHg
(9.3 kPa)

Put both gases together in either
container

110 mmHg
(14.6 kPa)

The pressure is now 40 + 70 = 110 mmHg
or 5.3 + 9.3 = 14.6 kPa

Figure 32.1 Partial pressures

PARTIAL PRESSURE

Take two closed cylinders of equal volume at the same temperature.
Let cylinder 1 contain CO_2 at a pressure of 40 mmHg (5.3 kPa)
(Figure 32.1).

Let cylinder 2 contain O_2 at a pressure of 70 mmHg (9.3 kPa).

Put both gases together in either container

The pressure is now 40 + 70 = 110 mmHg (or 5.3 + 9.3 = 14.6 kPa).
Therefore the CO_2 exerts 40 parts of the 110 parts pressure and O_2
exerts 70 parts of 110 parts pressure in the shared container. Thus each
gas exerts a part pressure (a partial pressure) against the walls of the
container. Partial pressure of a gas in a mixture of gases is defined as
that pressure it would exert were it alone in the same space or container. Partial pressure is denoted by the letter P and the partial

pressures of CO_2 and O_2 are PCO_2 and PO_2. Partial pressure is measured in mmHg or kilopascals (kPa) – the derivation of the latter is described on p. 331.

If a gas is above a liquid in a closed container some of the gas enters the liquid. Eventually equilibrium is established, where as many molecules of gas are entering as leaving the liquid. If the pressure of the gas above the liquid is increased, more molecules of gas start to enter the liquid until the pressures in the gas over and in the liquid are again equal and a new equilibrium is established. Therefore, at the same temperature, the higher the partial pressure of the gas applied to the liquid the more gas enters and raises the partial pressure of gas within the liquid.

With reference to CO_2 entering the blood vessels, the higher its partial pressure the more CO_2 enters the plasma and the greater is the production of H_2CO_3.

Reactions to right and left ($\rightleftharpoons$)

$$CO_2 + H_2O \longrightarrow H_2CO_3$$

When more CO_2 enters the blood it causes an increased value of the CO_2 in the left-hand side of the equation which therefore becomes unbalanced. To restore equilibrium the additional CO_2 combines with H_2O to form more H_2CO_3 which lies on the right-hand side of the equation, and the reaction is said to move to the right. Often it is indicated by a single arrow or by a thicker arrow pointing towards the right if both arrows are retained.

$$CO_2 + H_2O \rightarrow H_2CO_3$$
or $\qquad CO_2 + H_2O \rightleftharpoons H_2CO_3$

If blood with a higher concentration of H_2CO_3 arrives at the lungs where the CO_2 level is low, then the H_2CO_3 splits up into CO_2 and H_2O, the CO_2 being expired to the atmosphere. The reaction is said to move to the left and is depicted

$$CO_2 + H_2O \leftarrow H_2CO_3$$
or $\qquad CO_2 + H_2O \leftrightharpoons H_2CO_3$

SOLUBILITY CONSTANT

Above it was stated (p. 304) that the amount of gas dissolved in a liquid depends on the partial pressure of the gas to which the liquid is exposed. Although this is true it is obvious that some gases are more soluble than others and all gases enter the liquid to a different extent for each mmHg (or kPa) rise in partial pressure. For example, 0.03 mmol CO_2 enters 1 litre of plasma at a temperature of 38 °C for every mmHg rise in pressure (in SI units 0.23 mmol CO_2 enters 1 litre of plasma at 38 °C per kilopascal (kPa) of pressure). This value, written 0.03 mmol l^{-1} $mmHg^{-1}$ (0.23 mmol l^{-1} kPa^{-1}), is known as the solubility constant S, and is another example of a proportionality constant (p. 296).

Therefore, the quantity of CO_2 dissolved in a liquid is proportional to the PCO_2, and is equal to $S \times PCO_2$ or $SPCO_2$. At a normal arterial PCO_2 of 40 mmHg (5.3 kPa) the quantity of CO_2 that dissolves in plasma is

$$S\ 40 = 0.03 \times 40 = 1.2 \text{ mmol } l^{-1}$$
$$\text{or } S\ 5.3 = 0.23 \times 5.3 = 1.2 \text{ mmol } l^{-1}$$

Replacing [H_2CO_3] by $SPCO_2$
The substitution of [H_2CO_3] by $SPCO_2$ is derived from the following reasoning:

(1) As previously stated, the amount of gas dissolved in a liquid depends on the partial pressure of the gas to which the liquid is exposed

$$\therefore \quad [\text{dissolved } CO_2] \propto PCO_2$$
$$\text{and } [\text{dissolved } CO_2] = \text{a constant } (S') \times PCO_2$$
$$= S'PCO_2$$

(2) The dissolved CO_2 is in equilibrium with the hydrated CO_2, that is H_2CO_3

$$\therefore \quad [\text{dissolved } CO_2] \propto [H_2CO_3]$$
$$\text{But, } [\text{dissolved } CO_2] \propto PCO_2$$
$$\therefore \quad [H_2CO_3] \text{ is also } \propto PCO_2$$

(3) If [dissolved CO_2] and [H_2CO_3] separately are proportional to PCO_2 then the two added together must also be proportional to PCO_2

$$\text{that is } [\text{dissolved } CO_2 + H_2CO_3] \propto PCO_2$$
$$\therefore \quad [\text{dissolved } CO_2 + H_2CO_3] = \text{a constant } (S) \times PCO_2$$
$$= SPCO_2$$

(Note that the constant S here in (3) above is different from the constant S' in (1) above).

(4) Because the equilibrium between dissolved CO_2 and H_2CO_3 is far to the left

$$CO_2 + H_2O \rightleftharpoons H_2CO_3$$

the concentration of dissolved CO_2 is about 1000 times greater than that of H_2CO_3. This predominant value of dissolved CO_2, has led to the term [dissolved $CO_2 + H_2CO_3$] being abbreviated to $[CO_2]$

Therefore $[CO_2]$ = [dissolved $CO_2 + H_2CO_3$]
∴ from (3) above $[CO_2]$ = $SPCO_2$

(5) The $[CO_2]$ can replace the $[H_2CO_3]$ in the Henderson–Hasselbalch equation, therefore

$$pH = pK + \log \frac{[HCO_3^-]}{0.03 \times PCO_2} \text{ (in mmHg)}$$

$$\text{or } pH = pK + \log \frac{[HCO_3^-]}{0.23 \times PCO_2} \text{ (in kPa)}$$

DIFFERENT WAYS OF EXPRESSING THE HENDERSON–HASSELBALCH EQUATION

Because the $[HCO_3^-]$ is mostly regulated by the kidneys, and $[H_2CO_3]$ by the lungs, the Henderson–Hasselbalch equation can also be expressed as

$$pH = pK + \log \frac{kidneys}{lungs}$$

Besides primarily controlling HCO_3^- retention or excretion the kidney is involved with the production and disposal of H^+ ions, which when produced exchange places with the Na^+ in the tubules. The Na^+ is retained and unites with HCO_3^- to form $NaHCO_3$, and preserves the bicarbonate. The H^+ ion in the tubules then:

(1) combines with HCO_3^- in the tubules to form H_2CO_3; and
(2) combines with HPO_4^{2-} radicals to form $H_2PO_4^-$ radicals.

The H^+ ions also combine with ammonia NH_3.

$$NH_3 + H^+ \rightarrow NH_4^+$$

to form ammonium ions which unite in the tubules with the sodium salts of strong acids. This replacement of Na^+ with NH_4^+ allows the Na^+ to be reabsorbed, and the ammonium salt of the strong acid is excreted.

Although the renal mechanisms involved in acid–base balance are complex and difficult to memorize, it is essential to remember that the response of the kidney to pH changes is relatively slow compared with that of the lungs.

$T[CO_2]$
The sample introduced into the acid–base laboratory is whole blood but the '$T[CO_2]$' (total $[CO_2]$) recorded in the printout is a measurement of the total carbon dioxide concentration in plasma. This plasma $T[CO_2]$ features in one variation of the Henderson–Hasselbalch equation (p. 307). Its actual value is unnecessary for routine clinical resuscitation provided the other measurements are available, but it is important to understand how it helps in calculating the bicarbonate.

How to obtain the value of $T[CO_2]$
$T[CO_2]$ can be measured, or derived as below.

The *total* $[CO_2]$, abbreviated $T[CO_2]$ (see also p. 308) in plasma consists of $[CO_2] + [HCO_3^-]$,

but $[CO_2] = [\text{dissolved } CO_2] + [H_2CO_3]$, that is $SPCO_2$

$\therefore$ bicarbonate $= T[CO_2] - SPCO_2$

now $pH = 6.10 + \log \dfrac{[HCO_3^-]}{[CO_2]}$

but the numerator $[HCO_3^-] = T[CO_2] - SPCO_2$

and the denominator $[H_2CO_3] = SPCO_2$

$\therefore pH = pK + \log \dfrac{(T[CO_2] - SPCO_2)}{SPCO_2}$

now $pK = 6.1$

and $S = 0.03$ (if PCO_2 is measured in mmHg) or 0.23 (if PCO_2 is measured in kPa)

$$\therefore \text{pH} = 6.1 + \log \frac{(T[CO_2] - 0.03\ PCO_2)}{0.03\ PCO_2}$$

$$\text{or} = 6.1 + \log \frac{(T[CO_2] - 0.23\ PCO_2)}{0.23\ PCO_2}$$

The arrows point to the three unknown values; if any two are known the third value is obtainable. If pH and PCO_2 are measured then the $T[CO_2]$, and hence the bicarbonate, can be estimated from

$$\text{bicarbonate} = T[CO_2] - SPCO_2$$

Relationship between $T[CO_2]$ and plasma bicarbonate
The total $[CO_2]$, usually written $T[CO_2]$ of the plasma consists of the sum of [dissolved CO_2], $[H_2CO_3]$ and [bicarbonate] (p. 307). Its value does not indicate the relative concentration of its constituents. However, if the PCO_2 and solubility coefficient of $CO_2(S)$ are known, the plasma bicarbonate can be calculated; in other words

$$\text{total } [CO_2] = [CO_2] + [H_2CO_3] + [\text{bicarbonate}]$$

written as

$$= [H_2CO_3] + [\text{bicarbonate}]$$
$$= PCO_2 \times S + [\text{bicarbonate}] \text{ the value of}$$
$$S \text{ depends on the units used (p. 305)}$$

If $T[CO_2]$ = 25.2 mmol/l, $\qquad S = 0.03$ and PCO_2 = 40 mmHg then 25.2 = 40 × 0.03 + [bicarbonate] $\therefore$ 25.2 = 1.2 + [bicarbonate] [bicarbonate] = 25.2 − 1.2 $\qquad\qquad$ = 24 mmol/l	If $T[CO_2]$ = 25.2 mmol/l, $\qquad S = 0.23$ and PCO_2 = 5.3 kPa then 25.2 = 5.3 × 0.23 + [bicarbonate] $\therefore$ 25.2 = 1.2 + [bicarbonate] [bicarbonate] = 25.2 − 1.2 $\qquad\qquad$ = 24 mmol/l

The value of the plasma bicarbonate concentration is calculated in this way in the blood gas machine, and to obtain the value the PCO_2 is first measured by the machine's PCO_2 electrode. The plasma bicarbonate is the value of the plasma bicarbonate calculated at the existing PCO_2 level in the blood specimen. Therefore, if a sample of blood is taken and the PCO_2 is 60 mmHg (8 kPa), then the plasma bicarbonate is measured when the PCO_2 is 60 mmHg (8 kPa).

STANDARD BICARBONATE
In the term 'standard bicarbonate' the key word is 'standard' because the bicarbonate level calculated is that which would be present when the blood is exposed to standard conditions, that is fully oxygenated at 37 °C and at a PCO_2 of 40 mmHg (5.3 kPa).

Plasma bicarbonate concentration can change due to either respiratory or metabolic causes. The standard bicarbonate is used in an attempt to find out what the bicarbonate concentration would be if the respiratory causes of change are removed. It therefore reflects metabolic causes of acid—base disturbances.

Clinical significance of plasma bicarbonate and standard bicarbonate
Consider an acute exacerbation of chronic bronchitis in which CO_2 retention rapidly develops. Due to the reaction

$$CO_2 + H_2O \rightleftharpoons H^+ + HCO_3^-$$

as the amount of CO_2 in the blood increases so as a *direct* result does the *plasma* bicarbonate. However, the *standard* bicarbonate (or the bicarbonate level measured in a sample of the patient's plasma equilibrated at a PCO_2 of 40 mmHg – 5.3 kPa) will not rise unless a metabolic alkalosis develops to compensate for the respiratory acidosis (p. 314).

Another example is a hyperventilating patient in the second stage of labour who reduces her PCO_2 to below normal. The reaction will tend to move to the left.

$$CO_2 + H_2O \rightleftharpoons H^+ + HCO_3^-$$

and the *plasma* bicarbonate will fall. The *standard* bicarbonate, however, will remain constant since it is measured at a PCO_2 of 40 mmHg (5.3 kPa), and a compensatory metabolic acidosis is unlikely to develop in the short interval before delivery.

It may be seen from the above examples that neither respiratory acidosis nor alkalosis can *directly* affect the value of the standard bicarbonate. They can only *indirectly* affect it by inducing metabolic changes to minimize the pH change. Therefore, if (a) the standard bicarbonate level is raised, a metabolic alkalosis exists, which may be primary, or merely compensating for a respiratory acidosis, or (b) the standard bicarbonate level is low, a metabolic acidosis exists, which may be primary, or merely compensating for a respiratory alkalosis.

That is all the information an isolated standard bicarbonate value provides; for further elucidation of the acid–base upset the pH and the PCO_2 are required to determine the overall acid–base status of the patient and whether there is a respiratory component in the acid–base derangement.

BASE EXCESS OR DEFICIT

If sufficient acid is added to a known quantity of alkali there comes a point where the acid is neutralized. This is the basis behind the assessment of 'base excess or base deficit', which refers to the surplus of fixed, non-volatile base or acid in the blood. The blood is exposed at 37 °C to a PCO_2 of 40 mmHg (5.3 kPa) and sufficient acid or base is added to restore the pH to 7.4. The amount of acid or base required to restore the pH of 1 litre of blood to 7.4 is termed base excess or deficit and is measured in mmol/l. When there is a sudden excess of non-volatile acid in the blood there is deficiency of blood base, or negative base excess or base deficit – all these terms therefore, have the same meaning; similarly, excess of ·blood base and base excess are synonymous. Any value of base excess or deficiency obtained should not be relied upon by itself when diagnosing an acid–base disturbance. The same criteria of its use and limitations should be applied as those suggested under 'standard bicarbonate' (p. 309).

It is frequently used as a guide to the amount of bicarbonate solution to be given to a patient with metabolic acidosis, to reduce it to acceptable limits (p. 251).

INFORMATION DERIVED FROM THE HENDERSON–HASSELBALCH EQUATION

From the previous reasoning it should be apparent that:

(1) pH depends on the bicarbonate/carbonic acid ratio;
(2) if the concentration of H_2CO_3 rises without an equivalent compensatory rise in the concentration of HCO_3^-
    $[H]^+$ rises, pH falls and the acidity is increased;
(3) if the concentration of H_2CO_3 falls without an equivalent compensatory fall in the concentration of HCO_3^-
    $[H]^+$ falls, pH rises and the acidity is decreased;
(4) if the concentration of HCO_3^- rises without an equivalent compensatory rise in the concentration of H_2CO_3
    $[H]^+$ falls, pH rises and the alkalinity is increased;

(5) if the concentration of HCO_3^- falls without an equivalent compensatory fall in the concentration of H_2CO_3
[H]$^+$ rises, pH falls and the alkalinity is decreased.

If both H_2CO_3 and HCO_3^- rise or fall proportionately the pH remains normal. This explains why alone a pH value within normal limits, without considering the values of the other reagents in the equation, can lead to a false assumption that all is well unless the values of the other variables are considered. On the following pages (314-20) the actual mechanisms by which alteration of the $[HCO_3^-]$/ $[H_2CO_3]$ ratio changes the pH are indicated. It is stressed, however, that such alterations are only apparent if they cannot be dealt with by compensatory mechanisms such as alveolar ventilation, buffer pairs and by renal excretion of unwanted ions. It is only possible here to give a general outline of the principles involved; to get a true picture the doctor must correlate laboratory findings with the clinical history and physical examination.

Percentage oxygen saturation (% oxygen saturation)
This is discussed here rather than in the section dealing with respiratory physiology (p. 208) because it is included in 'SAT' in Table 32.1, p. 290.
The oxygen saturation is the amount of oxygen the blood contains expressed as a percentage of the oxygen it would contain were it fully saturated.

$$\therefore \ O_2 \ saturation = \frac{O_2 \ content}{O_2 \ content \ when \ fully \ saturated} \times 100\%$$

One of the factors determining the oxygen saturation of blood is the tension of oxygen to which it is exposed. Plotting oxygen saturation as ordinate and oxygen tension as abscissa leads to the tracing of an oxygen dissociation curve (Figure 32.2).
Several interesting points which are important in resuscitation emerge from a study of this curve.

(1) At a PO_2 of 100 mmHg (13.3 kPa) blood is 97% saturated (typical PO_2 and saturation of arterial blood).
(2) At a PO_2 of 40 mmHg (5.3 kPa) blood is 70% saturated (typical PO_2 and saturation of mixed venous blood).
(3) At a PO_2 of 26 mmHg (3.5 kPa) blood is 50% saturated (P_{50}).

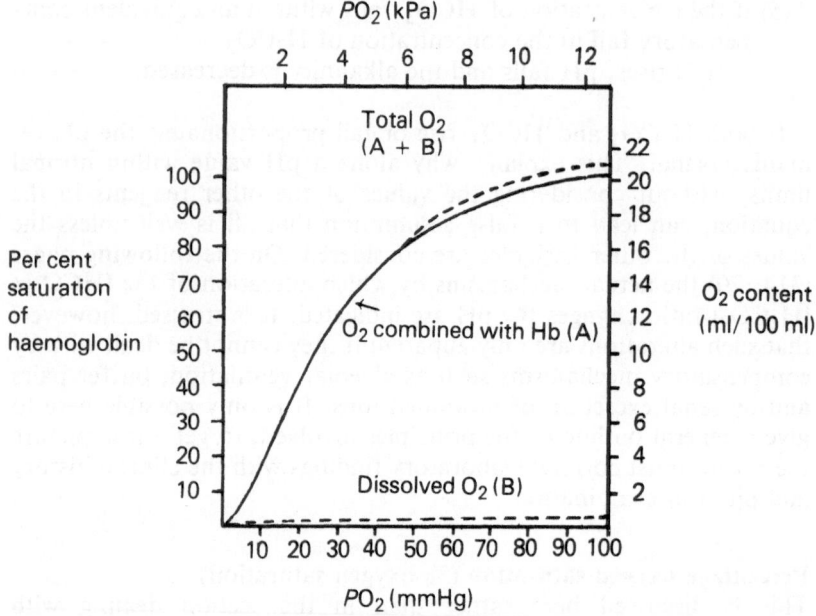

Figure 32.2 Oxygen dissociation curve

Therefore a fall of PO_2 from 100 mmHg (13.3 kPa) to 40 mmHg (5.3 kPa) which is usual in resting conditions, produces a fall in saturation of 27%.

A further fall of PO_2 of 14 mmHg (1.9 kPa) from 40 mmHg (5.3 kPa) causes a 20% fall in saturation, almost as great as that which results when the PO_2 falls from 100 mmHg (13.3 kPa) to 40 mmHg (5.3 kPa).

This effect is due to the shape of the oxygen dissociation curve because the higher values of the PO_2 fall on the flat part of the curve, whereas the lower PO_2 values fall on the steepest part of the curve. As a result a fall in oxygen tension down the steep part of the curve is far more dangerous than if it lies on the horizontal segment. On the other hand administration of oxygen to a person who is hypoxic due to hypoventilation will benefit more if his PO_2 lies in the steep section than if it lies on the horizontal limb of the curve because it will produce a disproportionate increase in the oxygen saturation.

In the elderly PaO_2 can sometimes be misleading. Take for example a PaO_2 of 80 mmHg (10.6 kPa), a value which immediately suggests the presence of hypoxia. However, studying the oxygen dissociation curve shows that this can give an oxygen saturation of 90%, so the patient does not need treatment on this evidence alone.

Pulmonary function and thus PaO_2 values slowly decline through life, even in people with no demonstrable lung disease. It is therefore worth remembering when deciding to take an old person off a ventilator that when breathing air a PaO_2 of 75–85 mmHg (10–10.6 kPa) is probably normal for that particular patient.

Acceptable values for the 'normal' PaO_2, according to age when breathing air, can be calculated from the formula

$$PaO_2 \text{ mmHg} = 102 - 0.33 \times \text{age (years)}$$

$$\text{or } PaO_2 \text{ (kPa)} = 13.6 - 0.044 \times \text{age (years)}$$

When the PAO_2 has been calculated the alveolar–arterial oxygen difference can be derived. Provided the values determining the PaO_2 are stable, then a decrease in the value of $P(A-a)O_2$ difference suggests that the shunt is decreasing, and the patient's condition should begin to improve; an increased $P(A-a)O_2$ difference suggests deterioration.

33

Changes in pH and their interpretation

Respiratory acidosis

Due to the compensating mechanisms of the buffers, lungs and kidneys any primary alteration in the value of either component of the $[HCO_3^-]$ $[H_2CO_3]$ ratio invokes a compensatory change in the other component, thus reducing the extent of the initial change in the pH. For example, in a respiratory acidosis with a PCO_2 of 80 mmHg (10.6 kPa), if there were no compensatory rise in HCO_3^-, the pH would be 7.1; in other words

$$pH = pK + \log \frac{[HCO_3^-]}{[H_2CO_3]}$$

$$= pK + \log \frac{24}{80 \times 0.3} = \log \frac{24}{2.4} \text{ (if } CO_2 \text{ is measured in mmHg),}$$

$$\text{or} = pK + \log \frac{24}{10.6 \times 0.23} = \log \frac{24}{2.4} \text{ (if } PCO_2 \text{ is measured in kPa)}$$

$$= \log 10 = 1$$

$$\therefore pH = 6.1 + 1$$

$$= 7.1$$

From the above it can be seen that a fall in pH of 0.3, from 7.4 to 7.1, is caused by doubling the PCO_2.

A compensatory rise in bicarbonate to 48 mmol/l would restore the ratio of $[HCO_3^-]/[H_2CO_3]$ to 20; in other words $48/2.4 = 20$, and the pH would again be normal at 7.4. Usually, however, there is incomplete compensation, that is a rise in bicarbonate to a level lower than 48 mmol/l; this allows some change in pH but less than that expected if there had been no compensation.

Summary
If CO_2 rises, more H_2CO_3 is formed and the reaction moves to the right to try to re-establish equilibrium.

$$H_2O + CO_2 \rightleftharpoons H_2CO_3$$

that is   primary change – H_2CO_3 rises

and so $\dfrac{[HCO_3^-]}{[H_2CO_3]}$ ratio falls, and pH falls.

Under normal circumstances the body compensates by increasing the depth and rate of respiration, and by improving the alveolar ventilation the excess CO_2 is blown off thus preventing a significant build-up of H_2CO_3. It is only when such an increase in alveolar ventilation is not possible that the H^+ ion concentration rises and causes the findings characteristic of a respiratory acidosis.

Laboratory findings
PCO_2 raised above 40 mmHg (5.3 kPa). pH will be below normal unless a respiratory acidosis is compensating for a metabolic alkalosis.

Respiratory alkalosis
In a respiratory alkalosis the PCO_2 could fall to 20 mmHg (2.7 kPa). Theoretically compensatory renal excretion of bicarbonate could eventually reduce the bicarbonate part of the equation to 12 mmol/l which would restore the $[HCO_3^-]/[H_2CO_3]$ ratio to

$$\frac{12}{20 \times 0.3} \text{ or } \frac{12}{2.7 \times 0.23} = \frac{12}{0.6} = 20$$

with no change in pH. In actual fact compensation is incomplete and the pH remains elevated.

Summary
If CO_2 falls more H_2CO_3 dissociates and the reaction moves to the left to try to re-establish equilibrium

$$H_2O + CO_2 \rightleftharpoons H_2CO_3$$

that is the primary change is a fall in H_2CO_3 and so the $[HCO_3^-]/[H_2CO_3]$ ratio rises, and pH rises.

Laboratory findings
PCO_2 low. pH raised unless the alkalosis is compensating for a metabolic acidosis.

Metabolic or non-respiratory acidosis
Metabolic acidosis is due to an increase in the blood concentration of acids which cannot be excreted through the lungs. They are the normal breakdown products of materials such as sulphur- and phosphorus-containing compounds, and are usually adequately buffered. In metabolic disorders such as diabetic ketosis the buffering power is overloaded since H^+ ions are generated faster than they can be excreted by the kidney; therefore bicarbonate is used up quicker than it can be regenerated so that the bicarbonate part of the $[HCO_3^-]/[H_2CO_3]$ ratio falls below the normal value of 24.

If the bicarbonate falls to 12 mmol/l full compensation occurs if the ensuing hyperventilation causes the PCO_2 to fall to 20 mmHg (2.7 kPa). Then the ratio of $[HCO_3^-]/[H_2CO_3]$ would be

$$\frac{12}{0.3 \times 20} \text{ or } \frac{12}{2.7 \times 0.23} = \frac{12}{0.6} = 20,$$

giving a pH of 7.4. By hyperventilation the body compensates for the loss of bicarbonate, caused by the increase in H^+ ions from the excess acids, in an attempt to reduce the $[H_2CO_3]$ and restore the $[HCO_3^-]/[H_2CO_3]$ ratio and pH to normality. As a result the H_2CO_3 concentration falls but insufficiently to prevent the pH from falling due to the original disproportionate loss of bicarbonate.

Summary
If a strong acid is introduced into plasma there is a reaction between the HCO_3^-, and the H^+ of the strong acid to form H_2CO_3 which is weakly dissociated.

So, primary change – HCO_3^- falls. H_2CO_3 tends to rise initially, but hyperventilation then causes it to fall though not to the same extent as the fall in HCO_3^-. The combined effect is that the $[HCO_3^-]/[H_2CO_3]$ ratio falls.

The above theoretical values of $[HCO_3^-]/[H_2CO_3] = 12/0.6 = 20$ are the same as those quoted on p. 315 under respiratory alkalosis. It is, therefore, necessary to be able to differentiate between a metabolic acidosis and a respiratory alkalosis when compensation has become well established. This is possible because clinically compensation is never complete, so that in a metabolic acidosis when the H_2CO_3 falls the hyperventilation and consequent fall of H_2CO_3 is never enough to prevent some alteration in pH. Therefore, in metabolic acidosis the pH is lowered because $[H_2CO_3]$ falls proportionally less than does the $[HCO_3^-]$. In a respiratory alkalosis the initial fall in $[H_2CO_3]$ is proportionally greater than the compensating fall in bicarbonate, so the pH rises.

Laboratory findings
In uncompensated metabolic acidosis pH, standard bicarbonate and base excess fall, and PCO_2 is within normal limits. In compensated metabolic acidosis the PCO_2 falls, therefore reducing the fall in pH which would otherwise occur.

Metabolic alkalosis
Metabolic alkalosis occurs after the ingestion of alkalis or the vomiting of gastric juice with loss of H^+ ions. The bicarbonate part of the $[HCO_3^-]/[H_2CO_3]$ ratio rises and the lungs therefore decrease ventilation so that the $[H_2CO_3]$ component rises. However, compensation is incomplete, the $[HCO_3^-]$ increases proportionately more than the $[H_2CO_3]$, and so the pH rises.

Summary
Primary change – $[HCO_3^-]$ rises, and so $\dfrac{[HCO_3^-]}{[H_2CO_3]}$ rises, and pH rises

Laboratory findings
pH, standard bicarbonate and base excess raised. PCO_2 normal unless compensation has taken place.

Although it may appear that acid–base disturbances automatically fall into one of the above four categories the extent to which the components alter in the Henderson–Hasselbalch equation depends on the rate at which the variations occur, the efficiency of the compensatory mechanisms and the time allowed for compensation to occur.

Mixed disorders
Mixed pictures occur when one type of disorder changes into another as in salicylate intoxication. For example, in this disorder there is an initial hyperventilation which gives rise to a respiratory alkalosis. The PCO_2 falls, the bicarbonate remains fairly steady and the pH rises. Later a metabolic acidosis supervenes. The H^+ ion concentration, the

[H$_2$CO$_3$] produced by the buffers and the PCO_2 rise, and the bicarbonate falls with a consequent fall in pH.

In assessing the results obtained from acid–base investigations it is mandatory to take into account the clinical history of the disease which will often help the investigator to anticipate and correlate the findings and thereby influence the management of restoration of the acid–base balance.

Clinical interpretation of the acid–base readout

An understanding of acid–base readouts and their interpretation is needed in order to start appropriate corrective treatment should a disorder exist. A popular approach is to look at, in the following order, the values of

(1) PaO_2
(2) pH
(3) $PaCO_2$
(4) Standard HCO$_3^-$.

A pH *less* than 7.4 denotes the presence of an *acidosis*. *If also*
(1) the $PaCO_2$ is > 40 mmHg (5.3 kPa), an element of respiratory acidosis is present.

Cause: CO$_2$ retention due to hypoventilation, such as in chronic bronchitis and emphysema or sedative drug overdose.

Effect: $PaCO_2$ ↑ → pH↓

Treatment: Controlled oxygen therapy (p. 68), IPPV if $PaCO_2$ continues to rise.

(2) the $PaCO_2$ is < 40 mmHg (5.3 kPa), the acidosis is not respiratory in origin but is due to the presence of excess of non-volatile acids or more rarely a deficit of base. The standard HCO$_3^-$ is low.

The lowered $PaCO_2$ is the compensatory effect of the patient blowing off CO$_2$ in an attempt to reduce the non-respiratory (metabolic) acidosis.

Cause (1): Excess non-volatile acid for example in diabetes, chronic renal failure and shock.

Treatment: Give base in form of NaHCO$_3$, the amount of which can be determined by formula (p. 251):

$$\frac{\text{Body weight (kg)} \times \text{base deficit (mmol/l)}}{4}$$

Cause: (2) Deficit of base, for example in pancreatic fistula.

A pH *greater* than 7.4 denotes the presence of an *alkalosis*. *If also*
(1) the $PaCO_2$ is < 40 mmHg (5.3 kPa), an element of respiratory
alkalosis is present.

Cause: Hyperventilation, for example due to pain caused by taking
of blood sample, hysteria, fear; seen initially in salicylate poisoning.

Effect: $PaCO_2 \downarrow \rightarrow$ pH↑

Treatment: Relieve pain and anxiety; breathing in and out of a
paper bag may relieve distressing paraesthesiae, especially in the
obstetric patient and the hysteric; salicylate poisoning is treated by
forced alkaline diuresis (p. 32).

(2) the $PaCO_2$ is > 40 mmHg (5.3 kPa), an element of non-
respiratory alkalosis is present due to excessive loss of acid or excessive intake of alkali. The standard HCO_3^- is raised.

The raised $PaCO_2$ is the compensatory effect of the patient retaining CO_2 in an attempt to reduce the non-respiratory (metabolic)
alkalosis.

Cause: Vomiting of gastric juice; ingestion or infusion of alkali.

Effect: HCO_3^-↑ $\rightarrow$ pH↑ $\rightarrow$ $PaCO_2$↑ (compensatory mechanism).

Treatment: Give saline if vomiting; the need for intravenous acid
therapy is rare.

WITH LOW $PaCO_2$

A $PaCO_2$ < 40 mmHg (5.3 kPa) with a low PaO_2 indicates a
respiratory alkalosis due to hypoxia. In an attempt to raise his PaO_2
concentration the patient hyperventilates, washes out CO_2 and so
lowers his $PaCO_2$.

Cause: Hypoxia

Effect: $PaO_2 \downarrow \rightarrow PaCO_2 \downarrow \rightarrow$ pH↑

Treatment: Increase FiO_2 (p. 68); IPPV if necessary.

Using a flow diagram

An alternative approach to acid–base interpretation is by way of a
flow diagram.

A minimum of three factors must be known if acid–base changes
are to be elucidated: (1) the pH to determine the overall state of acidity
or alkalinity; (2) $PaCO_2$ which reflects changes in respiration; and (3)
a factor which reflects metabolic changes (standard bicarbonate or
base excess).

A flow diagram can be drawn, and the nature of a change in the
acid–base balance elucidated by asking the appropriate questions
(Figure 33.1).

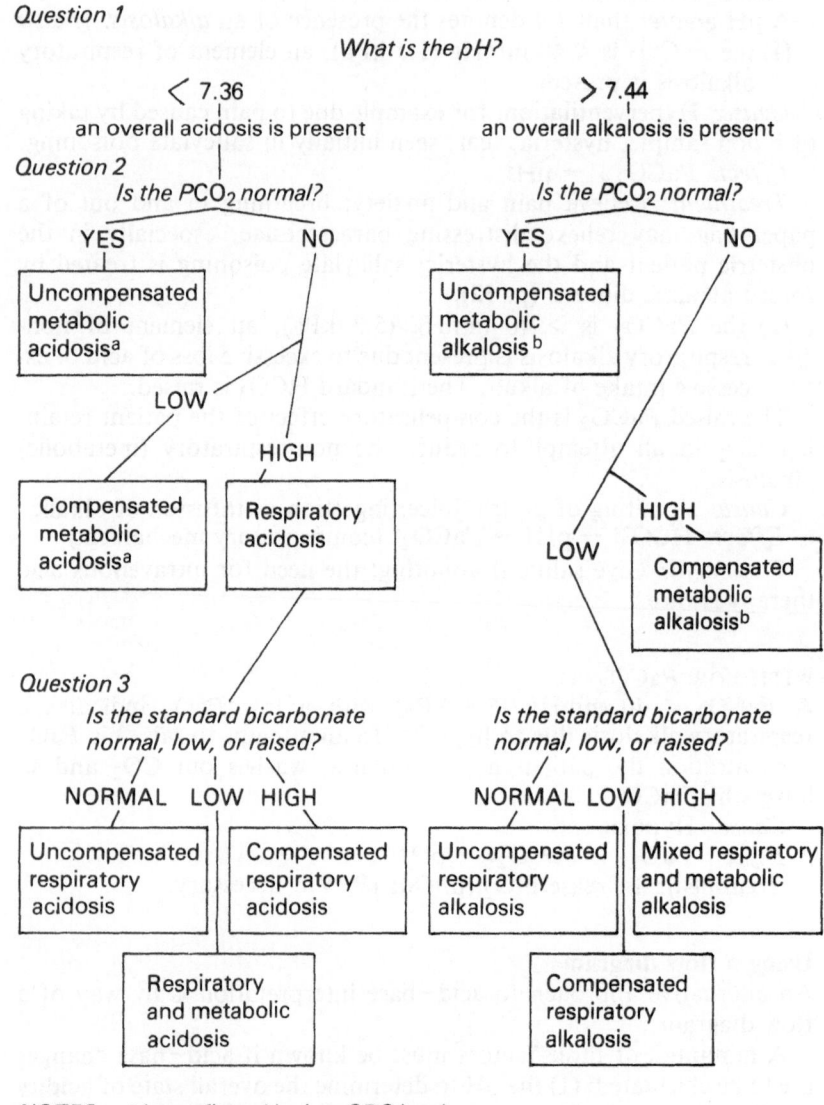

Figure 33.1

34

SI units used in resuscitation – moles, pascals and joules

The mole

AVOGADRO'S NUMBER

Many find the concept of the mole difficult to understand. However, an analogy can be drawn between ordering a dozen eggs and being given 12. 'Dozen' is therefore a number with a value of 12; a mole too is a number, but it has the rather forbidding value of 6.02×10^{23}. Consequently, if one asked for a mole of eggs, the number of eggs one would expect to receive would be 6.02×10^{23}. This number is known as *Avogadro's number* or *Avogadro's constant,* and the amount or mass of substance which contains Avogadro's number of particles is known as 1 mole. It does not matter whether the particles are atoms, molecules or ions. For example:

(a) 1 mole of sodium metal (Na) contains
6.02×10^{23} particles (*atoms*) of sodium;
(b) 1 mole of chlorine gas (Cl_2) contains
6.02×10^{23} particles (*molecules*) of chlorine gas.

But, one molecule of chlorine gas (Cl_2) consists of two particles (atoms) of chlorine (Cl).

$$Cl_2 = Cl + Cl$$

∴ 1 mole of chlorine molecules contains 2 moles of chlorine atoms.
(c) 1 mole of sodium chloride (NaCl) molecules contains
6.02×10^{23} Na^+ particles (*ions*) and
6.02×10^{23} Cl^- particles (*ions*);
∴ 1 mole of NaCl molecules contains
1 mole Na^+ ions and 1 mole Cl^- ions.

To repeat, it must be clearly understood that the mole refers to a specific number of particles, either atoms, molecules or ions. This can be illustrated by the following analogy.

If one sticky treacle toffee (TT) is placed in contact with one sticky peppermint toffee (PT) they stick together to form one sticky treaclepeppermint toffee (TTPT).

$$1 \text{ TT} \quad + \quad 1 \text{PT} \quad \rightarrow \quad 1 \text{ TTPT}$$
$$(1 \text{ particle}) \quad (1 \text{ particle}) \quad (1 \text{ particle})$$

Next, replace each toffee with Avogadro's number of toffees or moles of toffee

$$6.02 \times 10^{23} \text{ TT} + 6.02 \times 10^{23} \text{ PT} \rightarrow 6.02 \times 10^{23} \text{ TTPT}$$
$$\text{or} \quad 1 \text{ mole TT} \quad + \quad 1 \text{ mole PT} \quad \rightarrow \quad 1 \text{ mole TTPT}$$

Every sticky treaclepeppermint toffee combination is now regarded as one (and not two) differently named particles of a new substance.

Similarly,

$$Na^+ \qquad + \quad Cl^- \qquad \rightarrow \quad NaCl$$

$$1 \text{ mole } Na^+ + 1 \text{ mole } Cl^- \rightarrow 1 \text{ mole NaCl}$$
$$(\text{ions}) \qquad (\text{ions}) \qquad (\text{molecules})$$

Note that on combining, the particles change their name from ion to molecule. Although 1 molecule is composed of 2 atoms it is only 1 particle.

Reversing the process, every sticky treaclepeppermint toffee combination can be pulled apart to give 1 particle of treacle toffee and 1 particle of peppermint toffee

$$1 \text{ mole TTPT} \quad \rightarrow \quad 1 \text{ mole TT} \quad + 1 \text{ mole PT}$$
$$\text{and} \qquad 1 \text{ mole NaCl} \quad \rightarrow \quad 1 \text{ mole } Na^+ \qquad 1 \text{ mole } Cl^-$$
$$(\text{molecule}) \qquad (\text{ion}) \qquad (\text{ion})$$

Therefore the use of moles give a clear picture of the *proportions* in which the reagents are related without mentioning their weights. It is argued that it is much clearer to all concerned to say that a patient is in need of 0.15 moles Na^+ ions and 0.15 moles Cl^- ions rather than 3.45 (23×0.15) g Na^+ ion and 4.325 (35.5×0.15) g Cl^- ion. Consequently the student is often taught that the concept of moles is a convenient way of expressing the amounts of the individual constituents of an intravenous solution and the quantity required to correct some electrolyte deficiency without using units of weight such as the gram.

However, for the student one important question remains: 'How do you know how much NaCl there is in a mole of NaCl?' He is told either that a mole of NaCl contains Avogadro's number of molecules or else it contains 58.5 g of NaCl. Paradoxically, the mole was introduced to avoid using weights but the measurement of the amount of substance in the mole does involve the use of weights – the wheel has turned the full circle.

THE GRAM ATOM

In order to measure out 1 mole of a substance it is obviously impossible to count 6.02×10^{23} particles. However, it is known that this number of atoms is present in 1 *gram atom* of any element. The term gram atom is the relative atomic mass of an element (that is the old 'atomic weight') expressed in grams. For example,

> 1 gram atom of C weighs 12 g $\equiv$ 1 mole of C
> (atomic weight)
>
> 1 gram atom of Na weighs 23 g $\equiv$ 1 mole of Na
>
> 1 gram atom of Cl weighs 35.5 g $\equiv$ 1 mole of Cl

and because 1 atom of Na^+ + 1 atom of Cl^- combine to form
(1 particle) + (1 particle)
1 molecule of NaCl,
(1 particle);

$23 \text{ g } Na^+$ + $35.5 \text{ g } Cl^-$ combine $\longrightarrow$ 58.5 g NaCl
that is
6.02×10^{23} ions + 6.02×10^{23} ions $\longrightarrow 6.02 \times 10^{23}$ molecules
or 1 mole Na^+ + 1 mole Cl^- $\longrightarrow$ 1 mole NaCl

Similarly, take glucose $C_6H_{12}O_6$
Relative atomic mass in grams of

$$
\begin{array}{llll}
C = 12 & \therefore C_6 = 12 \times 6 = & 72 \text{ g} \\
H = 1 & \therefore H_{12} = 1 \times 12 = & 12 \text{ g} \\
O = 6 & \therefore O_6 = 16 \times 6 = & \underline{96 \text{ g}} \\
& & \underline{180 \text{ g}}
\end{array}
$$

$\therefore$ 6 moles of C + 12 moles H + 6 moles O $\rightarrow$ 1 mole $C_6H_{12}O_6$
   atoms   atoms   atoms   molecules

Therefore, to measure the quantity of matter in a substance in moles it is necessary to know the actual composition, that is the true formula, and the relative atomic masses in grams (atomic weights in grams).

Because the total amount of substance is the sum of all the atomic masses depicted by the formula, the mole is often appropriately regarded as consisting of the formula mass of a substance whether it be an atom, an ion or a molecule.

It is relatively easy to convert mg/ml or mg% to moles per litre and vice versa (p. 325), and to determine the contents of the various kinds of intravenous transfusions that may be needed in resuscitative therapy (p. 326). Conversion, however, requires an understanding of the basic units of concentration.

Units of concentration

When a substance is present in solution its concentration may be expressed either as mass concentration or as amount of substance concentration.

MASS CONCENTRATION

The SI unit for mass is the kilogram, with the symbol kg. The unit of volume usually used is the litre, with the symbol l. Concentration is then expressed as kg/l, g/l, mg/l, μg/l, etc.

Above, the litre is used because it is extremely useful but it is not a derived SI unit; for volume this is the cubic metre, with the symbol m^3. So the SI unit of concentration is expressed as kg/m^3 which is perhaps less clear than the equivalent concentration g/l. The association between concentration expressed as kg/m^3 and g/l is derived below

1 kg	= 1000 g = 10^3 g
Now (a) 1 decimetre (dm)	= 1/10 of 1 metre (m)
i.e. 1 metre (m)	= 10 decimetres (dm) = 10 dm
∴ 1 m^3	= $(10 \text{ dm})^3$ = 10^3 dm^3
(b) 1 centimetre (cm)	= 1/10 of 1 decimetre (dm)
i.e. 1 decimetre (dm)	= 10 centimetres (cm) = 10 cm
and 1 litre	= $(10 \text{ cm})^3$
	= 1 dm^3
i.e. 1 dm^3	= 1 litre
∴ 10^3 dm^3	= 10^3 l

Returning to the concentration kg/m³, substitution shows

$$1 \text{ kg/m}^3 \quad = \quad \frac{10^3 \text{g}}{10^3 \text{l}} \quad = \quad 1 \text{ g/l}$$

To most people 1 g/l gives a clearer concept of concentration than does 1 kg/m³ and it is easy to understand why the litre is not always superseded by the SI units.

AMOUNT OF SUBSTANCE CONCENTRATION
The amount of substance concentration is expressed as the molar concentration in moles per litre (mol/l), either:

> millimoles per litre (mmol/l)
> micromoles per litre (μmol/l)
> nanomoles per litre (nmol/l)

A mole is the formula mass of the substance (p. 324).

RELATIONSHIP BETWEEN THE TWO TYPES OF CONCENTRATION
Conversion of the values of mass concentration to amount of substance concentration is basically simple. The necessary steps are shown below.

Conversion of grams or milligrams % to moles per litre etc. (g%, mg% to mol/l)
1 mole of a substance contains its formula weight

∴ the number of moles (mol) of substance present

$$= \frac{\text{the actual mass in grams}}{\text{formula mass in grams}}$$

and the number of millimoles (mmol) of substance present

$$= \frac{\text{actual mass in milligrams}}{\text{formula mass in grams}}$$

Now concentration = moles per litre or milligrams per litre; if, say, concentration of blood glucose = 90 mg%

then 90 mg% = 90 mg/100 ml = 900 mg/1000 ml
= 900 mg/l

	No. of atoms	Atomic mass
Formula mass in grams of glucose $C_6H_{12}O_6$ =	6	$\times$ 12 = 72 g
	12	$\times$ 1 = 12 g
	6	$\times$ 16 = $\underline{96\ g}$
		180 g

Now number of millimoles per litre $= \dfrac{\text{actual mass in mg}}{\text{formula mass in g}} = \dfrac{900}{180} = 5$

$\therefore$ 90 mg/100 ml glucose = 5 mmol/l

INTRAVENOUS SOLUTIONS

Mass concentration and amount of substance concentration are both frequently stated on the labels of intravenous fluids. Examples of such labelling and the means of interconversion of the different types of concentration are illustrated below.

Example 1: 0.9% NaCl
Sodium chloride solution BP or USP 0.9% w/v containing approximately the following millimoles of ions per litre: sodium: 150, chloride: 150.

0.9% w/v means 0.9 g/100 ml which is 9 g/l.

Formula mass of NaCl = 23 + 35.5 g
$\qquad\qquad\qquad\qquad$ = 58.5 g

Molar concentration $= \dfrac{\text{actual mass/l}}{\text{formula mass}}$

$\therefore$ molar concentration $= \dfrac{9}{58.5}$ mol/l of NaCl in 0.9% saline

$\qquad\qquad\qquad\qquad = \dfrac{9 \times 1000}{58.5}$ mmol/l

$\qquad\qquad\qquad\qquad$ = 150 mmol/l

Now 1 mol NaCl $\rightleftharpoons$ 1 mol Na^+ + 1 mol Cl^-
$\qquad\qquad\qquad\qquad\qquad$ (ions) $\qquad\qquad$ (ions)

or $\quad$ 1 mmol NaCl $\rightleftharpoons$ mmol Na^+ + 1 mmol Cl^-
$\qquad\qquad\qquad\qquad\qquad\quad$ (ions) $\qquad\qquad\quad$ (ions)

$\therefore$ 150 mmol NaCl $\rightleftharpoons$ 150 mmol Na^+ + 150 mmol Cl^-
$\qquad\qquad\qquad\qquad\qquad\quad$ (ions) $\qquad\qquad\qquad$ (ions)

Hence NaCl 0.9% w/v contains approximately 150 mmol Na^+ ions and 150 mmol Cl^- ions per litre.

Example 2: 0.18% NaCl and dextrose 4%

Sodium chloride (0.18% w/v) + dextrose (4% w/v) injection BP or USP containing approximately the following millimoles of ions per litre: sodium: 30; chloride 30; and anhydrous dextrose 40 g/litre (equivalent to 164 calories).

First, consider the NaCl:

0.18% w/v means 0.18 g/100 ml = 1.8 g/l
$$= 1800 \text{ mg/l}$$

No. of millimoles NaCl/l $= \dfrac{\text{actual mass in mg/l}}{\text{formula mass in g}}$

$$= \frac{1800}{23 + 35.5} = \frac{1800}{58.5} = 30/1 \text{(approximately)}$$

Now 1 mmol NaCl $\rightleftharpoons$ 1 mmol Na$^+$ + 1 mmol Cl$^-$
 (ions) (ions)

∴ 30 mmol NaCl $\rightleftharpoons$ 30 mmol Na$^+$ + 30 mmol Cl$^-$
 (ions) (ions)

Hence, NaCl 0.18% w/v contains approximately 30 mmol Na$^+$ ions and 30 mmol Cl$^-$ ions per litre.

Second, consider the dextrose

Dextrose 4% w/v = 40 g/l
1 g dextrose = 4.1 calories
∴ 40 g dextrose = 164 calories = 164 × 4.2 joules (p.000)

molar concentration of dextrose $= \dfrac{\text{actual mass in g/l}}{\text{formula mass in g}}$

$$= \frac{40}{180} \text{ mol/l}$$

$$= \frac{40 \times 1000}{180} \text{ mmol/l}$$

$$= 222 \text{ mmol/l}$$

Example 3: 8.4% NaHCO₃

Na	=	23
H	=	1
C	=	12
O₃ = 3 × 16	=	48
		84

1 mol/l NaHCO$_3$ is equal to a concentration of 84 g/l NaHCO$_3$

1 mol/l NaHCO$_3$ is equivalent to a concentration of 8.4 g/100 ml NaHCO$_3$, which is an 8.4% solution;

∴ 100 ml of 8.4% solution NaHCO$_3$ contains 8.4 g NaHCO$_3$, which is equivalent to 1/10 mol = 0.1 mol NaHCO$_3$.

∴ 100 ml 8.4% solution NaHCO$_3$ contains 0.1 × 1000 = 100 mmol Na HCO$_3$;

∴ 1 ml 8.4% solution NaHCO$_3$ contains 1 mmol NaHCO$_3$

Thus it is immaterial whether the doctor directs, say, 75 mmol NaHCO$_3$ or 75 ml 8.4% NaHCO$_3$ to be given to the patient; they are both the same.

Units of pressure
Until the introduction of SI units, pressure was usually measured in milligrams of mercury (mmHg). The introduction of the pascal (Pa) and kilopascal (kPa) has caused some confusion and it will certainly take years for the kilopascal to replace the mmHg, especially in the minds of the older doctors and nurses. Perhaps the kilopascal will never supersede the mmHg in certain measurements because the values obtained in kilopascals are sometimes less neat and more difficult to remember and manipulate than are those in mmHg. For example, a blood pressure of 100/80 mmHg is equivalent to 13.3/10.6 kPa whereas a PO_2 of 100 mmHg equals 13.3 kPa, and a PCO_2 of 40 mmHg is equivalent to 5.33 kPa. However, as SI units of pressure and its components, length and force, are found in medical books, publications and pathology reports they must, of course, be understood. It may perhaps, seem unnecessary to describe the steps taken to derive the kilopascal from basic SI units such as the kilogram, metre and second. However, an elementary but sound knowledge of how to use these three basic units as building blocks will ensure a greater understanding of the kilopascal and of other units from which it is derived, such as the newton and pascal.

DERIVATION OF THE KILOPASCAL
Three pieces of information are necessary:

    (1) The basic SI unit for
        (a) length is the metre, with the symbol m,
        (b) mass is the kilogram, with the symbol kg,
        (c) time is the second, with the symbol s.

(2) The term 'rate of change of something' means that the 'something' is divided by time. For example velocity = rate of change of distance, that is velocity = $\dfrac{\text{distance}}{\text{time}}$.

(3) An expression $x = \dfrac{n^{+1}}{d^{+1}}$

has a numerator (n^{+1}) and a denominator (d^{+1})

By convention the numerator can be multiplied by the denominator provided the sign preceding the power is changed.

Thus

$$x = \frac{n^{+1}}{d^{+1}} \text{ can be rewritten}$$

$$x = n^{+1} d^{-1}$$

Again by convention the powers which have a value of $+1$ are omitted,

$$\therefore \quad x = n^{+1} d^{-1}$$

becomes $\quad x = nd^{-1}$

similarly $\quad x = \dfrac{n}{d^2}$ can be rewritten and becomes

$$x = nd^{-2}$$

OTHER DERIVATIONS
Velocity

For example velocity (v) = $\dfrac{\text{distance}}{\text{time}}$

The SI units for distance, which is length, is the metre, and that for time is the second

$$\therefore \text{ velocity} = \frac{\text{length}}{\text{time}}$$

$$v = \frac{m}{s} \text{ (metres per second); this can be written } v = ms^{-1}$$

Acceleration

Similarly acceleration a = rate of change of velocity, but velocity

$$v = \frac{m}{s} = ms^{-1}$$

Thus acceleration $a = \frac{ms^{-1}}{s}$ (metres per second per second).

This can be rewritten $a = ms^{-2}$

Force
Force is mass $\times$ acceleration. The SI unit for mass is the kilogram, but acceleration $= ms^{-2}$

$\therefore$ force $=$ kilograms $\times$ acceleration

$= kg \times ms^{-2} = kgms^{-2}$ (kilogram metre per second per
second)

Newtons
The derived SI unit for force is the newton and so

$$\text{force in newtons (N)} = kgms^{-2}$$

Thus 1 newton (N) is that force which, when it pushes or pulls a mass of 1 kg gives it an acceleration of 1 metre per second per second, or

$N = 1 \ kgms^{-2}$

Pressure
Pressure P is defined as force per unit area. Area is equal to length $\times$ length (or breadth), that is $length^2$. The SI derived unit for area is therefore metres squared (m^2)

$$\therefore P = \frac{N}{m^2} = Nm^{-2}$$

That is, pressure is measured in newtons per square metre.

Pascal
The unit of pressure is the pascal and 1 pascal is the pressure exerted by a force of 1 newton per square metre, that is 1 pascal (Pa) $= 1 \ Nm^{-2}$. However, the pascal is too small a unit of pressure to be of much practical use in medicine, so the unit chosen is one which is a thousand times the value of the pascal, namely the kilopascal (kPa).

Kilopascal
1000 pascals $= 10^3$ pascals

$\therefore$ 1000 pascals $= 1$ kilopascal
and $\therefore$ 1 kPa $= 10^3$ newtons per square metre
$= 10^3$ Nm^{-2}

Conversion factors
Those who are unfamiliar with the use of the kilopascal may find it useful to remember that in Great Britain force is still measured when purchasing vegetables, for instance, in pounds weight. In other words, 1 lb weight = mass of 1 lb $\times$ acceleration due to gravity which is equal to 32 feet per second per second.

Because weight is a force, 1 lb weight is better written 1 lb force, with the symbol lbf; in other words 1 lb weight is 1 lbf, and pressure

$$= \frac{\text{lb weight}}{\text{area in sq. in}} \quad \text{or} \quad \frac{\text{lb force units}}{\text{area in sq. in.}}$$

= lb weight per square inch or 1lb force per square inch
= lb/in^2 or lbf/in^2

The two ways of expressing pressure are therefore

(1) Pressure = lb weight per square inch = lb/in^2
    or lb force per square inch = lbf/in^2
(2) Pressure = newtons per square metre = N/m^2 = pascals

Therefore, pascals and kilopascals are the derived SI units which express pressure and are now frequently used in preference to pounds weight per square inch or pounds force per square inch. The pascal is approximately equal to 1.45×10^{-4} pounds force per square inch (lbf/in^2).

The kilopascal is approximately equal to $1.45 \times 10^{-1} = 0.145$ lbf/in^2, and is often used to replace pressure equivalent to that exerted by a column of water or a column of mercury.

Equivalent values are

1 cmH$_2$O	= 98.1 Pa
	or 0.0981 kPa
1 mmHg	= 133.3 Pa
	or 0.1333 kPa
1 kPa	= 7.5 mmHg

Therefore to convert mmHg into kilopascals the value in mmHg should be divided by 7.5; in other words

$$100 \text{ mmHg} = \frac{100}{7.5} = 13.3 \text{ kPa}$$

$$\text{a } PCO_2 \text{ of 30 mmHg} = \frac{30}{7.5} = 4 \text{ kPa}$$

In clinical matters to do with resuscitation the use of the kilopascal is often restricted to blood gas measurements. Central venous pressure, the pressure component of compliance and inflation pressure used in ventilation (p. 163) are usually still measured in cm water (cmH_2O).

Unit of mechanical work or energy (joule)

When a force moves an object it does work on that object. The greater the distance through or along which the force moves the object, the greater is the work done.

$\therefore$ work done is force $\times$ distance moved

The unit of force is the newton (p. 330), and 1 newton (N) = 1 $kgms^{-2}$

Therefore the unit of work is N $\times$ m and it is called the joule (with the symbol J).

$\therefore$ 1 joule = 1 Nm (referred to as the newton metre)
$\qquad\qquad$ = $kgms^{-2} \times$ m
$\qquad\qquad$ = kgm^2s^{-2}

The joule is defined accordingly as the work done or energy expended when a force of 1 newton acts through a distance of 1 metre.

The joule is also the unit of electrical energy, the magnitude of which must be carefully selected on the 'joules stored' dial of the defibrillator before the current is passed through the heart (p. 12).

The joule has replaced the calorie as a unit of heat energy, 1 calorie being equal to approximately 4.2 joules (p. 327).

Bibliography

Chapter 5
Ward, C.S., *Anaesthetic Equipment: Physical Principles and Maintenance* (London: Baillière Tindall, 1975)

Chapter 21
Mushin, W.W., Rendell-Baker, L., Thompson, P.W., and Mapleson, W.W., *Automatic Ventilation of the Lungs, 3rd Edition* (Oxford, London, Edinburgh and Melbourne: Blackwell Scientific Publications, 1979)

Chapter 26
Comroe, J.H., *Physiology of Respiration,2nd Edition* (Chicago: Year Book Medical Publishers Incorporated, 1974)
West, J.B., *Respiratory Physiology – The Essentials* (Oxford, London, Edinburgh and Melbourne: Blackwell Scientific Publications, 1974)

Chapter 32
Adams, A.P. and Hahn, C.W.E., *Principles and Practice of Blood–Gas Analysis*, (London: Franklin Scientific Projects, 1979)
Davenport, H.W., *The ABC of Acid–Base Chemistry, 6th Edition* (Chicago and London: University of Chicago Press, 1974)
Robinson, J.R., *Fundamentals of Acid – Base Regulation, 5th Edition* (Oxford and Edinburgh: Blackwell Scientific Publications, 1975)

Index

suction 184–6, 206
suxamethonium 194–200
  dangers 196–9

tachycardia 16, 17, 21
  paroxysmal supraventricular
    16, 18
  ventricular 8, 12, 19, 20
temperature
  core 40, 41, 44
  regulation see heatstroke,
    hyperpyrexia, hypothermia
  shell 40, 41
tension pneumothorax 89, 91–4
thiopentone 187–91
  dangers 188–90
thrombolytic therapy for
    pulmonary embolism 23
thyroid crisis 47–8
thyrotoxicosis 47
tidal volume
  definition 121–3
  effective 127
tissue flow, in shock 245
tongue, in relief of respiratory
    obstruction 203, 205
tracheal puncture 97
transfusion, blood 265–9
tricyclic antidepressants, treatment
    of poisoning 34

unconscious patient, care of 76,
  85–7

valve
  expiratory 135, 156
  non-return 133
vasoconstriction, in shock 250–1
venous return 231–2, 235
ventilation
  in asthma 63
  in cardiac arrest 8–12, 13
  controlled 142–6, 151–2
  intermittent positive pressure
    (IPPV) 65, 90, 92, 140, 152,
    156–61, 182–3, 198–9
  manual 148
  in multiple injuries 73–4
  neonatal 114–15
  –perfusion characteristics
    214–22, 223
  spontaneous 138–42, 151
  terminology 121–32
  see also ventilators
ventilators 162–70
  indications for use 166–9
ventricular failure, left 25–6,
  37–8
ventricular fibrillation 7, 8, 12, 15
violent patients, control of 56
vomiting, induced, in poisoning
  30

wasp stings 38–9
Wright's respirometer 122